FOUNDATIONS OF ĀYURVEDA, VOLUME II

Core principles & the human body in Āyurveda

(सिद्धान्त & शारीर - *Siddhānta & Śhārīra*)

Vaidya (Dr.) Jessica Vellela, BAMS
Vaidya (Dr.) Prasanth Dharmarajan, PhD (Ayu)

ĀYU COUNCIL
A PUBLIC BENEFIT CORPORATION

8 The Green Ste A
Dover, DE 19901

https://www.ayucouncil.org

FOUNDATIONS OF ĀYURVEDA, VOLUME II
Core principles & the human body in Āyurveda (सिद्धान्त & शारीर - *Siddhānta* & *Śhārīra*)

Authors
Jessica Vellela
Prasanth Dharmarajan

First Edition

Notice - Disclaimer

Knowledge and best practices in the field of Āyurveda regularly change as new research and experience broaden the understanding of the subject. Adaptable changes with research methods, professional practice and/or management protocols may become necessary. Every effort has been made to ensure that the content provided in this publication is accurate and complete at the time of publishing. However, this is not an exhaustive treatment of the subject. No liability is assumed for losses or damages due to the information provided. Interpretation and application of information from this publication is solely the responsibility of the reader. Always consult an appropriate professional with any questions related to legal, medical or other issues.

Previous editions copyrighted 2017, 2018, 2019.

ISBN: 978-1-950876-06-8

Printed in the United States of America

To all of our teachers,

and their teachers,

and the teachers before them

Special thanks to the

SVASTHA ĀCHĀRYA STUDENTS

who helped make this book and

higher standards of Āyurveda a reality.

अनेनोपदेशेन नानौषधिभूतं जगति किंचिद्द्रव्यमुपलभ्यते तां तां युक्तिमर्थे च तं तमभिप्रेत्य ॥

च. सू. २६।१२

Anenopadeśhena nānauṣhadhibhūtaṃ jagati kiṅciddravyamupalabhyate tāṃ tāṃ yuktimarthe cha taṃ tamabhipretya ||

Ca. Sū. 26/12

"Like it was just mentioned in the preceding verse, there is nothing which exists in this world that cannot be used for curative effects (as a medicine) when one's logical thought power is able to determine the correct application."

reiterated by:

Su. Sū. 41/5

AH Sū. 9/10

Table of Contents: Unit I

Chapter 1 : Introduction 1
Classical introductions 2
Who should study? 3
How does the science work? 3
What are the basic variables? 3
Summing it all up 4
Darśhana 4
How to use this volume 7
Chapter 2 : Overview of siddhānta 12
Sṛshṭi utpatti 13
Satkārya vāda 13
Kārya-Kāraṇa bhāva 14
Nava kāraṇa dravya, Dravya saṅgraha 14
Dravya 15
Pañcha tanmātra 16
Pañcha mahābhūta 17
Mūrti-Amūrti 17
Chetanā-Achetanā 18
Jaṅgama-Audbhida-Pārthiva 18
Sāmānya-Viśheṣha siddhānta 19
Samavāya 19
Samavāyi 20
Saṁyoga-Vibhāga 20
Vṛddhi-Kṣhaya 21
Guṇa 21
Karma 22
Rasa 22
Vīrya 23
Vipāka 23
Prabhāva 24
Loka-puruṣha sāmya 24
Āyu 25
Tri-daṇḍavat 25
Puruṣha 26
Tridoṣha, Tri-sthūṇa 26
Doṣha 27
Agni 27
Pāka, pāchana 28
Koṣhṭha 28
Saptadhātu 29
Upadhātu 29
Dhātu-mala 30
Mala, Trimala 30

Chaya-Prakopa-Praśhamana 31
Āśhraya-Āśhrayi Bhāva 31
Gati 32
Prakṛti 32
Tri-guṇa 32
Mānasika doṣha 33
Trayopastambha 33
Kāla 34
Ṛtu 34
Ṛtu-sandhi 35
Avasthā 35
Diśha (Dik) 35
Tri deśha 36
Avara-Madhyama-Uttama 36
Chapter 3 : Dravya 41
Dravya 41
Paribhāṣhā 42
Bheda 43
Mechanics of dravya 43
Pañcha mahābhūta 45
Pañcha Mahābhūta Overview 46
Pṛthvi guṇa and karma 47
Ap or Jala guṇa and karma 48
Tejo or Agni guṇa and karma 49
Vāyu guṇa and karma 50
Ākāśha guṇa and karma 51
Mahābhūta composition 52
Guṇa 52
Paribhāṣhā 53
Bheda 53
Vaiśheṣhikā 54
Sāmānya 54
Ātmaguṇā 59
Karma 61
Paribhāṣhā 61
Bheda 61
Rasa 62
Paribhāṣhā 62
Bheda 63
Origin of rasa 65
Rasa and pañcha mahābhūta 65
Rasa and doṣha 66
Rasa and guṇa 67
Rasa and karma 69
Vīrya 69
Paribhāṣhā 69
Bheda 70

Vipāka ... 70
Paribhāṣhā ... 71
Bheda ... 71
General mechanics of *dravya, rasa, vīrya* and *vipāka* ... 72
Prabhāva ... 73
Paribhāṣhā ... 73
Chapter 4 : Tridoṣha siddhānta ... 79
Deha ... 79
Śharīra ... 80
Kāya ... 80
Puruṣha ... 81
Charaka's perspective ... 81
Suśhruta's perspective ... 82
Paryāya ... 82
Tridoṣha ... 83
Origin of tridoṣha siddhānta ... 83
Nirukti ... 83
Paribhāṣhā ... 84
Paryāya and technical terms ... 86
Tridoṣha bheda ... 86
Tridoṣha and pañcha mahābhūtas ... 87
Tridoṣha and guṇas ... 88
Tridoṣha and special features ... 91
Chapter 5 : Agni ... 97
Agni as pitta ... 98
Paribhāṣhā ... 99
Bheda ... 100
Jaṭharāgni ... 100
Bhūtāgni ... 101
Dhātvagni ... 102
States of agni ... 103
Normal ... 103
Abnormal ... 104
Key Principles ... 106
Koṣhṭha ... 106
Dhātu poṣhaṇa nyāya ... 107
Āhāra parināma bhāvas ... 108
Duration for conversion ... 109
Dhātu pariṇāma ... 110
Step 1: Intake of *āhāra* ... 110
Step 2: Āhāra pāka ... 112
Step 3: Dhātu pariṇāma ... 115
Outputs of conversion ... 117
Doṣhas: as dhātus or malas? ... 117
Dhātus: Supportive tissues ... 117
Malas: Waste products ... 117
Āma ... 117

Vegas: Relieving reflexes 118
Chapter 6 : Dhātu sāmya 123
Nirukti & Paribhāṣhā 123
Nirukti 123
Paribhāṣhā 124
The opposite state: Dhātu vaiṣhamya 125
Causes for dhātu sāmya 126
Āhāra 126
Agni 126
Rasa 127
Changes in states 127
Chapter 7 : Doṣha 133
How doṣhas function in the body 133
States of doṣhas 134
Recognizing states of doṣhas 135
Doṣha vṛddhi and kṣhaya kāraṇa 136
Sama doṣha 137
Prākṛta doṣha lakṣhaṇas 138
Vaiṣhamya doṣha 141
Vṛddha doṣha lakṣhaṇa 141
Kṣhīna doṣha lakṣhaṇa 144
Doṣha sthāna 146
Doṣha bheda 149
Pañcha vāta 150
Pañcha pitta 155
Pañcha kapha 158
Chapter 8 : Dhātu 165
Paribhāṣhā 165
Dhātu vṛddhi and kṣhaya kāraṇa 166
Prākṛta dhātu lakṣhaṇa 167
Vṛddha dhātu lakṣhaṇa 169
Kṣhīna dhātu lakṣhaṇa 175
Dhātus and pañcha mahābhūtas 181
Upadhātu and dhātumala 181
Chapter 9 : Mala 188
Prākṛta mala lakṣhaṇa 189
Vṛddha mala lakṣhaṇa 190
Kṣhīna mala lakṣhaṇa 191
Chapter 10 : Ojas 197
Paribhāṣhā: Definitions 197
Are *ojas* and *bala* the same? 198
Ojo guṇa and karma 199
Ojo bheda 202
Ojo sthāna 202
Channels carrying ojas 203
Factors responsible for ojas and bala 203
Ojo kṣhaya kāraṇa 204

Ojo kṣhaya lakṣhaṇas 207
Chapter 11 : Srotas 213
Paribhāṣhā and paryāya 213
Definition #1: General overview 213
Definition #2: Primary function 214
Definition #3: Detailed functions 214
Definition #4: Anatomical features 215
Synonyms 216
Bheda 217
Potential for infinite srotases 217
13 systems of srotases 218
Other classifications of srotases 219
Sroto mūla and duṣhṭi 220
Prāṇavahā srotas 221
Udakavahā srotas 221
Annavahā srotas 222
Rasavahā srotas 222
Raktavahā srotas 222
Māṁsavahā srotas 222
Medovahā srotas 223
Asthivahā srotas 223
Majjavahā srotas 223
Śhukravahā srotas 223
Mūtravahā srotas 223
Purīṣhavahā srotas 224
Svedavahā srotas 224
Sroto mūla and duṣhṭi (Input networks) 225
Sroto mūla and duṣhṭi (Transformation networks) 226
Sroto mūla and duṣhṭi (Output networks) 229
Sroto duṣhṭi bheda 230
Sroto duṣhṭi nidāna 231
Samānya nidāna 231
Viśheṣha nidāna 232
Sroto duṣhṭi viśheṣha nidāna 236
Chapter 12 : Doṣha-dūṣhya sammūrchhana 243
Paribhāṣhā 243
Doṣha 243
Dūṣhya 243
Sammūrchana 244

Table of Contents: Unit II

Chapter 13 : Classical perspectives and definitions 255
Śhārīra and śharīra 255
Paribhāṣhā 255
Chapter 14 : Āyu (Life span) 261
Vayas 261
Chapter 15 : Garbha vijñāna (Embryology) 268
Ṛtu kāla (Fertile period) 268
Assessment of śhukra and ārtava 269
Garbhotpatti (Procreation) 270
Chapter 16 : Prasūti vijñāna (Pregnancy) 277
Garbhiṇi (Mother) 277
Garbha (Fetus) 279
Prasava kāla (Labor and delivery) 280
Sūtikopachara (Care of the mother after delivery) 282
Chapter 17 : Bāla prakaraṇa (Management of birth and childhood) 287
Chapter 18 : Prakṛti 294
Nirukti & Paribhāṣhā 294
Nirukti 294
Paribhāṣhā 295
Bheda 298
Śharīrika prakṛti 298
Mānasika prakṛti 299
Bhautika Prakṛti 300
Śharīrika prakṛti lakṣhaṇas 304
Charaka's perspective 304
Suśhruta's perspective 309
Chapter 19 : Śharīra saṅkhya avayava 320
Organization and measurement 320
Śharīra saṅkhya avayava 321
Chapter 20 : Aṣhṭa vidha sāra 330
Assessing sāra 330
Sāra lakṣhaṇas 334
Chapter 21 : Saṁhanana 348
Understanding saṁhanana 348
Chapter 22 : Nidrā (Sleep) 357
Paribhāṣhā and paryāya 357
Definition #1: Suśhruta's perspective 358
Definition #2: Charaka's perspective 358
Definition #3: Vāgbhaṭa's perspective 358
Bheda 359
Rātri and divā svapna 359
Five types of sleep based on onset 360
Seven types of sleep based on onset 361

Normal sleep process ... 363
Role of hṛdaya in sleep ... 363
Role of triguṇa in sleep ... 364
Normal physiology of sleep ... 364
State of suspended animation ... 364
Dreams ... 365
General recommendations for sleep ... 365
Outcomes ... 365
Chapter 23 : Manas, indriya, sattva-rajas-tamas ... 371
Paribhāṣhā and paryāya ... 371
Definition ... 372
Synonyms ... 372
Role of manas in āyu ... 373
Mano sthāna ... 374
Importance of the hṛdaya ... 374
Mano guṇa ... 376
Tri-guṇas ... 376
Mano guṇas ... 381
Mano karma ... 381
Mano viṣhaya ... 382
Indriya ... 384
Jñānendriya ... 385
Karmendriya ... 387
Pañcha pañchaka ... 388
Chapter 24 : Ātma ... 396
Ātma ... 396
Paryāya ... 396
Understanding ātma ... 397
Existence of ātma ... 398
Ātma activates manas ... 402
Ātma bheda ... 403
Adhyātma dravya-guṇa saṅgraha ... 404
Transmigration of ātma ... 404
Chetanā adhiṣhṭhāna ... 404
Responsibilities of ātma ... 405
Attachment of ātma ... 405
Detachment, rebirth and mokṣha ... 406
Buddhi ... 408
Smṛti ... 409
Dhṛti ... 409
Ahaṅkāra ... 410
Chapter 25 : Mṛtyu (Death) ... 416
Paribhāṣhā and paryāya ... 416
Āyu as a function of mṛtyu ... 418
Kāla and akāla mṛtyu ... 420
Ariṣhṭa (riṣhṭa) lakṣhaṇas ... 422
Nirukti & Paribhāṣhā ... 423

UNIT I

सिद्धान्त

Siddhānta

(Core principles)

Chapter 1 : Introduction

KEY TERMS

anādi	dhātu	Pūrva-mīmāṁsā	sthāna
Āstika darśhana	guru-śhiṣhya parampara	ṣhaḍ darśhana	Upaniṣhad
ātma	Kāyachikitsā	sampradāya	Uttara-mīmāṁsā
bhāva	Nāstika darśhana	Sāṅkhya	vāda
chatuṣhka	Nyāya	siddhānta	Vaiśheṣhika
darśhana	Padārtha Vijñāna	sṛṣhṭi utpatti	Yoga

The core principles and theoretical foundations of Āyurveda are contained in a set of laws collectively known as *siddhānta* (theory). The study of this information is a specialized area called Āyurveda Samhitā & Siddhānta and its advanced study, research and investigation in India falls under a non-clinical department available at Postgraduate and PhD levels (Central Council of Indian Medicine Notification, 2012, March 19).

Throughout this volume, the core knowledge of *siddhānta* will be covered along with a critical review of statements from multiple classical authors and relevant commentaries. *Siddhānta* include universal principles and timeless laws that likely provided support to the claim of Āyurveda being eternal and present since the beginning of creation since these are constant laws demonstrated in nature. That which is found in nature will be present in the manifested reality as long as that reality or matter exists.

In some instances, variations may be seen in statements from different classical authors on certain topics in *siddhānta*. These variations in perspectives should all be analyzed to provide a broader understanding of how the principle may operate under varying conditions, in different environments or with other variables at play. This is one of the keys to taking theoretical knowledge and successfully applying it in practice.

The term *siddhānta* derives from the Sanskrit *dhātu* √ *sidh*, defined as:

√ sidh	to go, move
	to drive off, scare away, repel, restrain, hinder
	to punish, chastise
	to ordain, instruct
	to turn out well or auspiciously

As a weak form of the *dhātu* √ *sādh*, the term *siddhānta* can also derive meanings as:

√ sādh	**to be accomplished or fulfilled or effected or settled, be successful, succeed**
	to hit a mark (loc.)
	to attain one's aim or object, have success
	to attain the highest object, become perfect, attain beatitude
	to be valid or admissible, hold good
	to be proved, demonstrated or established, result from
	to be set right, (esp.) be

	healed or cured
	to be well cooked
	to conform to a person's will, yield to (gen.)
	to fall to a person's (gen.) lot or share
	to come into existence, originate, arise

The term *siddhānta* itself refers to:

siddhānta	established end, final end or aim or purpose
	demonstrated conclusion of an argument
	settled opinion or doctrine, dogma, axiom, received or admitted truth
	any fixed or established or canonical text-book or received scientific treatise on any subject

Siddhānta is defined as a statement which has been thoroughly and exhaustively assessed and tested, and is found to be true (Cha. Vi. 8/3). Today, this can be equated to applying the scientific method to a hypothesis and proving it into a demonstrated and accepted theory.

In classical texts from Āyurveda and other philosophical schools, many synonyms have been used for the term *siddhānta*. Today, these continue to be used by scholars throughout India. The common synonyms include *vāda* (law) and *bhāva* (tenet) which are terms that may follow the name of a certain *siddhānta*. They can be translated as theory, law or tenet.

TEST YOURSELF

Learn, review and memorize key terms from this section.

bhāva

dhātu

siddhānta

vāda

CLASSICAL INTRODUCTIONS

Each classical author takes their own approach to introducing the science and presenting *siddhānta* throughout their treatise. By considering their *sampradāya* (school of thought), purpose, time period and available literature and knowledge, the specific reasons for their methodologies may become more obvious. The classical authors typically recorded information in the most concise and efficient way possible. The well developed Āyurvedic vocabulary and terminologies stand as evidence that they were capable of conveying meanings succinctly and clearly for use within the scope of their science and practice.

For all works, remember that none are written for introductory level instruction. All major treatises were meant to be used as tools under direct guidance of a qualified and skilled teacher. Once the student was fully capable in the science they would then be able to navigate, read and interpret the treatises independently.

Next, let's review each of the major authors individually to understand their perspective and methodology for introducing the science and *siddhānta*.

Who should study?

Suśhruta begins his 186-chapter treatise, the *Suśhruta Samhitā*, by dedicating the first four chapters to preparation for training and specifying who should study Āyurveda to maintain the integrity of the science. In Su. Sū. 1/, he recounts the story of how Divodāsa Dhanvantari became the teacher of a group of students including Suśhruta. This is followed by a very broad overview of the scope of the study.

Su. Sū. 2/ provides detailed instructions on how to select appropriate students and initiate them into study. It also provides guidelines for new students on ethical behavior, expectations, and responsibilities which were expected to be strictly maintained during their study period which could last several years or more, depending on their learning abilities.

In Su. Sū. 3/, the student is then introduced to the layout of the text, its *sthānas* (chapters) and purpose. More expectations are given for the student's behavior to reinforce their commitment to completing studies. In chapter four, the student is reminded that even upon completing studies and earning the title of Vaidya, they should strive to continue expanding their knowledge through learning related disciplines within Āyurveda and in allied Vedic sciences.

Of all classical treatises, the *Suśhruta Samhitā* is the only one to start the work with an introduction to the subject directed towards the student. Being one of the oldest surviving classical works, this demonstration is significant for many reasons and very likely that it would be effective and popular today.

How does the science work?

In clear contrast to Suśhruta's introduction to the subject, Charaka focuses the first four chapters of his treatise on laying the ground rules for how the science of Āyurveda works. Remember that Charaka's *Sūtra-sthāna* has a special arrangement of *chatuṣhkas* (quadrates, or set of four chapters), and the first four chapters form the *Bheṣhaja chatuṣhka*, or the quadrate on therapeutics and medicinal formulations.

A good portion of the most critical *siddhānta* are included in Cha. Sū. 1/ along with the key therapeutic ingredients of the time. By laying out the text in this way, Charaka reinforces the fact that he intends to write the work for a reader who is already fully competent in the subject and practice of Āyurvedic medicine, and that this work is meant as a thorough review of known material in the specialized field of *Kāyachikitsā* (Internal medicine).

Chapter 30, the final chapter of Charaka's *Sūtra-sthāna* is actually more of a basic introduction to the science and a summary of expectations for practicing. The fact that this is reiterated at the end of *Sūtra-sthāna* speaks to the point that the text is directed to a reader who is already thoroughly familiar with the material. This serves more as a review rather than an introduction.

What are the basic variables?

Vāgbhaṭa, the author who is credited with two classical treatises, provides another perspective on introducing the subject through his methods of consolidation and reorganization of previous works. The *Aṣhṭāṅga Hṛdaya* begins its very succinct recapitulation of the science by reviewing the variables which mainly include the qualitative and quantitative principles.

While the first chapter sets the stage for how the science's principles can be applied, the second and third chapters quickly move into recommendations and guidelines for daily health maintenance and seasonal and annual care. The text reads much more like direct instructions on what to do and how to do it so that the Vaidya can successfully care for themselves and others. Like Charaka,

Vāgbhaṭa is not writing to a novice reader, and although the instructions in *Aṣhṭāṅga Hṛdaya* are very direct, systematic and concise, they do not teach each concept at a fundamental level through the actual text. Any explanations required to fully convey the meaning were to be provided by the student's teacher in the *guru-śhiṣhya parampara* (direct instruction in class).

Summing it all up

The later work of Bhāvamiśhra titled *Bhāva Prakāśha*, provides another valuable approach to introducing the science. With so much information available to this 16th century author, it was possible to restructure and reorganize the content in a much cleaner way compared to earlier treatises. The result is a very well laid out and comprehensive presentation of the first few chapters that explain the science in an orderly, sensible summary.

BP Pū. 1/ begins by recounting a very detailed compilation of the origins of the science starting from a mythological perspective. BP Pū. 2/ then describes the concept of *sṛṣhṭi utpatti*, the origin of the universe and life, as it was accepted at the time. The terms and perspective used in this chapter are greatly influenced by the philosophy and religion of the time and culture. Although many of these philosophical terms are also seen in Āyurveda, they take on varied meanings depending on the field of science where they are applied. From BP Pū. 3/ on, the science of Āyurveda and its many *siddhānta* are laid out in progressive order through the evolution and stages of human life.

TEST YOURSELF

Learn, review and memorize key terms from this section.

chatuṣhka

guru-śhiṣhya parampara

Kāyachikitsā

sampradāya

sṛṣhṭi utpatti

sthāna

DARŚHANA

The evolution of Āyurveda over millennia has been influenced by philosophies, religions, cultures, political, social and other factors. Although the classical authorities like Charaka clearly state that Āyurveda is *anādi* (eternal), history and remaining evidence today tell a bigger story. Records of continual development of the science of Āyurveda make it clear that the practical application of the science has most definitely evolved and adapted to meet changing demands over time.

From its earliest records, Āyurveda has drawn parts of its knowledge and understanding of the life from six philosophical schools, collectively known as the *ṣhaḍ darśhana* (six philosophical schools). These philosophies were recorded in the last section of the Vedas called the Upaniṣhads. This knowledge was the prevalent foundation for philosophical and scientific thought during the time of Charaka and Suśhruta.

While *ṣhaḍ* means six, *darśhana* is a term with a variety of meanings and it may be interpreted differently according to context. The term *darśhana* comes from the Sanskrit *dhātu* √ *dṛśh* which has a number of interpretations according to the Monier-Williams dictionary:

√ dṛśh	**to see, behold, look at, regard, consider**
	to see, ie wait on, visit
	to see with the mind, learn, understand
	to notice, care for, look into, try, examine
	to see by divine intuition, think or find out, compose, contrive (hymns, rites, etc); to be seen, become visible, appear
	to be shown or manifested, appear as, prove
	to show, demonstrate
	to produce (money) ie pay
	knowing, discerning

The term *darśhana* refers to:

darśhana	showing
	seeing, looking at
	knowing
	exhibiting, teaching
	ocular perception, the eye-sight
	inspection, examination
	view, doctrine, philosophical system (six in number, ie, Pūrva-mīmāṁsā, Uttara-mīmāṁsā, Nyāya, Vaiśheṣhika, Sāṅkhya, Yoga).

Based on this, the term *darśhana* can be interpreted in several ways. In a historical sense, it refers to one or more philosophical schools of thought, especially the *ṣhaḍ darśhana*. In a more active, applied way, it indicates a perspective or viewpoint, especially when that understanding leads to a methodology and ultimately graduates into its own system or science. And in terms of planning ahead, it can help provide a framework based on its methodology for advancement of the science through research and development.

Each of these interpretations can be seen in the history and evolution of Āyurveda and its *siddhānta*. While the base knowledge of the science was built on the *ṣhaḍ darśhana*, its trial, error, research, development and advancement over time happened because of the transformation of the initial *ṣhaḍ darśhana* into the Āyurvedic *darśhana*. This transformation can also be seen to encompass the various schools of thought, or *sampradāya* within the entire field of Āyurveda. Today, these philosophical foundations form a cornerstone of introductory study for Āyurvedic professionals in India under the subject of Padārtha Vijñāna.

The *ṣhaḍ darśhana* are traditionally grouped together under the umbrella of *Āstika darśhana* ("Continuity" philosophies) because each of them adheres to specific fundamental beliefs. They all follow the Vedas as the supreme source of knowledge, and accept a common explanation for the generation of life in the universe. These tenets include birth, death and the continuity of the *ātma*, or persistent spirit.

Interestingly, it is important to note that Āyurveda also drew concepts from another category of *darśhana*, the *Nāstika darśhana* ("Non-Continuouity" philosophies). The tenets held by these philosophical schools did not recognize some of the key *Āstika* concepts like the Vedas or the existence of *ātma* and continuity of life beyond death. Assuming or believing that a religious, spiritual or personal belief system must be connected to Āyurveda for it to work is not a primary focus within the scope of professional Āyurvedic studies. The science is capable of demonstrating its own abilities in research, development and advancement separately from the influences of socio-

The *ṣhaḍ darśhana*, authors, and major contributions to Āyurveda include:

Darśhana	Author	Major contributions to Āyurveda
Pūrva-mīmāṃsā	Jaimini	• *Mokṣha*
Uttara-mīmāṃsā	Vyāsa	• *Pūrva karma* • *Antarātma*
Nyāya	Goutama	• Stronger influence in Charaka's work, especially in Vimāna-sthāna • *Pramāṇa siddhānta* • *Tantrayukti* • *Kārya abhinivṛtti ghaṭaka*
Vaiśheṣhika	Kanada	• *Padārtha siddhānta*
Sāṅkhya	Kapila	• *Trividha pramāṇa* • Suśhruta's *trividha duḥkha* • Recognition of *puruṣha* in *sṛṣhṭi utpatti* • *Pariṇāma vada* • *Satkārya vada* • *Triguṇa siddhānta*
Yoga	Patānjali	• *Pramāṇa siddhānta* • *Nidra* • *Smṛti* • *Abhyāsa* • Charaka's description of Yoga in Śhārīra-sthāna

Typically, the *Nāstika* schools were considered inferior by popular culture, society and religions, yet Āyurveda continued to recognize that truth could be found in all systems.

Over the last several millennia, the Āyurvedic *darśhana* and *sampradāya* have developed well enough to stand on their own as a complete, independent body of science. religious pressures. It is a body of knowledge which can adapt to different cultures, environments and time periods and its *darśhana* can be utilized to demonstrate this progress on its own.

Today, the question is where can Āyurveda go from here. Should it be a science perpetually stuck in its history and attachments, or can it develop to help transform the understanding of health and meet the increasing demands of society today? This is a critical juncture for the establishment of Āyurveda on a global scale and a topic which has been addressed by some of the finest scholars in India. Read the article, *Need of new research methodology for Āyurveda*, by MS Baghel for a deeper review.

TEST YOURSELF

Learn, review and memorize key terms from this section.

anādi

Āstika darśhana

ātma

darśhana

Nāstika darśhana

Nyāya

Padārtha Vijñāna

Pūrva-mīmāṁsā

ṣhaḍ darśhana

Sāṅkhya

Upaniṣhad

Uttara-mīmāṁsā

Vaiśheṣhika

Yoga

HOW TO USE THIS VOLUME

Following this introduction, chapter two of this volume provides an overview of the classical *siddhānta*. Each *siddhānta* is listed with a basic explanation and examples wherever possible. In the following chapters, major *siddhānta* are elaborated with thorough explanations, comprehensive reviews and comparisons from multiple classical sources.

Unit II then explores classical concepts of *śhārīra* (the study of the human body), with a thorough review of understanding the human body in Āyurveda. This builds to complete the full picture of life with a review of *sṛṣhṭi utpatti*, which brings all the components together in the formation of life and the universe.

One of the reasons that Āyurveda has been challenging to understand and apply fully is that it requires having a large base of foundational knowledge to connect all of the pieces and create a complete, functioning system. All volumes in this textbook series have been designed to present material in digestible portions and continuously build on a comprehensive learning process. From a student's perspective, this presents all of the information required to move forward in one place and encourages regular study and review. From a practical standpoint, some of the most pertinent information of the science is available in quick reference style. In later chapters, the concepts are presented in detail using tables and charts wherever possible. These are intended to be used as quick reference desk guides in practice, until they are fully memorized.

Chapter 1: Review

ADDITIONAL READING

Read and review the references listed below to expand your understanding of the concepts in this chapter. Write down the date that you complete your reading for each. Remember that consistent repetition is the best way to learn. Plan to read each reference at least once now and expect to read it again as you continue your studies.

References marked with (skim) can be read quickly and do not require commentary review.

CLASSICS		1st read	2nd read
Charaka	Cha. Sū. 1-4/ (skim) Cha. Vi. 8/3		
Suśhruta	Su. Sū. 1-4/		
Aṣhṭāṅga Hṛdaya	AH Sū. 1-3/ (skim)		
Bhāva Prakāśha	BP Pū. 2-4/ (skim)		

JOURNALS & CURRENT RESOURCES

Baghel, M. S. (2011). Need of new research methodology for Āyurveda. Ayu, 32(1), 3–4. http://doi.org/10.4103/0974-8520.85711

QUESTIONS & ANSWERS

Record your questions for this chapter here for further research and discussion.

Question:

Answer:

Question:

Answer:

Question:

Answer:

SELF-ASSESSMENT

1. Which of the following scientific theories or laws could be considered *anādi*?
   a. For every action, there is an equal and opposite reaction
   b. Gravity
   c. Law of conservation of energy
   d. All of the above
   e. None of the above

2. Which of the following meanings of the Sanskrit *dhātu* √ *sidh* is least relevant to the practical application of *siddhānta*?
   a. to be well cooked
   b. to demonstrate conclusion
   c. to ordain, instruct
   d. to punish, chastise
   e. None of the above

3. A common synonym for *siddhānta* is
   a. *abhyāsa*
   b. *bhāva*
   c. *darśhana*
   d. *sampradāya*
   e. Sāṅkhya

4. The preparation and indoctrination of students into the long-term, committed study of Āyurveda was best conveyed through the classical work of
   a. Bhāvamiśhra
   b. Charaka
   c. Nyāya
   d. Suśhruta
   e. Vāgbhaṭa

5. How can *darśhana* be translated?
   a. view
   b. perspective
   c. belief
   d. sight
   e. All of the above

6. All of the following are *ṣhaḍ darśhana* which contributed to Āyurveda except
   a. Nyāya
   b. Pūrva-mīmāṁsā
   c. Sāṅkhya
   d. Uttara-mīmāṁsā
   e. Yoga

7. Today, followers of *Nāstika darśhana* would most likely adhere to
   a. Atheism
   b. Catholicism
   c. Hinduism
   d. Islam
   e. New Age Spirituality

8. In *Need of new research methodology for Āyurveda*, by MS Baghel, the author explains that the current format of Āyurvedic research provides a direct benefit to
   a. Electronic health records (EHR)
   b. Evidence-based medicine
   c. Future students
   d. Homeopathy
   e. Pharmaceutical interests

9. Practical application of Āyurveda outside of India can be strongly supported by a foundational study of
   a. the *Charaka sampradāya* only
   b. *ṣhaḍ darśhana*
   c. *siddhānta*
   d. *sṛṣhṭi utpatti*
   e. Vedic history

10. *Bhāva Prakāśha* presents a clear, well organized introduction to the science of Āyurveda because
    a. It contains the Nighaṇṭu section.
    b. It is organized in fewer sections than the older *saṁhitās*.
    c. It uses a reductionist approach to presenting the subject by explaining *sṛṣhṭi utpatti* at the beginning of the text.
    d. It was one of the earliest, original texts of Āyurveda that was regularly updated.
    e. It was one of the most recently composed treatises and had a large body of knowledge to draw upon.

CRITICAL THINKING

1. Find three examples where the classical authors provide similar information across the introductory sections of different texts.

2. Compare and contrast the four texts described in the section on classical introductions. Out of the four, rate their ease of use and explain your reasoning.

3. Define *siddhānta* in your own words, and describe your understanding of its role in Āyurveda.

4. Considering the history and evolution of Āyurvedic *siddhānta*, what would be appropriate for the science and profession to focus on today? Analyze benefits and drawbacks of investing research time and effort into understanding historical origins versus developing future perspectives and methodologies.

5. In *Need of new research methodology for Āyurveda*, by MS Baghel, what is the author's viewpoint on Āyurveda and Evidence-based Medicine? What does he recommend for Āyurveda in his article?

References

"Central Council of Indian Medicine Notification." (2012, March 19). Retrieved from https://ccimindia.org/ayurveda-pg-reg.php.

Chapter 2 : Overview of siddhānta

KEY TERMS

achetanā
agni
ākāśha
amla
amūrti
ap
āśhraya
āśhrayi
asthi
ātma
audbhida
avara
avasthā
āyu
chaya
chetanā
chikitsā
deśha
dhātu
dhātu-mala
diśha
doṣha
dravya
gandha
gati
guṇa
gurvādi
hṛdaya
jala
jaṅgama
kāla
kapha
karma
kārya-kāraṇa bhāva
kaṣhāya
kaṭu
koṣhṭha
kṣhaya
lavaṇa
loka
madhyama
madhura
mahābhūta
majja
mala
māṁsa
manas
manasika doṣha
medas
mūrti
mūtra
nava kāraṇa dravya
pañcha mahābhūta
pañcha tanmātra
pārthiva pitta
prabhāva
prakopa
prakṛti
praśhamana
pṛthvi
purīṣha
puruṣha
rajas
rakta
rasa
ṛtu
ṛtu-sandhi
rūpa
śhabda
ṣhaḍ darśhana
sāmānya
samavāya
samavāyi
sāmya
saṁyoga
saṅgraha
śharīra
satkārya vāda
sattva
siddhānta
śhīta
sparśha
sṛṣhṭi utpatti
śhukra
sveda
tamas
tanmātra
tejas
tikta
trayopastambha
tri-daṇḍavat puruṣha
tri-deśha
tri-guṇa
upadhātu
uṣhṇa
uttama
varṣha
vāta
vāyu
vibhāga
vipāka
vīrya
viśheṣha
vṛddhi

In this chapter, each *siddhānta* will be listed and explained in a basic and introductory manner. In many cases, the *siddhānta* will have much more underlying detail which must also be fully learned and understood in order to be applied. Those details will follow in entire chapters dedicated to their thorough review. Note that the *siddhānta* covered here do not include those from *chikitsā*, or therapeutics, which will be covered in a separate volume.

The *siddhānta* are listed in order of their manifestation or creation in the world as they are normally explained classically and seen practically. For example, in order for the world as we know it to exist, an environment, or what is usually considered the universe, should be present first. Upon manifestation of this universe, matter became present which provided a foundation to the myriad forms of life now seen. Of all these forms, the human being takes precedence in the study of Āyurveda as it is the subject of focus. Classically, a human being is also called *karma puruṣha* or *chikitsā puruṣha*, which refers to the individual as the field of scope for application of therapeutics.

Each of the following listings begins with a heading of the classical Sanskrit name of the *siddhānta* and any common variations. Just below the Sanskrit name, the translation of the *siddhānta* name in its nearest English equivalent is presented, if available.

The heading is followed by the individual Sanskrit terms of the *siddhānta* with their nearest English equivalents. The translations of individual terms include generic meanings from the Monier-Williams Sanskrit dictionary and specific uses for the context of the field of Āyurveda. Advanced students will notice that certain terms have many more meanings which are not listed here. Those additional meanings have not been included to focus this introduction on the core foundational interpretations within the scope of Āyurveda.

Finally, the *siddhānta* is discussed in a brief, introductory explanation. At the end of each *siddhānta* section, pertinent references are listed. These include classical, abbreviated references and volume and chapter numbers from this series of textbooks which cover the topic in detail.

SṚṢHṬI UTPATTI

Creation of life

sṛṣhṭi	nature, procreation, creation, life, universe
utpatti	producing as an effect or result, giving rise to, generating as a consequence

The concept of *sṛṣhṭi utpatti* refers to the creation of life, as the first of three stages, followed by *sthiti* (existence and maintenance of life) and *laya* (death, destruction, and dissolution). *Sṛṣhṭi utpatti* ties together the origins of life from the *ṣhaḍ darśhana* into the field of Āyurveda. This level of knowledge and understanding is one of the most challenging concepts to prove or test in many branches of classical and modern science. Its tenets explain the sources for other key concepts in Āyurveda and lay the foundations for the functioning of matter in its gross, observable form. It describes the processes and steps that allow the five human senses to detect and recognize the presence of matter and reality. A thorough understanding of *sṛṣhṭi utpatti* requires a solid basis in all Āyurvedic concepts that can be physically manifested and recognized in material environments.

Additional references

BP Pū. 2/	Vol 2: Chapter 25

TEST YOURSELF

Learn, review and memorize key terms from this section.

ṣhaḍ darśhana __________

sṛṣhṭi __________

utpatti __________

sthiti __________

laya __________

SATKĀRYA VĀDA

Matter exists

sat	being, existing, occurring, happening, being present; truth
kārya	to be made or done or

	practiced or performed; to be caused to do
vāda	law, principle, rule

The *satkārya vāda* states that any *dravya* (matter) that is produced must be generated from *dravya* which already exists. The ability to produce any *dravya* lies latent within its inputs.

TEST YOURSELF

Learn, review and memorize key terms from this section.

sat

---

kārya

---

vāda

---

dravya

KĀRYA-KĀRAṆA BHĀVA

Cause and effect

kārya	to be made or done or practiced or performed; to be caused to do
kāraṇa	cause, reason, the cause of anything; instrument, means

Kārya-kāraṇa bhāva states that there is always a cause for any effect. When combined with the *satkārya vāda,* these two *siddhānta* can be interpreted as the first law of thermodynamics, the law of conservation of energy. This states that "Energy can neither be created nor destroyed, it can only be transformed."

Additional references

Cha. Vi. 8/68-78

TEST YOURSELF

Learn, review and memorize key terms from this section.

kārya

---

kāraṇa

---

bhāva

NAVA KĀRAṆA DRAVYA, DRAVYA SAṄGRAHA

The nine causes of matter

nava	nine
kāraṇa	doing, making, effecting, causing
dravya	a substance, thing, object; matter; the ingredients or materials of anything
saṅgraha	holding together, collecting, gathering, conglomeration, accumulation; inclusion, comprehension; drawing together, making narrower

The *nava kāraṇa dravya* states that there are nine causes, or constituent components, required for any *dravya* to exist. These nine include the *pañcha mahābhūta* (five gross elements) and four additional, independent components:

Ākāśha	Space, ether
Vāyu	Air, wind

Tejas	Fire, light
Ap / Jala	Water
Pṛthvi	Earth
Ātma	Persistent spirit
Manas	Mind
Kāla	Time
Diśha (*Dik*)	Direction

Additional references

Cha. Sū. 1/48

TEST YOURSELF

Learn, review and memorize key terms from this section.

nava ______

kāraṇa ______

dravya ______

saṅgraha ______

pañcha mahābhūta ______

ākāśha ______

vāyu ______

tejas ______

ap / jala ______

pṛthvi ______

ātma ______

manas ______

kāla ______

diśha (dik) ______

DRAVYA

Matter

dravya	a substance, thing, object; matter; the ingredients or materials of anything; medicinal substance or drug

Dravya is considered any substance or matter which exists and can be recognized by the sense organs. It is classically defined by Charaka as the base which connects and holds *guṇa* (characteristics) and *karma* (actions) in *samavāya* (perpetual attachment).

It is often used to refer to Āyurvedic medicines or therapeutic processes in more specific contexts and is commonly translated as "drug(s)" in Indian Āyurvedic literature. There are several classification methods for *dravya* to clarify its utility and purpose, and allow it to be applied practically.

Additional references

Cha. Sū. 1/51
Cha. Sū. 1/68-73
Cha. Sū. 26/10

Vol 2: Chapter 3

TEST YOURSELF

Learn, review and memorize key terms from this section.

dravya

guṇa

karma

PAÑCHA TANMĀTRA

The five subtle elements

pañcha	five
tanmātra	subtle element

The *pañcha tanmātra* are the subtle forms of the five gross elements which are not directly recognizable by the five sense organs. Each subtle form corresponds to only one gross form, and through their special relationship, they are able to convey information between their connected gross and subtle states. The pair also shares their special relationship with one sense organ thus allowing the information they carry to be recognized by that single sense organ. The *pañcha tanmātra* were generated as part of the process of *sṛṣhṭi utpatti* in a specific, sequential order where the first generated the second, and so on.

The order of generation is:

Śhabda tanmātra	Subtle element of sound
↓	↓
Sparśha tanmātra	Subtle element of touch
↓	↓
Rūpa tanmātra	Subtle element of sight
↓	↓
Rasa tanmātra	Subtle element of taste
↓	↓
Gandha tanmātra	Subtle element of smell

Additional references

BP Pū. 2/19-21 Su. Śhā. 1/4	Vol 2: Chapter 22

TEST YOURSELF

Learn, review and memorize key terms from this section.

pañcha

tanmātra

śhabda

sparśha

rūpa

rasa

gandha

PAÑCHA MAHĀBHŪTA

The five gross elements

pañcha	five
mahā	great, gross
bhūta	element

The *pañcha mahābhūta* (five gross elements) include those which are directly knowable, recognizable or understandable by each of the five sense organs. Each element corresponds to a specific sense organ and has a special relationship with that sense organ so that it can be detected. Produced as an outcome of the *pañcha tanmātra*, the *pañcha mahābhūta* also developed in succession. Variations in classical opinions exist about their specific make-up, but all authors agree that each individual *mahābhūta* (gross element) contains a predominance of the *bhūta* (element) which bears its name. This significant observation means that there is variability in the content and proportion of all matter.

The order of generation is:

Ākāśha mahābhūta	Gross element of space or ether
↓	↓
Vāyu mahābhūta	Gross element of air
↓	↓
Tejo mahābhūta	Gross element of light
↓	↓
Ap / Jala mahābhūta	Gross element of water
↓	↓
Pṛthvi mahābhūta	Gross element of earth

Additional references

Cha. Sū. 1/	Vol 2: Chapter 3
Cha. Sū. 26/10	
Cha. Śhā. 1/	
Su. Sū. 46/	

TEST YOURSELF

Learn, review and memorize key terms from this section.

pañcha

____

mahā

____

bhūta

____

ākāśha

____

vāyu

____

tejas

____

ap / jala

____

pṛthvi

____

MŪRTI-AMŪRTI

Formed-Formless

mūrti	any solid body or material form, anything which has definite shape or limits such as mind and the four elements *pṛthvi* (earth), *ap* (water), *tejas* (fire), *vāyu* (air), but not *ākāśha* (ether)
amūrti	shapelessness, absence of shape or form, formless

Mūrti (formed) and *amūrti* (formless) *dravya* are those which have definite form or shape, and those which do not, respectively. This classification is most commonly applied to the *pañcha mahābhūtas* and the *doṣhas*. The *pañcha mahābhūta* which was generated first, *ākāśha*, is *amūrti*. The remaining four *mahābhūtas* are all *mūrti* since they have increasing levels of mass. With the *doṣhas*, *vāta* is considered *amūrti* because of its predominance in *ākāśha* and *vāyu*, while *pitta* and *kapha* are *mūrti*.

Additional references

Cha. Sū. 1/ Cha. Sū. 26/10 Cha. Śhā. 1/ Su. Sū. 46/	Vol 2: Chapter 4

TEST YOURSELF

Learn, review and memorize key terms from this section.

mūrti

amūrti

pañcha mahābhūta

doṣha

CHETANĀ-ACHETANĀ

Sentient-Insentient

chetanā	aware, conscious, sentient, intelligent
achetanā	without consciousness, inanimate

All *dravya* must fall under *chetanā* (sentient) or *achetanā* (insentient). *Chetanā dravya* possess sense organs while *achetanā dravya* do not. These are generally considered human beings who have *chetanā* (consciousness) which resides in the *hṛdaya* (heart). It also includes animals and plants.

Additional references

Cha. Sū. 1/48 (Chakr.)

TEST YOURSELF

Learn, review and memorize key terms from this section.

chetanā

achetanā

hṛdaya

JAṄGAMA-AUDBHIDA-PĀRTHIVA

Animal-Vegetable-Mineral

jaṅgama	moving, locomotive (as opposed to stationary), living
audbhida	coming forth, springing forth, breaking through, issuing from
pārthiva	earthen, earthy, earthly, being in or relating to or coming from the earth

All *dravya* can also be classified under one of these three categories. The subcategory of minerals also includes metals. Each of the subcategories also has finer classification methods based on the specific characteristics of the *dravya*. The *jaṅgama-audbhida-pārthiva* classification is most commonly used for Āyurvedic medicines, therapeutic formulations and substances.

Additional references

Cha. Sū. 1/68

TEST YOURSELF

Learn, review and memorize key terms from this section.

jaṅgama

audbhida

pārthiva

dravya

SĀMĀNYA-VIŚHEṢHA SIDDHĀNTA

Similar-Opposite

sāmānya	equal, alike, similar, in general, in common, the connection of different objects by common properties
viśheṣha	distinction, difference between, particularity, individuality, essential difference

Sāmānya-viśheṣha states that "like increases like, opposites decrease." It is perhaps one of the most important fundamental *siddhānta* in Āyurveda. It is universally seen in practice that any *dravya* with similar characteristics will increase or accumulate when combined. And *dravya* with dissimilar characteristics will decrease or diminish when combined, by causing a net effect of canceling each other out. In certain classical translations, *sāmānya* is often translated as "generic concomitance" while *viśheṣha* is translated as "variant factor."

Additional references

Cha. Sū. 1/44-45

TEST YOURSELF

Learn, review and memorize key terms from this section.

sāmānya

viśheṣha

siddhānta

dravya

SAMAVĀYA

Perpetual attachment

samavāya	perpetual co-inherence, inner or intimate relation, constant and intimate union, inseparable concomitance

Samavāya states that certain aspects of *dravya* are always attached to that *dravya*. This perpetual attachment exists because of the nature of the *dravya* and its *guṇa* and *karma*. The *samavāya* relationship is permanent. In certain classical translations, *samavāya* is translated as "inseparable concomitance."

Additional references

Cha. Sū. 1/50

TEST YOURSELF

Learn, review and memorize key terms from this section.

samavāya

dravya

guṇa

karma

SAMAVĀYI

That which is perpetually attached

samavāyi	closely connected or united, concomitant, inherent in, having or consisting of a combination

Samavāyi refers to the specific feature of a *dravya*, usually its *guṇa* or *karma*, which is perpetually attached because of a *samavāya* relationship. In certain classical translations, it may be referred to as that which is "concomitant" or a "concomitant factor."

Additional references

Cha. Sū. 1/51

TEST YOURSELF

Learn, review and memorize key terms from this section.

samavāyi

dravya

guṇa

karma

SAṀYOGA-VIBHĀGA

Combination-Separation

saṁyoga	conjunction, combination, connection
vibhāga	disjunction, division, separation, distinction, difference

Saṁyoga is the act of combining or joining things together. It is the process which results in the combination or attachment. *Vibhāga* is the opposite and is the act of separating things resulting in division or distinction.

Additional references

Cha. Sū. 1/44 – 45
Cha. Sū. 1/52

TEST YOURSELF

Learn, review and memorize key terms from this section.

saṁyoga

vibhāga

VṚDDHI-KṢHAYA
Increase-Decrease

vṛddhi	growth, extension, increase, augmentation, advancement
kṣhaya	loss, waste, wane, diminution, destruction, decay, wasting or wearing away

Vṛddhi-kṣhaya is the act of increasing or decreasing of the *dravya* or its components through *sāmānya-viśheṣha*. When *dravya* undergo *sāmānya*, the result is *vṛddhi* by *saṁyoga*. When *dravya* undergo *viśheṣha*, the result is *kṣhaya* by *vibhāga*.

Additional references

Cha. Sū. 1/44-45 Vol 2: Chapter 6
AH Sū. 1/13.5

TEST YOURSELF

Learn, review and memorize key terms from this section.

vṛddhi

kṣhaya

dravya

sāmānya

viśheṣha

saṁyoga

vibhāga

GUṆA
Characteristic

guṇa	a quality, peculiarity, attribute or property, a property or characteristic of all created things

Guṇa may refer to an entire group of characteristics or individual sets of single characteristics. *Guṇa* can also be used as an umbrella term which refers to the entire concept. At the highest level, the groups of *guṇas* include:

Vaiśheṣhikā	the *sārtha* or *viśheṣha guṇas*
Sāmānyā	the *gurvādi* or *samānya*, and *parādi guṇas*
Ātmaguṇā	the *buddhi* and *prayatna guṇas*

Each group contains a specific list of *guṇas* which are used individually to describe a certain quality or characteristic. The *samānya* or *gurvādi guṇas* are by far the most common. They include ten pairs of opposite *guṇas* which are used heavily in clinical practice.

Guṇas are considered the objects of the sense organs. They exist within *dravya* with a *samavāyi* relationship.

Additional references

Cha. Sū. 1/49 Vol 2: Chapter 3
Cha. Sū. 1/51

TEST YOURSELF

Learn, review and memorize key terms from this section.

guṇa

dravya

gurvādi guṇas

samānya guṇas

samavāyi

TEST YOURSELF

Learn, review and memorize key terms from this section.

karma

dravya

samavāyi

saṁyoga

vibhāga

KARMA
Action

karma	act, action, performance

Karma refers to action, specifically curative efforts within the context of Āyurveda. Like *guṇa*, it also exists within *dravya* with a *samavāyi* relationship. It is the cause for *saṁyoga* and *vibhāga*. The act or performance of *karma* is done to achieve a specific goal. Its actualization happens by *karma* alone, and does not require any additional force or effort. Specifically, *guṇa* is not involved in the actual performance of *karma* even though they often seem closely related.

Additional references

Cha. Sū. 1/49 Cha. Sū. 1/52	Vol 2: Chapter 3

RASA
Flavor

rasa	taste, flavor; the sap or juice of plants, juice of fruit, any liquid or fluid; the best or finest or prime part of anything, essence

Rasa is the perceived flavor or taste of any substance when put directly in contact with the tongue. It is generally accepted to be classified as six types:

Madhura	Sweet
Amla	Sour
Lavaṇa	Salty
Kaṭu	Pungent (or spicy)
Tikta	Bitter
Kaṣhāya	Astringent

Additional references

Cha. Sū. 26/28	Vol 2: Chapter 3
Cha. Sū. 1/65	
Su. Sū. 42/	
AH Sū. 1/14-17	

TEST YOURSELF

Learn, review and memorize key terms from this section.

rasa __________

madhura __________

amla __________

lavaṇa __________

kaṭu __________

tikta __________

kaṣhāya __________

VĪRYA

Potency

vīrya	potency, efficacy (of medicine); strength, power, consequence

Vīrya is potency of the *dravya* to produce an effect in the body while the *dravya* is in contact with the body. This occurs during the process of digestion. *Vīrya* is generally classified as *śhīta* (cold) or *uṣhṇa* (hot), as these two often demonstrate the most prominent outcomes of substances. In general, *dravyas* follow a standard rule where a certain *rasa* typically results in a specific *vīrya*. However, there are several exceptions to these rules.

Additional references

Cha. Sū. 26/64-66	Vol 2: Chapter 3

TEST YOURSELF

Learn, review and memorize key terms from this section.

vīrya __________

dravya __________

śhīta __________

uṣhṇa __________

VIPĀKA

Post-digestive effect

vipāka	cooking, ripening, maturing; maturing of food (in the stomach), digestion conversion of food into a state for assimilation

Vipāka is the final action of the *dravya* which directly affects one specific *doṣha*. In general, *dravya* follow a standard rule where a certain *rasa* typically results in a specific *vipāka*, but there are exceptions to these rules.

Additional references

Cha. Sū. 26/66	Vol 2: Chapter 3
Cha. Sū. 26/57-58	

TEST YOURSELF

Learn, review and memorize key terms from this section.

vipāka

dravya

doṣha

rasa

PRABHĀVA

Special effect

prabhāva	might, power, majesty, dignity, strength, efficacy

Prabhāva is the umbrella term for any *dravya* which does not follow standard rules in its *rasa*, *vīrya* and *vipāka*. Any *dravya* which exhibits a special effect or unexpected outcome based on its *rasa, vīrya* and *vipāka* profile is stated to be capable of producing its special effect through *prabhāva*. This is explained classically by comparing two *dravya* which have similar *rasa*, *vīrya* and *vipāka* profiles, yet only one of the two is capable of effecting a specific curative action. This special effect is called *prabhāva*.

Of all components of *dravya*, *prabhāva* is always considered the strongest. Whenever present, it will produce its effect(s) and supercede *rasa*, *vīrya* and *vipāka*.

Additional references

Cha. Sū. 26/67-72 Vol 2: Chapter 3

TEST YOURSELF

Learn, review and memorize key terms from this section.

prabhāva

dravya

rasa

vīrya

vipāka

LOKA-PURUṢHA SĀMYA

Macrocosm-Microcosm Similarities

loka	the earth or world of human beings, the wide space or world
puruṣha	a man, male, human being, a person, mankind
sāmya	equality, likeness, sameness, identity with

Loka-puruṣha sāmya is classically stated as *"Puruṣho'ayaṁ loka-saṁmitaḥ"* in Cha. Śhā. 5/3 by Punarvasu Ātreya. Literally translated, the teacher is saying "I, a human being, am the world's equivalent." The meaning of this statement is that whatever is found in the external world can be seen in human beings and vice versa. An infinite number of correlations can be made between the two.

Additional references

Cha. Śhā. 5/3-8
Cha. Śhā. 4/13
Su. Sū. 21/8
Su. Sū. 6/8

TEST YOURSELF

Learn, review and memorize key terms from this section.

loka

____

puruṣha

____

sāmya

____

ĀYU

Vitality

āyu	life, lifespan, quantity and quality of life

Āyu (vitality) is defined as the *saṁyoga* of *śharīra* (the body), *indriya* (the sense organs), *sattva* (determination) and *ātma*. It is the state of being alive, duration and quality of life. When *āyu* is present in *puruṣha*, he is considered *chetanā*.

Additional references

Cha. Sū. 1/42 Vol 2: Chapter 4, 13

TEST YOURSELF

Learn, review and memorize key terms from this section.

āyu

____

saṁyoga

____

śharīra

____

indriya

____

sattva

____

ātma

____

puruṣha

____

chetanā

____

TRI-DAṆḌAVAT

Three pillars of the living world

tri	three
daṇḍavat	like a stick, rod or pole

Tri-daṇḍavat states that the *saṁyoga* of *sattva*, *ātma* and *śharīra* sustain or support the world. These three act as the basis for all life.

Additional references

Cha. Sū. 1/46 Vol 2: Chapter 4

TEST YOURSELF

Learn, review and memorize key terms from this section.

tri

____

daṇḍavat

____

saṁyoga

____

sattva

____

ātma

____

śharīra

____

PURUṢHA
Human being

puruṣha	a man, male, human being, a person, mankind

Puruṣha is included in the context of the *tri-daṇḍavat siddhānta* because he is *chetanā* and the result of the *saṁyoga* of *sattva*, *ātma* and *śharīra*. *Puruṣha* is the reason for the existence of the science of Āyurveda and in therapeutic contexts may be referred to as *karma puruṣha* or *chikitsā puruṣha*.

Additional references

Cha. Sū. 1/47 Vol 2: Chapter 4

TEST YOURSELF

Learn, review and memorize key terms from this section.

puruṣha

chetanā

karma puruṣha

chikitsā puruṣha

TRIDOṢHA, TRI-STHŪṆA
Three doṣhas, three supports

tri	three
doṣha	vitiator, alteration, affection, morbid element, disease; equilibrium controller
sthūṇa	a post, pillar

The *tridoṣhas* are the three main constituents of the physical body responsible for health in their normal state, and responsible for deviation from health when abnormal. The three include *vāta, pitta* and *kapha*, and each has five *bhedas* (classifications) which are applied practically and clinically.

According to Suśhruta, they are also called the *tri-sthūṇa* (three pillars). This indicates their importance in supporting the health of the body.

Additional references

Cha. Sū. 1/59-61 Vol 2: Chapter 4
Su. Sū. 21/3
AH Sū. 1/6-7

TEST YOURSELF

Learn, review and memorize key terms from this section.

tri

doṣha

sthūṇa

vāta

pitta

kapha

DOṢHA

Vice, vitium

doṣha	vitiator, alteration, affection, morbid element, disease; equilibrium controller

The term *doṣha* is defined classically as:

doṣha दूष्यन्ति इति दोषाः

Dūṣhyanti iti doṣhāḥ

The *doṣhas* vitiate, pollute, or make impure.

Doṣhas tend towards disruptive behavior. This accelerates when they are supplied with the resources to produce their effects. However, when they are not supplied with such resources, their normal activities and behaviors work to maintain, support and promote the baseline health of an individual.

Additional references

Cha. Sū. 1/59-61
Su. Sū. 21/3
AH Sū. 1/6-7

Vol 2: Chapter 4

TEST YOURSELF

Learn, review and memorize key terms from this section.

doṣha

AGNI

Igniter

agni	fire, the god of fire, fire of the stomach, digestive faculty

Agni is a broad and complex concept that covers several key theories. Its English translations can vary significantly depending on its usage and context. The term *agni* derives from the Sanskrit *dhātu* √ *ag* (to move tortuously, wind) which is likely related to the Latin root ag, variant ig (to do, act, drive) and the Latin term ignire (to set on fire). *Agni* is the igniting power that sparks or initiates a process of combustion, cooking or transformation.

In the field of Āyurveda, *agni* most commonly refers to the capacity of the body to convert and transform consumed food into proper outputs, including *dhātus* (supportive systems) and *malas* (waste products). *Agni* can encompass a wide range of processes including digestion, metabolism, cellular transformation, conversion of any substance into another, and more.

There are three categories of *agnis* which manage conversion and transformation processes at various stages in normal digestion and metabolism. *Agni* has four states – one of which is normal and healthy while the remaining three tend toward varying manifestations of dysfunction. Each of the three dysfunctional states is predominantly afflicted by a single *doṣha*. Classically, these are considered the root causes for disease.

Additional references

Cha. Chi. 15/
AH Sū. 1/8

Vol 2: Chapter 5

TEST YOURSELF

Learn, review and memorize key terms from this section.

agni

doṣha

PĀKA, PĀCHANA

Cook

pāka — cooking, baking, roasting, boiling; digestion, assimilation of food; ripening, ripeness (of fruit or boil of the body); inflammation, suppuration

pāchana — causing to cook or boil, to cause to soften, digest, dissolve, suppurate; a styptic for closing wounds

Pāka and *pāchana* both derive from the Sanskrit *dhātu* √ *pach* (to digest, ripen, mature, bring to completion). In the context of Āyurveda, these occur after *agni* has ignited and initiated combustion processes.

Proper *pāchana* is vital to health. Errors in *pāchana* can occur due to an almost infinite number of causes and can generally be associated with a type of dysfunctional *agni*. In certain situations, these errors can result in the immediate or delayed formation of *āma* (undigested, incompletely digested or improperly digested consumed items).

Additional references

Cha. Chi. 15/ — Vol 2: Chapter 5

TEST YOURSELF

Learn, review and memorize key terms from this section.

pāka

pāchana

agni

āma

KOṢHṬHA

Gastrointestinal tract (mouth to anus)

koṣhṭha — the complete digestive tract from mouth to anus; alimentary canal; any one of the viscera of the body (particularly the stomach, abdomen)

Koṣhṭha can refer to two concepts. First, it is the physical, anatomical system which includes the pathway and related organs responsible for moving consumed food from mouth to anus. In this context, it can be compared to and roughly translated as the gastro-intestinal tract, or GIT. Second, it refers to the way in which an individual's digestive system functions and produces its output. The organs involved are not directly relevant in this type of assessment. Instead, *koṣhṭha* is categorized based on the ease by which consumed substances move through the digestive tract, and how well they undergo digestion.

In its functional assessment, *koṣhṭha* is classified into three types dominated by a single *doṣha*. The presentation of one's *koṣhṭha* can change for various reasons. However, the baseline or tendency towards a single type for any individual can almost always be determined through long-term assessment.

Additional references

AH Sū. 1/8 — Vol 2: Chapter 5

TEST YOURSELF

Learn, review and memorize key terms from this section.

koṣhṭha

____

doṣha

____

SAPTADHĀTU

Seven supportive systems

sapta	seven
dhātu	a supportive, constituent product generated by the body

The *saptadhātu* (seven supportive systems) are composed of the physical structures of the body and their proper functional purpose in a state of normal health. They are generated in a specific order of formation through complex processes of nutrient absorption via systemic channels after *pāchana*. The *saptadhātu* include:

Rasa	first "juice" of digested food
Rakta	juice converted to red, life-supporting fluid
Māṁsa	"meat" of the body
Medas	fat of the body
Asthi	bones and bony structures
Majja	fatty tissue filling the bones
Śhukra	reproductive components

In addition to supporting the physical body, the *saptadhātu* also produce *upadhātu* (secondary supportive systems).

Additional references

AH Sū. 1/13 AH Sū. 11/14	Vol 2: Chapter 8

TEST YOURSELF

Learn, review and memorize key terms from this section.

sapta

____

dhātu

____

rasa

____

rakta

____

māṁsa

____

medas

____

asthi

____

majja

____

śhukra

____

UPADHĀTU

Secondary supportive systems

upa-	(a prefix) towards, near to, with; secondary or subordinate
upadhātu	the secondary, supportive systems and constituents of the body

The *upadhātu* (secondary supportive systems) of the body are produced by the *saptadhātu*. While both the *saptadhātu* and *upadhātu* support the body, their main distinction is that *upadhātu* do not produce further supportive systems or products. Instead, their primary purpose is to carry out a specific function.

A single *dhātu* may produce one or more *upadhātu*.

Additional references

Cha. Chi. 15/17 Vol 2: Chapter 8
AH Sū. 11/1c
BP Pū. 3/210

TEST YOURSELF

Learn, review and memorize key terms from this section.

saptadhātu

upadhātu

DHĀTU-MALA

Waste products of the supportive systems

dhātu	a supportive, constituent product generated by the body
mala	dirt, filth, dust, impurity, any bodily excretion or secretion

The *dhātu-mala* (waste products of the supportive systems) include the minor waste products normally generated by each *dhātu*. These are generated as part of regular functioning of the body and normal processes of combustion and transformation. Each *dhātu* is stated to be responsible for producing one or more specific *dhātu-mala* only.

Additional references

Cha. Chi. 15/18-20 Vol 2: Chapter 8
Su. Sū. 46/529
AH Śhā. 3/63
BP Pū. 3/209

TEST YOURSELF

Learn, review and memorize key terms from this section.

dhātu

mala

MALA, TRIMALA

Waste products, Three waste products

mala	dirt, filth, dust, impurity, any bodily excretion or secretion

The *trimala* include the major waste products normally generated by the body and the primary functions of *agni*. These include:

Mūtra	Urine
Purīṣha	Stool
Sveda	Sweat

Additional references

AH Sū. 1/13 Vol 2: Chapter 9

TEST YOURSELF

Learn, review and memorize key terms from this section.

mala

mūtra

purīṣha

sveda

CHAYA-PRAKOPA-PRAŚHAMANA

Accumulation–Aggravation–Normalization

chaya	collecting, accumulating of the *doṣhas*
prakopa	excess, superabundance, vitiation, effervescence, excitement, raging (of diseases)
praśhamana	calming, pacifying, curing, healing, tranquilizing

Chaya (accumulation), *prakopa* (aggravation) and *praśhamana* (normalization) are the three *doṣha avasthās* (stages of *doṣhas*) where the *doṣhas* undergo slight increase, great increase and then return to normal level. These changes can be recognized and measured in quantity and quality.

Additional references

Cha. Sū 17/62
AH Sū. 12/22-23

Vol 2: Chapter 7

TEST YOURSELF

Learn, review and memorize key terms from this section.

doṣha

avasthā

chaya

prakopa

praśhamana

ĀŚHRAYA-ĀŚHRAYI BHĀVA

Container-Inhabitant

āśhraya	dwelling, asylum, place of refuge, shelter; that to which anything is annexed, or with which anything is closely connected, or on which anything depends or rests
āśhrayi	dwelling in, resting on, inhabiting, following

Āśhraya-āśhrayi bhāva (container-inhabitant) states that the *āśhraya* (container) provides a place for the *āśhrayi* (inhabitant) to reside. This relationship is known to occur normally in certain locations of the body in healthy conditions. It may also occur as an abnormal outcome of unhealthy conditions.

Additional references

AH Sū. 11/26-27

TEST YOURSELF

Learn, review and memorize key terms from this section.

āśhraya

āśhrayi

bhāva

GATI
Movement

gati	going, moving, manner or power of going

Gati (movement) can refer to any type of movement and is used specifically with the *doṣhas* to describe their direction when functioning normally or abnormally. In general, normal situations, gati is usually described as upward, downward or sideways. It is most often used to describe movements of *vāta*.

Additional references

Vol 2: Chapter 3, 4

TEST YOURSELF

Learn, review and memorize key terms from this section.

gati

____

doṣha

____

PRAKṚTI
Baseline constitution

prakṛti	"making or placing before or at first," the original or natural form or condition of anything, original or primary substance, cause, origin, nature, character, constitution

Prakṛti (baseline constitution) is the first, primary, natural state of any individual. It is not necessarily healthy or unhealthy. It can be considered in the context of *śharīrika* (the physical body) or *mānasika* (the mind) with each having seven and three subtypes, respectively. *Prakṛti* may be considered an individual's baseline state of normal health and being. It is set at conception and during gestation and does not change until the end of life. *Prakṛti* is typically dominated by one or more *doṣhas*.

Additional references

Cha. Vi. 6/5, 8/95-100 AH Sū. 1/10	Vol 2: Chapter 17

TEST YOURSELF

Learn, review and memorize key terms from this section.

prakṛti

____

śharīrika

____

mānasika

____

doṣha

____

TRI-GUṆA
Behavioral determinants

tri	three
guṇa	(in Sāṅkhya phil.) an ingredient or constituent of *prakṛti*, chief quality of all existing beings (ie *sattva*, *rajas*, and *tamas*; ie goodness, passion, and darkness, or virtue, foulness, and ignorance)

The *tri-guṇa* (behavioral triad) is a theory which originates from Sāṅkhya philosophy.

During the initial creation of life, the *tri-guṇa* are generated as part of the materialization of the universe and they contribute to producing physical substance including one's ability to interact with the world through *jñānendriya* (sense organs), *karmendriya* (action organs) and *manas* (the mind). The *tri-guṇa* function as the main methods for understanding the characteristics of an individual's behavior, personality, disposition and mental state. They are categorized as *sattva* (determination), *rajas* (initiation) and *tamas* (inertia) and always work together interdependently.

Additional references

Cha. Śhā. 4/36-39 Vol 2: Chapters 22-24

TEST YOURSELF

Learn, review and memorize key terms from this section.

tri-guṇa

---

sattva

---

rajas

---

tamas

MĀNASIKA DOṢHA

Mental vice

mānasika	of the mind, relating to the mind
doṣha	vitiator, alteration, affection, morbid element, disease; equilibrium controller

The *doṣhas* of *manas* (the mind) consist of two of the three *tri-guṇa* – *rajas* and *tamas*. In their healthy state, they contribute to the overall health and happiness of the individual. In their unhealthy state, they are responsible for abnormal, unhealthy behavior and mental state. They tend to drive an individual to misunderstand the truth, make inappropriate decisions and act in detrimental ways.

Additional references

Cha. Vi. 6/5 Vol 2: Chapter 23
AH Sū. 1/21

TEST YOURSELF

Learn, review and memorize key terms from this section.

mānasika

---

doṣha

---

manas

---

tri-guṇa

---

rajas

---

tamas

TRAYOPASTAMBHA

Three supports (of vitality)

traya	triple, threefold, consisting of three, of three kinds, triad
upastambha	stay, support, strengthening, base; support of life (as food, sleep, and government of passions)

The *trayopastambha* (three supports of vitality) include proper use of food, sleep and sexual activity. When utilized and applied judiciously, these three promote a long, happy and healthy life in all aspects.

Additional references

Ca Sū. 11/34-35 AH Sū. 7/52	Vol 3: Chapter 1

TEST YOURSELF

Learn, review and memorize key terms from this section.

traya

____

upastambha

____

KĀLA
Time

kāla — a fixed or right point of time, a space of time, time (in general)

Kāla is defined classically as "*Kāla punaha parinamamuchyate.*" It is the cause for all transformation and encompasses the concept of time. It is classified in Āyurveda from the shortest calculable moment, called *nimeṣha* (the blink of an eye or about half a second) up to large periods of practical use, such as *varṣha* (one year) and beyond. Many more classifications exist outside of these which are not practically applied in Āyurveda.

Additional references

Cha. Sū. 6/ Cha. Sū. 11/37-43 Su. Sū. 6/	Vol 3: Chapter 4

TEST YOURSELF

Learn, review and memorize key terms from this section.

kāla

____

varṣha

____

ṚTU
Season

ṛtu — a period, division or part of a year, a season of varying length

In classical Āyurvedic literature, a *ṛtu* (season) is a period of time that lasts approximately two months in which specific seasonal characteristics manifest themselves in the external environment. The six classical *ṛtu* described in classical Āyurvedic literature are intended for the Indian subcontinent. The term *ṛtu* can be used to indicate seasons of other durations (three months, four months, etc) and can be used to appropriately refer to seasons in any geographical region.

Additional references

Cha. Sū. 6/ AH Sū. 3/	Vol 3: Chapter 4

TEST YOURSELF

Learn, review and memorize key terms from this section.

ṛtu

____

ṚTU-SANDHI

Seasonal transition

ṛtu	a period, division or part of a year, a season of varying length
sandhi	critical juncture, joint

A *ṛtu-sandhi* (seasonal transition) is the transition from one *ṛtu* to the next. It is generally a two-week period where the characteristics of one *ṛtu* noticeably fade out while the characteristics of the next *ṛtu* become predominant. It is a period of mild instability where adjustments must be made to daily routines. The *doṣhas* are naturally prone to fluctuate, exacerbate and manifest signs of their presence especially during these seasonal transitions.

Additional references

AH Sū. 3/	Vol 3: Chapter 4

TEST YOURSELF

Learn, review and memorize key terms from this section.

ṛtu

---

sandhi

AVASTHĀ

Stage

avasthā	state, condition, situation, stage, degree

An *avasthā* is a stage, or period of time in which a specific event occurs. It is not necessarily bound by a specific timeframe or limit of time and may continue as long as its notable characteristics are present. It can be applied in a variety of concepts and its name is often modified to include a descriptor appropriate to its use in a specific context.

TEST YOURSELF

Learn, review and memorize key terms from this section.

avasthā

DIŚHA (DIK)

Direction

diśha	quarter or region pointed at, direction, cardinal point

Variations in the name of this term arise due to grammatical rules, usage and *sandhi* in particular. Each variation refers to the same meaning. Direction can classically be indicated in 10 ways: N, NE, E, SE, S, SW, W, NW, above and below. It is one of the primary concepts which can be used when considering *dravya* and its attributes. Classical interpretations based on *diśha* are known to be relevant to the Indian subcontinent.

TEST YOURSELF

Learn, review and memorize key terms from this section.

diśha (dik)

---

dravya

TRI DEŚHA

Three types of environments

tri	three
deśha	point, region, spot, place, part, portion, province, country, kingdom

The *tri-deśha* (three types of environments) states that there are three main types of external environments which are classified primarily based on their water content. The *ānupa deśha*, or wet environment, is very watery and contains many lakes, rivers and water bodies, often with a high level of humidity. The *jāngala deśha*, or dry environment is the opposite, and is recognized by its desert-like characteristics. *Sādhārana deśha*, or a moderate environment, is neither too wet nor too dry. *Tri-deśha* must always be considered when assessing concepts in practice. It is particularly relevant in assessing an individual's state of *svastha* (health).

Additional references

Cha. Ka. 12/ Su. Sū. 35/42 AH Sū. 1/23 BP Pū. 4/81-88	Vol 3: Chapter 3

TEST YOURSELF

Learn, review and memorize key terms from this section.

tri

---

deśha

ānupa

---

jāngala

---

sādhārana

AVARA-MADHYAMA-UTTAMA

Low-Medium-High (Comparative analysis)

avara	low, the worst of a group
madhyama	medium, the middle of a group
uttama	high, the best of a group

These three comparatives are used to analyze members of a group when performing assessments. They may be used to compare one member of a group to another, or one individual's current state to a known or estimated baseline.

TEST YOURSELF

Learn, review and memorize key terms from this section.

avara

---

madhyama

---

uttama

Chapter 2: Review

ADDITIONAL READING

Read and review the references listed below to expand your understanding of the concepts in this chapter. Write down the date that you complete your reading for each. Remember that consistent repetition is the best way to learn. Plan to read each reference at least once now and expect to read it again as you continue your studies.

Use the additional references throughout this chapter and record what you've completed.

CLASSICS	1st read	2nd read
Charaka		
Suśhruta		
Aṣhṭāṅga Hṛdaya		
Bhāva Prakāśha		

QUESTIONS & ANSWERS

Record your questions for this chapter here for further research and discussion.

Question:

Answer:

Question:

Answer:

Question:

Answer:

SELF-ASSESSMENT

1. The law of conservation of energy can be explained by which of the following *siddhānta*?
   a. *Kārya-kāraṇa bhāva* and *satkārya vāda*
   b. *Loka-puruṣha sāmya*
   c. *Sāmānya-viśheṣha* and *saṁyoga-vibhāga*
   d. *Sāmānya-viśheṣha* and *vṛddhi-kṣhaya*
   e. *Satkārya vāda*

2. Which of the following is not one of the *nava kāraṇa dravya*?
   a. *ātma*
   b. *dik*
   c. *kāla*
   d. *manas*
   e. *sattva*

3. The *amūrti doṣha* is
   a. *kapha*
   b. *pitta*
   c. *rajas*
   d. *tamas*
   e. *vāta*

4. Which of the following is not a *doṣha*?
   a. *pitta*
   b. *rajas*
   c. *tamas*
   d. *vāta*
   e. None of the above

5. Changing of one's *prakṛti* indicates
   a. death
   b. disease
   c. growth
   d. maturation
   e. mental imbalance

6. Which *tri-guṇa* is not a *mānasika doṣha*?
   a. *rajas*
   b. *sattva*
   c. *śhīta*
   d. *tamas*
   e. *uṣhṇa*

7. The concept of *kāla* calls one year a _________ and divides it into _________.
   a. *ṛtu*; six *ṛtu-sandhi*
   b. *ṛtu*; two *ṛtu-sandhi*
   c. *varṣha*; six *ṛtu*
   d. *varṣha*; ten *diśha*
   e. *varṣha*; three *ṛtu*

8. Moving upward, downward or sideways is described by
   a. *gati*
   b. *praśhamana*
   c. *sāmānya-viśheṣha*
   d. *tri-daṇḍavat*
   e. All of the above

9. Which *dravya* is *acetana*?
   a. *audbhida*
   b. *jaṅgama*
   c. *pārthiva*
   d. All of the above
   e. None of the above

10. The concept of *avasthā* is measured by
    a. *agni* and *koṣhṭha*
    b. *kāla*
    c. *saptadhātu*
    d. *tri-deśha*
    e. *upadhātu*

CRITICAL THINKING

1. Memorize all classical names of the concepts listed in this chapter along with their nearest English equivalents.

2. Properly recite and write the transliterated names of the concepts in this chapter.

3. Identify three *siddhānta* from this chapter which are easy to relate to concepts from Western science. Identify three which are new to you, or that you have not seen in any other scientific methodology or paradigm.

4. Choose any *siddhānta* which is a new concept for you, and explain it in your own words.

5. Combine at least 5 *siddhānta* and explain how they must work together to produce a valid result, output or event.

Chapter 3 : Dravya

KEY TERMS

adho gati
agneya
ākāśha
amla
anurasa
ap
avastha pāka
dhātu
pradūṣhaṇa
doṣha
praśhamana
drava
dravya
gaṇa
gandha
guṇa
guru
gurvādi guṇa
hima
kāla
karma
kaṣhāya
kaṭhina
kaṭu
khara
laghu
lavaṇa
madhura
mānasika guṇa
manda
mṛdu
pañcha mahābhūta
pichchhila
prabhāva
pṛthvi
rasa
rūkṣha
rūpa
śhabda
sāmānya guṇa
samavāya
samavāyi
saṁyoga
sāndra
sara
saumya
śhīta
śhlakṣhṇa
snigdha
sparśha
sthira
sthūla
sūkṣhma
svādu
svasthavṛtta
tejas
tīkṣhṇa
tikta
udaka
ūrdhva gati
uṣhṇa
vaiśheṣhikā guṇas
varga
vāyu
vibhāga
vipāka
vīrya
viśhada
viśheṣha guṇa
viśheṣha karma
yukti

DRAVYA

Dravya is the term used to refer to matter in general, as well as specific, individual substances, especially when used with an additional descriptor term. Each *dravya* acts as the *āśhraya* (container or housing) for its additional components which identify its specific features, characteristics and actions. These additional components are bound to each *dravya* by their *samavāya* relationship, or perpetual attachment. They include:

Guṇa	Characteristic
Karma	Action
Rasa	Flavor
Vīrya	Potency
Vipāka	Post-digestive effect
Prabhāva	Special effect

The additional components of every *dravya* are shown in the following diagram.

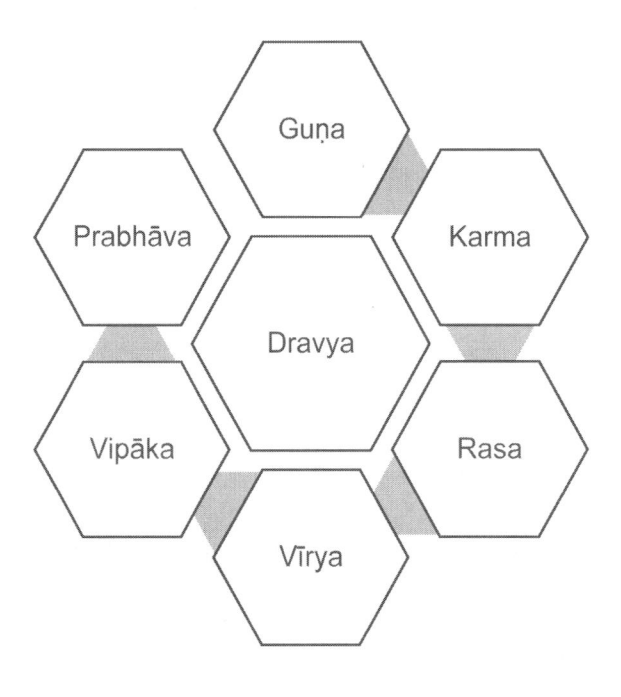

In classical literature, each *dravya*, especially in the context of medicaments, clinical application and therapeutic processes, had been tested and well-understood by scholars of the science in their time. The surviving literature stands as a record to the deep, thorough knowledge that was in practice at the time in various locations. The literature demonstrates highly sophisticated levels of practical knowledge which were clearly localized and customized to specific geographical regions and demographics.

And even though much of the information is still valid and practically applicable today, classical literature has yet to be updated for modern cultures and societies, especially those outside of the Indian subcontinent. Testing new *dravya* for different people of various geographical regions is greatly needed if Āyurveda is to continue as a living science today.

Paribhāṣhā

Classical literature provides a thorough, comprehensive explanation of *dravya*. A full review of the definitions will help clarify the concept.

Definition #1:
Dravya as the cause for karma and guṇa

यत्राश्रिताः कर्मगुणाः कारणं समवायि यत् ।
तद्द्रव्यं ... ॥

च. सू. १।५१

Yatrāśhritāḥ karmaguṇāḥ kāraṇaṁ samavāyi yat | Taddravyaṁ ... ||

Cha. Sū. 1/51

Tad (That) *dravyaṁ* (dravya, or matter) *yatra-āśhritāḥ* (is that abode or dwelling place) *karma-guṇāḥ* (of karma and guna), *kāraṇaṁ* (and the cause) *samavāyi yat* (for these being perpetually attached).

Dravya is that matter which holds *karma* and *guṇa* in a perpetual state of attachment.

This can be considered as *dravya* acting as the substrate, or required base for *guṇa* and *karma*. Without the presence of *dravya*, *guṇa* and *karma* cannot exist.

Note that Chakrapāṇi comments on this statement to clarify that the term *guṇa* includes *rasa*, *vīrya, vipāka* and *prabhāva*. All of these components should be considered when referring to *dravya*.

Definition #2:
Dravya's main feature

द्रव्यलक्षणं तु 'क्रियागुणवत् समवायि कारणम्' इति ।

सु. सू. ४०।३

Dravyalakṣhaṇaṁ tu 'kriyāguṇavat samavāyi kāraṇam' iti |

Su. Sū. 40/3

Dravya lakṣhaṇaṁ tu (The main, natural feature of d*ravya* is) '*kriyāguṇavat samavāyi kāraṇam*' (to be the cause for perpetual attachment of *kriyā* [*karma*] and *guṇa*) *iti* (and so, it is understood in this manner).

Definition #3:
Dravya is the most important

द्रव्यमेव रसादीनां श्रेष्ठं, ते हि तदाश्रयाः ।

अ. हृ. ९।१

Dravyameva rasādīnāṁ śhreṣhṭhaṁ, te hi tadāśhrayāḥ |

AH Sū. 9/1

Dravyameva (And so, dravya is truly) *śhreṣhṭhaṁ* (the best, most important of) *rasādīnāṁ* (all its components including *rasa*, *guṇa*, *karma*, *vīrya*, *vipāka*, *prabhāva*) *te hi* (because) *tad* (that itself [the dravya] is) *āśhrayāḥ* (the main home, location, abode or base matter).

The key point is that dravya is truly the chief among all its components (*rasa*, etc) because it provides the foundational base while the components reside within it. All of its components are dependent upon the *dravya* and cannot exist without it.

Bheda

Many types of classification methods are described by various authors. These methods can be used individually or jointly to better understand how a specific *dravya* operates. Certain methods are more appropriate for certain *dravya*. More than one classification method may be used to describe any *dravya*.

Classification #1:
Based on source

तत् पुनस्त्रिविधं प्रोक्तं जङ्गम-औद्भिद-पार्थिवम् ।

च. सू. १।६७.५

Tat punastrividhaṁ proktaṁ jaṅgama-audbhida-pārthivam |

Cha. Sū. 1/67.5

Tat punastrividhaṁ proktaṁ (The three types [of *dravya*] come from):

Jaṅgama	Animal origin
Audbhida	Vegetable origin
Pārthiva	Metallic and mineral origin

Dravya can be classified into three types – that which comes from animal, vegetable or metallic/mineral origin.

In similar classifications, other authors have used the term *sthāvara* as a synonym for *audbhida*.

Classification #2:
Based on gross constituents

सर्वं द्रव्यं पाञ्चभौतिकमस्मिन्नर्थे; ।

च. सू. २६।१०

Sarvaṁ dravyaṁ pañchabhautikaṁasminnarthe |

Cha. Sū. 26/10

Sarva (All) *dravya* (matter) *pañchabhautikaṁ asminn-arthe* (consists of all five gross elements).

Based on this classification, all *dravya* can be categorized by their *pañchabhautika* predominance or composition.

Classification #3:
Based on active constituents

तच्चेतनावदचेतनं च, ।

च. सू. २६।१०

Tachchetanāvadachetanaṁ ca |

Cha. Sū. 26/10

Tat (That [*dravya*] is) *chetanāvad* (sentient) *cha* (and) *achetanaṁ* (insentient).

Dravya can be classified as sentient or insentient.

Mechanics of dravya

Charaka and Suśhruta both detail the mechanics of *dravya* and explain how it works with its components *guṇa*, *karma*, *rasa*, *vīrya*, *vipāka* and *prabhāva*. Charaka provides a detailed explanation in Cha. Sū. 26/13 that *dravya* acts in one of three ways:

Dravya-prabhāva
: Dravya effects its final outcome through its own special effect or nature

Guṇa-prabhāva
: Dravya produces a special effect as its outcome is based off its characteristics

Dravya-guṇa-prabhāva
: Dravya acts in both ways.

In order for the acting *dravya* to have its desired effect, it must take place within the scope of the proper *kriyā*.

Kāla	The specific action or outcome should occur at or within a certain period of time.
Adhikaraṇa	The specific action or outcome occurs at a certain place or location. In context of therapeutic outcome, this is typically a location in the śharīra and/or manas.
Yukti	The outcome is produced through application of logical thought process.
Abhipretya	The outcome is targeted, purposeful and intended to produce a specific therapeutic action.

In Cha. Sū. 26/13 and Śhu. Sū. 40/5, both authors describe the mechanics of the *dravya's* action and provide specific terminology to describe the process of using the dravya for therapeutic effect.

Karma	This is the specific action which takes place and describes the effect produced by the dravya.
Vīrya	This is the effectual potency of the *dravya* after it has performed its action.
Adhikaraṇa	This is the location where the *dravya* acts in the *śharīra* and/or *manas*.
Kāla	This is the time period in which the *dravya* acts to produce its effect.
Upāya	This is the means or way by which the *dravya* effects its result.
Phala	This is literally the "fruit" of the action. It is the positive, targeted therapeutic outcome or the result achieved.

It is clear that there are many components and mechanics that participate in the action of a *dravya*. And among the components of *dravya* (*guṇa*, *karma*, *rasa*, *vīrya*, *vipāka* and *prabhāva*), even more features have been attributed to each one to classify them, identify how they function and asses their outcome. It must be remembered that although these subsequent features appear to belong to the components, they actually belong to the *dravya* itself. The *dravya* is what makes the final action and effects possible, while the components and features are detailed to help the student and practitioner apply each appropriately. Charaka specifies this point clearly in Cha. Sū. 26/36.

Ultimately, the purpose of using any *dravya* in Āyurveda is to produce therapeutic action.

TEST YOURSELF

Learn, review and memorize key terms from this section.

dravya ____________________

guṇa ____________________

karma ____________________

rasa ____________________

vīrya ____________________

vipāka ____________________

prabhāva ____________________

samavāya
samavāyi
kāla
yukti

PAÑCHA MAHĀBHŪTA

The *pañcha mahābhūta* are the five gross elements. They are listed in the "*Pañcha Mahābhūta* Overview" table with their common terminology and significant features from classical authors. Notice that the Sanskrit terms for each *mahābhūta* change based on their use as nouns or adjectives.

Use the references below the table to read more about each *mahābhūta* and understand the intention of the classical presentation in context of the original text.

Each *mahābhūta* can be compared to one of the five gross elements of earth, water, fire, air and space. Names of each of these gross elements refer to the predominance of the *mahābhūta* but they do not imply that the *dravya* is composed of only that *mahābhūta*. All of the other *mahābhūtas* are also present in each *dravya* in minor proportions. The specifics of this composition will be described at the end of this section.

The *viśheṣha guṇa* of each *mahābhūta* refers to the specific attribute by which human sense organs can detect its presence. The *rasa* of each is specified classically as a general, primary *rasa* that is generally present and secondary *rasa* which is slightly discernable. The *viśheṣha karma* is the *mahābhūta*'s natural tendency to move in a certain direction – either up or down. And the *mānasika guṇa* provides insight into each *mahābhūta*'s natural predominance of the *tri-guṇa* (*sattva*, *rajas* and *tamas*). Each of these topics and their significance in this relationship will be discussed in the following sections.

Following the "*Pañcha Mahābhūta* Overview," there are five detailed tables of each *mahābhūta*'s *guṇa* and *karma*. A comparison from classical authors demonstrates that there are multiple perspectives on these specific details. This is seen commonly throughout the classics and can be considered a sign of the development of the science of Āyurveda.

In each table, the *guṇa* and *karma* are presented side-by-side to connect the concepts of inherent qualities with their outcomes as recognizable actions. The reader should be aware of the fact that they are not presented this way in classical literature. Also, remember that while *guṇa* and *karma* appear related, they are not directly responsible for the result of the dravya. Instead, it is the base *dravya* which maintains the *samavāya* relationship that is the true cause for all final outcomes.

A set of exercises follows each table to help explore these connections more deeply.

Pañcha Mahābhūta Overview

Mahābhūta (noun form)	*Bhautika dravya* (adjective form)	Gross element	*Viśheṣha guṇa*	*Rasa*	*Viśheṣha karma*	*Mānasika guṇa*
Pṛthvi mahābhūta	*Pārthiva dravya*	Earth	*Gandha*	*Madhura* (*prayas*); *Kaṣhāya* (*īṣhat*)	*Adho gati*	*Tamas*
Ap or *Jala mahābhūta*	*Āpya dravya*	Water	*Rasa*	*Madhura* (*prayas*); *Kaṣhāya, amla, lavaṇa* (*īṣhat*)	*Adho gati*	*Sattva, Tamas*
Tejo or *Agni mahābhūta*	*Taijasa* or *āgneya dravya*	Fire	*Rūpa*	*Kaṭu* (*prayas*); *Amla, lavaṇa* (*īṣhat*)	*Ūrdhva gati*	*Sattva, Rajas*
Vāyu mahābhūta	*Vāyavya* or *vāyavīya dravya*	Air	*Sparśha*	*Kaṣhāya* (*prayas*); *Tikta* (*īṣhat*)	*Ūrdhva gati*	*Rajas*
Ākāśha mahābhūta	*Ākāśha-ātmaka, ākāsīya, nābhasa dravya*	Space or ether	*Śhabda*	*Avyakta* (unmanifest)		*Sattva*

Classical references:

Rasa: Su. Sū. 41/4
Prayas means that the *rasa* is generally present in this *mahābhūta*
Īṣhat means that the *rasa* is slightly present in this *mahābhūta*

Viśheṣha karma: Cha. Sū. 26/41
Su. Sū. 41/6
AH Sū. 9/11

Mānasika guṇa Su. Śhā. 1/20

Pṛthvi guṇa and karma

Pṛthvi guṇa Feature	Cha. Sū. 26/11	Su. Sū. 41/4.1	AH Sū. 9/6	BP Pū. 6/201	*Pṛthvi karma* Produces	Cha. Sū. 26/11	Su. Sū. 41/4.1	AH Sū. 9/6	BP Pū. 6/201
Guru Heavy	✓	✓	✓	✓	*Gaurava* Heaviness	✓	✓		
Kaṭhiṇa Hard	✓	✓			*Saṅghāta* Compactness	✓	✓		
Manda Slow	✓	✓			*Bala* Strength		✓		
Sthira Stable	✓	✓	✓		*Sthairya* Stability	✓	✓		
Viśhada Clear	✓								
Sāndra Dense	✓	✓							
Sthūla Large	✓	✓	✓		*Upachaya* Growth	✓	✓		

Exercise: Now choose a *dravya* that is predominant in *pṛthvi mahābhūta*. Describe three of its *guṇa* and related *karma*, and explain how these can be demonstrated through practical example.

Dravya:			
Guṇa #1:		*Karma* #1:	
Example:			
Guṇa #2:		*Karma* #2:	
Example:			
Guṇa #3:		*Karma* #3:	
Example:			

Ap or Jala guṇa and karma

Ap guṇa Feature	Cha. Sū. 26/11	Su. Sū. 41/4.2	AH Sū. 9/6	BP Pū. 6/201	*Ap karma* Produces	Cha. Sū. 26/11	Su. Sū. 41/4.2	AH Sū. 9/6	BP Pū. 6/201
Drava Flowing	√		√		*Kleda* Moisture		√	√	
Snigdha Oily	√	√	√	√	*Sneha* Grease	√	√	√	
Śhīta Cold	√	√	√		*Hlādana* Refreshing		√		
Manda Slow	√	√	√		*Bandha* Binding	√	√	√	
Mṛdu Soft	√	√			*Mārdava* Softness	√			
Pichchhila Slimy	√	√			*Prahlāda* Delight	√		√	
Guru Heavy	√	√	√						
Sāndra Dense		√	√						
Timita Wet		√			*Upakleda* Dampness	√			
Sara Flowing		√			*Viṣhyanda* Flowing	√	√	√	

Exercise: Now choose a *dravya* that is predominant in *ap mahābhūta*. Describe three of its *guṇa* and related *karma*, and explain how these can be demonstrated through practical example.

Dravya:			
Guṇa #1:		*Karma* #1:	
Example:			
Guṇa #2:		*Karma* #2:	
Example:			
Guṇa #3:		*Karma* #3:	
Example:			

Tejo or Agni guṇa and karma

Tejo Guṇa Feature	Cha. Sū. 26/11	Su. Sū. 41/4.3	AH Sū. 9/6	BP Pū. 6/201	*Tejo Karma* Produces	Cha. Sū. 26/11	Su. Sū. 41/4.3	AH Sū. 9/6	BP Pū. 6/201
Uṣhṇa Hot	✓	✓	✓		*Dāha* Burning	✓	✓	✓	
Tīkṣhṇa Sharp	✓	✓	✓	✓	*Prakāśha* Brilliance	✓	✓	✓	
Sūkṣhma Minute	✓	✓	✓		*Prabhā* Radiance	✓	✓	✓	
Laghu Light	✓	✓			*Tāpana* Illumination		✓		
Rūkṣha Dry	✓	✓	✓		*Pāka, Pācana* Cooking, digesting	✓	✓	✓	
Viśhada Clear	✓	✓	✓		*Varṇa kara* Improves complexion	✓	✓	✓	
Khara Rough		✓			*Dāruṇa* Hard		✓		

Exercise: Now choose a *dravya* that is predominant in *tejo mahābhūta*. Describe three of its *guṇa* and related *karma*, and explain how these can be demonstrated through practical example.

Dravya:			
Guṇa #1:		*Karma* #1:	
Example:			
Guṇa #2:		*Karma* #2:	
Example:			
Guṇa #3:		*Karma* #3:	
Example:			

Vāyu guṇa and karma

Vāyu Guṇa Feature	Cha. Sū. 26/11	Su. Sū. 41/4.4	AH Sū. 9/6	BP Pū. 6/201	*Vāyu Karma* Produces	Cha. Sū. 26/11	Su. Sū. 41/4.4	AH Sū. 9/6	BP Pū. 6/201
Laghu Light	√	√	√		*Lāghava* Lightness	√	√	√	
Śhita Cold	√				*Glāni, Glapana* Exhaustion, tiredness	√	√	√	
Rūkṣha Dry	√	√	√	√	*Raukṣhya, Virūkṣhaṇa* Dryness	√	√	√	
Khara Rough	√	√			*Vicāra, Vicāraṇa* Agitation	√	√	√	
Viśhada Clear	√	√	√		*Vaiṣhadya, Vaiṣhandya* Clearness, clarity	√	√	√	
Sūkṣhma Minute	√	√							
Śhiśhira Cool		√							

Exercise: Now choose a *dravya* that is predominant in *vāyu mahābhūta*. Describe three of its *guṇa* and related *karma*, and explain how these can be demonstrated through practical example.

Dravya:			
Guṇa #1:		*Karma* #1:	
Example:			
Guṇa #2:		*Karma* #2:	
Example:			
Guṇa #3:		*Karma* #3:	
Example:			

Ākāśha guṇa and karma

Ākāśha Guṇa Feature	Cha. Sū. 26/11	Su.Sū. 41/4.5	AH Sū. 9/6	BP Pū. 6/201	*Ākāśha karma* Produces	Cha. Sū. 26/11	Su. Sū. 41/4.5	AH Sū. 9/6	BP Pū. 6/201
Mṛdu Soft	✓	✓			*Mārdava* Softness	✓	✓		
Laghu Light	✓		✓	✓	*Lāghava* Lightness	✓	✓	✓	
Rūkṣha Dry	✓								
Śhlakṣhṇa Smooth	✓	✓							
Viśhada Clear		✓	✓						
Sūkṣhma Minute		✓	✓		*Śhau-ṣhīrya* Hollow-ness	✓	✓	✓	
Vyavāyi Spreads then acts		✓							

Exercise: Now choose a *dravya* that is predominant in *ākāśha mahābhūta*. Describe three of its *guṇa* and related *karma*, and explain how these can be demonstrated through practical example.

Dravya:			
Guṇa #1:		*Karma* #1:	
Example:			
Guṇa #2:		*Karma* #2:	
Example:			
Guṇa #3:		*Karma* #3:	
Example:			

Mahābhūta composition

Each *mahābhūta* is named for a specific element because it contains a predominance of that element. Śhusruta explains this concept in Su. Sū. 41/3 where he states that any particular *mahābhūta* is named so because it is constituted primarily of that element, but also has a varying portion of the others (see Charaka's explanation in Cha. Śhā. 1/27-28).

In AH Śhā. 3/2, Vāgbhaṭa further explains that as the *bhūtas* are generated, each one contains a portion of its previous *bhūta*. With *ākāśha* being the first, it is completely composed of *ākāśha mahābhūta* with the *viśheṣha guṇa* of *śhabda*. Next, it generates *vāyu*, which is primarily composed of *vāyu mahābhūta*, with a smaller portion of *ākāśha mahābhūta*. Because of this combination of *bhūtas*, the *viśheṣha guṇa* is primary *sparśha* along with *śhabda*. And this continues all the way up through the remaining *bhūtas* (see also Cha. Śhā. 1/28 and Su. Sū. 42/3).

Because the number of possible combinations in proportions of *bhūtas* and their additional features is practically infinite, the *dravya* available can also be considered of limitless possibility.

TEST YOURSELF

Learn, review and memorize key terms from this section.

pañcha mahābhūta
___

pṛthvi
___

ap
___

tejas
___

vāyu
___

ākāśha
___

viśheṣha guṇa
___

viśheṣha karma
___

mānasika guṇa
___

gandha
___

rasa
___

rūpa
___

sparśha
___

śhabda
___

GUṆA

The term *guṇa* is used as both the categorical umbrella term for the entire concept and to indicate a single feature of any *dravya*. As the broad category for the concept, *guṇa* is that which allows a *dravya* to be recognized. It can be considered to include the adjectives or descriptors that characterize the *dravya* and how to recognize them. The broad term of *guṇa* encompasses several subgroups which include individual *guṇas* to describe a wide variety of features that can be used to assess many aspects of life and health from a clinical perspective.

Classically, the topic of *guṇa* is one which has significantly more variability among authors than other topics. Although it is rare, in certain cases major authors make contradictory statements about very fundamental theories. More frequently, individual authors add extra information to expand the scope of the topic. These inconsistencies should not be taken as invalid or incorrect knowledge by any means. Instead, it is critical that the student recognize the allowance for customization of the science when the proposed knowledge could be validated and proven as a law or theory within the boundaries of time, place and population.

In this textbook, the major and most significant opinions of classical authors have been included wherever possible to provide the reader with a broader picture of the topic in total. The more obscure, and less popular statements have not yet been included.

Paribhāṣhā

Definition #1:
Guṇa attracts

गुण आमन्त्रणे । गुण्यते आमन्त्र्यते लोक अनेन इति गुणः ।

वाच:

Guṇa āmantraṇe | Guṇyate āmantryate loka anena iti guṇaḥ |

Vācaḥ

Guṇa āmantraṇe (*Guṇa* is that which calls a person to something, or attracts a person to a thing).

Guṇa is that which attracts a person to a thing. *Guṇa* has the power to draw one's attention to something.

Definition #2:
Guṇa does not act

समवायी तु निश्चेष्टः कारणं गुणः ॥

च. सू. १।५१

Samavāyī tu niśhcheṣhṭaḥ kāraṇaṁ guṇaḥ |

Cha. Sū. 1/51

Kāraṇaṁ guṇaḥ (Guṇa is the cause) *tu niśhcheṣhṭaḥ* (which is without action) *samavāyī* (that is perpetually attached).

Guṇa is perpetually attached [to the *dravya*] and it is the cause [for recognizing the dravya] which does not act.

Bheda

The high-level classification of *guṇa* will be discussed first, followed by an in-depth review of each subcategory in the next section.

Classification #1:
Complete *guṇa* classification

सार्था गुर्वादयो बुद्धिः प्रत्नान्ताः परादयः । गुणाः प्रोक्ताः,

च. सू. १।४९

अनेन त्रिविधा अपि वैशेषिकाः सामान्याः आत्मगुणाश्चोद्दिष्टाः ।

चक्रपाणि

Sārthā gurvādayo buddhiḥ pratnāntāḥ parādayaḥ |
Guṇāḥ proktāḥ,

Cha. Sū. 1/49

Anena trividhā api vaiśheṣhikāḥ sāmānyāḥ ātmaguṇāscoddiṣhṭāḥ |

Chakrapāṇi

According to Charaka, the groups of *guṇas* are:

Sārthā	The five *viśheṣha guṇas* which include the objects detected by the five sense organs
Gurvādi	The *guru*, etc *guṇas* which include ten pairs of opposites
Buddhi	*Guṇas* which describe the intellect
Pratnāntā	*Guṇas* which describe the *ātma*
Parādaya	Ten *parādi guṇas* used to help describe clinical practice methodologies

According to Chakrapāṇi, *guṇas* are classified in three categories:

Vaiśheṣhikā	The five *viśheṣha guṇas* which include the objects detected by the five sense organs
Sāmānyā	The *guṇas* which are most commonly used in practice, including two subcategories of *gurvādi* and *parādi guṇas*
Ātmaguṇā	The *guṇas* which describe *ātma*

The *guṇa* classification is an area which has evolved over the course of development of Āyurveda. Classical authors including Charaka utilized knowledge and resources from the *ṣhaḍ darśhana* to develop various methodologies which were more appropriate for Āyurvedic practice. Later authors, like Chakrapāṇi, consolidated and condensed this knowledge to make it more specific and applicable to the practice of Āyurveda. Because of this refinement, multiple classification methods exist today.

In this series of textbooks, Chakrapāṇi's high-level structure will be used for the main organization of *guṇas*. Additional significant information provided by other authors will be included within this structure.

Vaiśheṣhikā

The *Vaiśheṣhikā guṇas* originate from the *ṣhaḍ darśhana* and the *sṛṣhṭi utpatti siddhānta*. Details of their manifestation are covered in Chapters 22 and 25.

The *Vaiśheṣhikā guṇas* include the five *viśheṣha guṇas*. These are the single, special means by which each individual sense organ can recognize one object. This group of *guṇas* is called *sārthā* by Charaka, literally meaning *sa* (with) + *artha* (the objects, of the senses).

The five *Vaiśheṣhikā guṇas* are:

Vaiśheṣhikā guṇas	Recognized through the	By the sense of
Śhabda	ear	hearing
Sparśha	skin	touch
Rūpa	eye	sight
Rasa	tongue	taste
Gandha	nose	smell

Sāmānya

The *sāmānya guṇas* are those which are common to everyone and regularly applied in practice. These include two subcategories of *gurvādi* and *parādi.*

Gurvādi guṇa

Gurvādi means *guru* (heavy) + *ādi* (etc) and refers to the group of twenty *guṇas* where *guru* is the first in the list. The twenty *guṇas* are composed of ten pairs of opposites. This group can also be called the *śharīrika guṇas* because one of their main purposes is to describe the human body for clinical assessment. However, their utility extends much beyond the body and this entire group is used to describe all aspects of things involved in clinical management processes, especially *dravya* and their therapeutic utility.

The *gurvādi guṇas* are one of the most extensive topics in the classics. Because of this, many authors have provided varying opinions on their structure, terminology and usage. The following chart provides a comprehensive review of the *guṇa* pairs and names. Variations include the different synonyms and pairings found in the classics. Based on the popularity and applicability today, the "Common pair" column lists the names that will be used throughout this textbook.

Common pair	Cha. Sū. 25/36 Śhā. 6/10	Su. Sū. 46/514	AH Sū. 1/18	BP Pū. 6/202
Guru-laghu Heavy-Light	√	√	√	√
Śhīta-Uṣhṇa Cold-Hot	√	√	*Hima-Uṣhṇa* Cold-Hot	√
Snigdha-Rūkṣha Oily-Dry	√	√	√	√
Manda-Tīkṣhṇa Slow-Sharp	√	*Tīkṣhṇa-Mṛdu* Sharp-Soft	√	*Tīkṣhṇa-Śhlakṣhṇa* Sharp-Smooth
Sthira-Sara Stable-Flowing	√	*Sara-Manda* Flowing-Slow	*Sthira-Chala* Stable-Moving	√
Mṛdu-Kaṭhina Soft-Hard	√	*Sugandha-Durgandha* Good smelling-Bad smelling	√	*Mṛdu-Karkaśha* Soft-Rough
Viśhada-Pichchhila Clear-Cloudy	√	√	√	√
Śhlakṣhṇa-Khara Smooth-Rough	√	*Śhlakṣhṇa-Karkaśha* Smooth-Rough		*Āśhu-Manda* Quick-Slow
Sūkṣhma-Sthūla Minute-Large	√	√	√	√
Sāndra-Drava Dense-Liquid	√	√	√	*Drava-Śhuṣhka* Liquid-Dry

Suśhruta describes three additional *guṇas* in Su. Sū. 46/521-524. Some authors opine that these three can be placed within the format of the twenty *gurvādi guṇas*, while others, including Chakrapāṇi, do not accept that and chose not to recognize the extra *guṇas*. The three include:

Vyavāyi — spreads through the entire body and then gets digested (acts), ex. *saindhava*, *bhanga*

Vikāsī — spreads through the entire body and loosens or detaches the structures which bind or hold the *dhātus* together

Āśhukārī — spreads immediately through the entire body like oil over the surface of water, ex. *madya* (alcohol)

Part of the debate includes controversy over whether these should be considered *guṇa* or *karma*.

The following table provides the definitions for each of the twenty *gurvādi guṇas*. These definitions have been listed in the Hemādri commentary of AH Sū. 1/18.

Guṇa	Definition (AH Sū. 1/18c)	Opposite	Definition
Guru Heavy	Yasya bṛmhaṇe karmaṇi śhakti sa guru *Guru* is found in the power of producing *bṛmhaṇa* (the action of creating heaviness, strength, heartiness).	*Laghu* Light	Laṅghane laghu *Laghu* is in *laṅghana* (the action of creating lightness).
Manda Slow	Śhamane manda *Manda* is in *śhamana* (the action of calming or slowing the *doṣhas*).	*Tīkṣhṇa* Fast, sharp	Śhodhane tīkṣhṇa *Tīkṣhṇa* is in *śhodhana* (the action of expelling the *doṣhas*).
Hima *(śhīta)* Cold	Stambhane hima *Hima* is in *stambhana* (the action of freezing the *doṣhas*).	*Uṣhṇa* Hot	Svedane uṣhṇa *Uṣhṇa* is in *svedana* (the action of melting the *doṣhas*).
Snigdha Oily	Kledane snigdha *Snigdha* is in *kledana* (the action of creating liquidity).	*Rūkṣha* Dry	Śhoṣhaṇe rūkṣha *Rūkṣha* is in *śhoṣhaṇe* (the action of creating dryness).

Guṇa	Definition (AH Sū. 1/18c)	Opposite	Definition
Śhlakṣhṇa Smooth	Ropaṇe śhlakṣhṇa *Śhlakṣhṇa* is in *ropaṇa* (the action of creating smoothness, healing).	*Khara* Rough	Lekhane khara *Khara* is in *lekhana* (the action of scraping).
Sāndra Dense	Prasādane sāndra *Sāndra* is in *prasādana* (the action of soothing, calming).	*Drava* Flowing	Viloḍane drava *Drava* is in vilodana (the action of stirring up, churning, agitating).
Mṛdu Soft	Śhlathane mṛdu *Mṛdu* is in *śhlathana* (the action of loosening, relaxing, weakening).	*Kaṭhina* Hard	Dṛḍhane kaṭhina *Kaṭhina* is in *dṛḍhane* (the action of making something fixed, firm, hard, strong, solid, massive).
Sthira Stable	Dhāraṇe sthira *Sthira* is in dhāraṇa (the action of holding, bearing, keeping, retaining, preserving, protecting).	*Chala* Moving	Preraṇe chala *Chala* is in preraṇa (the action of setting in motion, urging, exciting, impeling, activating).
Sūkṣhma Minute	Vivaraṇe sūkṣhma *Sūkṣhma* is in *vivaraṇa* (the action of uncovering, opening).	*Sthūla* Gross	Saṁvaraṇe sthūla *Sthūla* is in saṁvaraṇa (the action of covering, containing, shutting, closing).
Viśhada Clear	Kṣhālane viśhada *Viśhada* is in *kṣhālana* (the action of washing, wiping, cleaning off).	*Pichchhila* Cloudy	Lepane pichchhila *Pichchhila* is in *lepana* (the action of spreading over, smearing, plastering).

Additional definitions and detailed descriptions can be found in Su. Sū. 46/514+, and BP Pū. 6/202-211.

Suśhruta describes the *pañchabhautika* composition of *dravya* and their related *guṇas* in Su. Sū. 41/4 and 41/11. He also explains how to identify *guṇa* based on its *karma*, using *anumāna pramāṇa* in Su. Sū. 41/6. Later, in Su. Sū. 46/514-519, he explains the related *karmas* of each *guṇa*.

The most important *guṇas*, or those which generally have the most pronounced effect on human health, are explained in relation to *vīrya* in Cha. Sū. 26/64-65, and in AH Sū. 9/12-18.

Parādi guṇa

Parādi guṇas include ten *guṇas* which are primarily used to aid clinical management processes. These *guṇas* help to shape the thought patterns during clinical analysis and decision-making by providing ways to identify and prioritize factors in the complex frameworks of therapeutic management. These ten are described in Cha. Sū. 26/29-35.

Parādi guṇa	Definition Cha. Sū. 26/29-35
Paratva Superiority	The ability to identify the superior item in a group by using one's *yukti* based on measurements of *deśha*, *kāla*, *vaya*, *māna*, *vipāka*, *vīrya*, *rasa*, etc
Aparatva Inferiority	The ability to identify the inferior item in a group by using one's *yukti* based on measurements of *deśha*, *kāla*, *vaya*, *māna*, *vipāka*, *vīrya*, *rasa*, etc
Yukti Logical application	The ability to apply logical thought processes in multi-factorial events and determine the correct course of action or solution
Saṅkhya Enumeration	The ability to use mathematics, including statistics, quickly and accurately
Saṁyoga Combination	The ability to combine items which may result in three possible outputs where only one of each combined item, or both, participate to produce the momentary outcome
Vibhāga Separation	The ability to separate items using any of three methods: *vibhakti* (create a portion, divide), *viyoga* (subtract), or *bhāgaso graha* (remove a portion)
Pṛthaktva Distinction	The ability to recognize items as distinct from a group using any of three methods: *syād-asaṁyoga* (quick differentiation), *vailakṣhaṇya* (distinction based on characteristics or features), or *anēkata* (individuality)
Parimāṇa Measurement	The ability to measure accurately, using quantitative and qualitative means, in any type of measurement scale or system
Saṁskāra Conversion	The ability to understand how processing converts *dravya* into various states
Abhyāsa Repetition	The ability to maintain repetition with all things, routines and activities

Additionally, these ten *parādi guṇas* help shape the application of the scientific method in clinical practice.

Ātmaguṇā

The *Ātmaguṇā* group describes the features and characteristics that can be used to recognize the presence and functioning of *ātma* in an individual. These characteristics are especially useful in practice to help assess the mental state which can have a bearing on choosing appropriate management protocols. The *guṇas* included in this group are:

Ātmaguṇā	Definition (Cha. Śhā. 1/72)
Buddhi Intellect	The ability to utilize intellectual faculties appropriately
Icchā Desire, interest	The presence of desire, interest, eagerness, etc when appropriate
Dveṣha Dislike	The presence of dislike, disinterest, aversion, repulsion, etc when appropriate
Sukha Contentment	The presence of a normal feeling of contentment, happiness, satisfaction, etc when appropriate
Duḥkha Unhappiness	The presence of a normal feeling of unhappiness, discontent, sadness, etc when appropriate
Prayatna Effort	The presence of a normal desire to apply effort, discipline, work, etc to achieve a goal

TEST YOURSELF

Learn, review and memorize key terms from this section.

guṇa

vaiśheṣhikā guṇas

śhabda

sparśha

rūpa

rasa

gandha

gurvādi guṇa

sāmānya guṇa

guru

laghu

śhīta / hima

uṣhṇa

snigdha

rūkṣha

manda

tīkṣhṇa

sthira

sara

mṛdu

kaṭhina

viśhada
pichchhila
śhlakṣhṇa
khara
sūkṣhma
sthūla
sāndra
drava

KARMA

The term *karma* is used as both the categorical umbrella term for the entire concept and to indicate a specific action or effect of any *dravya*. As the broad category for the concept, *karma* is that which allows a *dravya* to have a specific effect. Generally, the intended effect of *karma* is for curative purposes. The broad term of *karma* does not include any subcategories directly in classics. However, certain references which can be considered as a means for practical classification of types of karma are included in this textbook.

Paribhāṣhā

Definition #1:
How karma works

संयोगे च विभागे च कारणं द्रव्यमाश्रितम् ।
कर्तव्यस्य क्रिया कर्म कर्म नान्यदपेक्षते ॥
च. सू. १।५२

Saṁyoge cha vibhāge cha kāraṇaṁ dravyamāśhritam |
Kartavyasya kriyā karma karma nānyadapekṣhate ||
Cha. Sū. 1/52

Saṁyoge cha vibhāge cha kāraṇaṁ (It is the cause or reason for *saṁyoga* and *vibhāga* and) *dravyam-āśhritam* (it takes shelter, or resides in *dravya*).

Kartavyasya kriyā karma (*Karma* is the *kriyā* of what has been done, or accomplished); *karma nānyadapekṣhate* (*karma* does not require any other factor for it to operate).

Definition #2:
For curative effort

प्रयत्नादि कर्म चेष्टितमुच्यते ॥
च. सू. १।४९

Prayatnādi karma cheṣhṭamuchyate ||
Cha. Sū. 1/49

Karma (Action) *uchyate* (is explained as) *cheṣhṭam* (the activities) *prayatnādi* (made for effort, etc, ie, curative effort).

It is explained that the performance of *karma* is for producing curative results.

Bheda

The classification method for *karma*, which is discussed here, is a classical statement from Charaka which can be inferred to apply to *karma* through *dravya*, based on the objectives listed. The purpose of *karma* is to affect a certain result based on action(s), and these categories are specific actions intended to provide curative results.

Classification #1:
According to intended effect

किंचिद्दोषप्रशमनं किंचिद्धातुप्रदूषणम् ।
स्वस्थवृत्तौ मतं किंचित्त्रिविधं द्रव्यमुच्यते ॥

च. सू. १।६७

Kiñchiddoṣhapraśhamanaṁ kiñchiddhātupradūṣhaṇam |
Svasthavṛttau mataṁ kiñchittrividhaṁ dravyamuchyate ||

Cha. Sū. 1/67

See also AH Sū. 1/16

Trividhaṁ dravyam uchyate (These three types of *dravya* are explained as):

Kiñchid doṣha praśhamanaṁ

Some types (of dravya) have the purpose or effect of doṣha praśhamanaṁ, or returning doṣha(s) to their normal state

Kiñchid dhātu pradūṣhaṇam

Some types (of *dravya*) have the purpose or effect of *dhātu pradūṣhaṇam*, or vitiating (aggravating, dirtying, ruining) the *dhātus*

Svasthavṛttau mataṁ kiñchit

Some types (of *dravya*) have the purpose or effect of *svastha-vṛtta*, or maintaining health

A thorough list of individual *karmas*, their definitions, actions and examples can be found in BP Pū. 5/212 and onward.

TEST YOURSELF

Learn, review and memorize key terms from this section.

karma

saṁyoga

vibhāga

doṣha praśhamana

dhātu pradūṣhaṇa

svasthavṛtta

RASA

The term *rasa* is widely used in Āyurveda and carries many varied meanings in different contexts. Here, within the scope and study of *dravya-guṇa śhastra*, *rasa* is the flavor or taste which can be immediately recognized when a *dravya* is placed on the tongue and it comes into direct contact with the sense of taste. *Dravya-guṇa śhastra* focuses on the study of *dravyas* within the context of therapeutic utility and application.

Rasa is a topic which is always studied and reviewed along with the other inseparable components of *dravya* including *guṇa, karma*, *vīrya, vipāka* and *prabhāva.* There are many inter-related rules that work with all of these components as they are all perpetually attached to *dravya*. In order to completely understand the concept of *rasa*, all of the other components within *dravya* must also be studied in tandem.

Paribhāṣhā

Definition #1:
Rasa and anurasa

व्यक्तः शुष्कस्य चादौ च रसो द्रव्यस्य लक्ष्यते ।
विपर्ययेणानुरसो रसो नास्ति हि सप्तमः ॥

च. सू. २६।२८

Vyaktaḥ śhuṣhkasya chādau cha raso dravyasya lakṣhyate |
Viparyayeṇānuraso raso nāsti hi saptamaḥ ||

Cha. Sū. 26/28

Vyaktaḥ (That which is perceptible or known through the senses) *śhuṣhkasya chādau cha* (in its dry and other [wet] state) *raso dravyasya lakṣhyate* (is known as the flavor of the *dravya*). *Viparyayeṇānuraso* (The reverse or opposite of this is *anurasa*); *raso nāsti hi saptamaḥ* (there is not another seventh *rasa*).

Rasa is the flavor which is recognized when a *dravya*, in its dry or wet state, comes into contact with the sense of taste (ie, the tongue). *Anurasa* is the reverse of *rasa* and it is not a separate seventh flavor.

Based on this short definition, *anurasa* is understood to be the secondary flavor of any *dravya*. It can be known to exist in a dravya by recognizing the opposite or unexpected effects of the *dravya* based on the main *rasa*. *Anurasa* can be deduced through this type of presentation.

Definition #2:
How it acts

रसो निपाते द्रव्याणां,

च. सू. २६।६५.५

Raso nipāte dravyāṇāṁ ||

Cha. Sū. 26/65.5

Raso (Flavor) *dravyāṇāṁ* (in the *dravya*) *nipāte* ([is felt when] falling down [onto the tongue]).

Rasa is the flavor perceived when the *dravya* contacts the tongue.

Bheda

The classification methods for *rasa* vary among authors but in general, the *ṣhaḍ rasa*, or six types of *rasa*, are universally recognized. The additional classification methods mentioned are also useful for achieving a deeper understanding of the mechanisms of *rasa* and how they work with *dravya*, especially in clinical situations. In practice, both clinically and in day-to-day usage, *rasa* is never used singly because the *pañchabhautika* composition of *dravyas* always contains a proportion of *mahābhūtas*, which in turn influences their behavior, actions, final outcome and effects (Cha. Vi. 8/138).

Classification #1:
Ṣhaḍ rasa

मधुराम्ललवणकटुतिक्तकषायाः ।

च. सू. २६।९

Madhurāmlalavaṇakaṭutiktakaṣhāyāḥ ||

Cha. Sū. 26/9

See also: Cha. Sū. 1/65, Su. Sū. 42/3

The *ṣhadrasa* include:

Madhura	Sweet, also called *svādu*
Amla	Sour
Lavaṇa	Salty
Kaṭu	Pungent, spicy, also called *ūṣhana*
Tikta	Bitter
Kaṣhāya	Astringent

The six types of *rasa* are sweet, sour, salty, pungent, bitter and astringent.

Classification #2:
Two types

द्विविधाः - सौम्या आग्नेयाश्च ।
मधुरतिक्तकषायाः सौम्याः; कटवम्ललवणा
आग्नेयाः ।

सु. सू. ४२।७

Dvividhāḥ - saumyā āgneyāśhcha |
Madhuratiktakaṣhāyāḥ saumyāḥ,
kaṭavamlalavaṇā āgneyāḥ ||

Su. Sū. 42/7

Dvividhāḥ - saumyā āgneyāśhcha (Two types - *saumya* and *agneya* [cooling and heating] include) *madhuratiktakaṣhāyāḥ saumyāḥ* (sweet, bitter and astringent as *saumya* [cooling]) *kaṭavamlalavaṇā āgneyāḥ* (pungent, sour and salty as *agneya* [heating]).

Because the world or universe is of *agneya* and *saumya*, similarly, *rasas* are of two types - *saumya* (cooling) and *agneya* (heating). Sweet, bitter and astringent are cooling; pungent, sour and salty are heating.

Saumya	Madhura Tikta Kaṣhāya
Agneya	Kaṭu Amla Lavaṇa

Classification #3:
Sixty-three types

भेदश्चैषां त्रिषष्टिविधविकल्पो
द्रव्यदेशकालप्रभावाद्भवति, तमुपदेक्ष्यामः
।

च. सू. २६।१४

Bhedaśhchaiṣhāṁ
triṣhaṣhṭividhavikalpo
dravyadeśhakālaprabhāvādbhavati,
tamupadekṣhyāmaḥ |

Cha. Sū. 26/14

See also Su. Sū. 42/12, AH Sū. 10/

Bhedaśhchaiṣhāṁ triṣhaṣhṭividha (Sixty-three types) *bhavati tamupadekṣhyāmaḥ* (are now explained) *vikalpo dravya* (as the divisions of *dravyas* by) *deśha* (geographical location), *kāla* (time), *prabhāvād* (special effect).

Dravyas can be divided into sixty-three types based on geographical location, time and the special effects (properties, actions, etc) of the *dravya*.

In the very next statement, Charaka also recognizes the fact that based on the combinations and permutations of *dravya* components (in terms of their *pañchabhautika* composition), the number of possible *rasa* variations is actually infinite (see Cha. Sū. 26/26, Cha. Vi. 1/8, AH Sū. 10/44).

Because so many combinations and permutations can present a very complex problem in terms of predicting outcome, Punarvasu Atreya states in Cha. Sū. 26/9 that the wise do not make recommendations based on multiple flavor combinations. This is a key point for clinical application. In complex presentations, single *rasas* are especially effective when utilized as primary agents of action.

Additionally, classification methods of *dravya* based on *rasa* have been mentioned by classical authors. Remember that although these are classified under a single *rasa*, they are always composed of all *rasas* in minor proportions. These classification methods serve as aids in clinical practice when applying *dravyas* therapeutically. Many examples of these groups can be found throughout the classical texts and they are commonly referred to as *gaṇa* or *varga* (group). See Cha. Vi. 6/139-144, Su. Sū. 42/11 and AH Sū. 10/22-32 for examples.

Origin of rasa

Rasa manifests in *dravya* for two reasons - the *pañchabhautika* composition of the *dravya*, and *udaka* (रसानां योनिरुदकं, *Rasānāṁ yonirudakaṁ*, Cha. Sū. 26/9). *Udaka* is water and in this context, can also be considered as *ap* or *jala mahābhūta*. Suśhruta explains that because of the manner in which the *pañcha mahābhūtas* are generated, and because of their special connection with a specific sense organ, *rasa* must be primarily composed of *ap* (तस्मादाप्यो रसः, *Tasmādāpyo rasaḥ*, Su. Sū. 42/3).

The process of manifesting *rasa* in *dravya* happens as rain condenses from the atmosphere, falls to earth and comes in contact with the *pañchabhautika* composition of the air and ground. While this moisture is in the atmosphere, it is said to be influenced by the properties of the moon, which by nature is *saumya*. The moon's nature of being cool, light and nourishing is then imparted to the *udaka*. At this unmanifested stage, the atmospheric water has *avyakta rasa*, or a flavor which is imperceptible to the sense of taste.

Once the atmospheric moisture condenses and begins to fall, it comes in contact and is influenced by the *pañcha mahābhūtas* that it comes into contact with in the air and on the ground. These qualities of the environment get absorbed into the water resulting in its specific *pañchabhautika* composition. Suśhruta adds that water which has a flavor is considered defective or impure. Whatever qualities the water carries then go on to affect all life in that local area. For individuals born and raised in a specific area, this local water in its normal state can act as key nourishment and promote health because of its unique *pañchabhautika* composition. As this water is consumed, it can then manifest the *ṣhaḍ rasas* in the individual and provide its nourishing effect. This explanation can be found in Cha. Sū. 26/39, Cha. Sū. 27/200, Su. Sū. 42/3 and Su. Sū. 45/11.

Additionally, the variation in *ṛtus* results in the predominance of specific *mahābhūtas* at certain times of the year. The effects of this can be recognized in the flavors of plants grown in different seasons. These variations throughout the year influence human health in subtle but important ways.

Rasa and pañcha mahābhūta

The *pañchabhautika* composition in any *dravya* has a definite influence on the *dravya*'s *rasa* and its other components. All classical authors have established a definite relationship between the predominance of *mahābhūtas* in a given *dravya* and the expected *rasa*. This relationship works both ways, so that any *dravya* which is recognized to have a specific *rasa* can be assumed to also have a predominance in those related *mahābhūtas*. However, certain exceptions to these rules do apply and those are explained through the rules of known *prabhāva*.

See Cha. Sū. 26/40, Su. Sū. 42/3, AH Sū. 10/1.

Rasa	*Pṛthvi*	*Ap*	*Tejas*	*Vāyu*	*Ākāśha*
Madhura Sweet	Su. AH	Su. AH Cha. - *Soma guṇa*			
Amla Sour	✓		✓		
Lavaṇa Salty		✓	✓		
Kaṭu Pungent, spicy			✓	✓	
Tikta Bitter				✓	✓
Kaṣhāya Astringent	✓			✓	

Additionally, recall that each *mahābhūta* has a specific *gati*, or direction of movement. This is primarily based on the mass of the dravya which is strongly determined by its *pañchabhautika* composition. Based on this relationship between the *pañchabhautika* composition and *rasa* of *dravyas*, the *gati* can also be predicted by the predominant *rasa*. Charaka explains this in Cha. Sū. 26/41.

Agni and *vāyu mahābhūtas* have the tendency to move upwards. This is called *ūrdhva gati*. *Pṛthvi* and *ap mahābhūtas* have the tendency to move downwards, called *adho gati*. Because *ākāśha* is stated to have *avyakta rasa* (imperceptible flavor), it is not capable of *gati*. When a *dravya* exists with predominant *mahābhūtas* with opposing *gati*, both can occur.

Rasa and doṣha

Rasas also share a common relationship with *doṣhas* based on their *pañcha mahābhūtas* and related *guṇa* and *karma*. The following table lists the effects of *rasa* on each of the *doṣhas*, according to Cha. Vi. 1/6. It is important to note that increasing refers to aggravating the *doṣha* and making it go out of its normal healthy boundaries by excessive quantity and/or quality. Likewise, decreasing the *doṣha* can refer to eliminating it by causing its removal from the body or pacifying it to reduce it quantitatively and/or qualitatively to return it to its normal boundaries. Continued decrease can then cause the *doṣha* to go below its normal healthy boundary.

These functions are represented through the practical application of *Vṛddhi-Kṣhaya siddhānta*.

Rasa	V	P	K
Madhura	↓↓↓	↓↓↓	↑↑↑
Amla	↓↓	↑↑	↑↑
Lavaṇa	↓	↑	↑
Kaṭu	↑↑↑	↑↑↑	↓↓↓
Tikta	↑↑	↓↓	↓↓
Kaṣhāya	↑	↓	↓

Suśhruta described which *rasas* specifically reduce the *doṣhas* in order of effectiveness, however, he has not mentioned which *rasas* increase or aggravate the *doṣhas*. This is explained in Su. Sū. 42/4-6. In AH Sū. 1/15, Vāgbhaṭa also explains the *rasas* which reduce *doṣhas* but has not given a specific order for the aggravating ones. *Bhāva Prakāśha* identifies a slight variation in relationship by stating that *kapha* is reduced by *rasas* in a different order - *tikta, kaṭu*, then *kaṣhāya*, in BP Pū. 6/171. Like Suśhruta and Vāgbhaṭa, he also does not provide a specific order for the *rasas* which increase the *doṣhas*.

Charaka also describes in Cha. Sū. 26/59-60 that certain *rasas* can be generally understood to have an evacuating or constipating effect on the digestive system's output. This is because of the *rasa*'s relationship with the *pañcha mahābhūtas* and their tendency toward *adho* or *ūrdhva gati*. *Madhura, amla* and *lavaṇa rasas* tend to have *adho gati* along with *snigdha guṇa*, and thus, are helpful for eliminating flatus, urine and stool. *Kaṭu, tikta* and *kaśhāya rasas*, however, tend towards *ūrdhva gati*, which combined with their *rūkṣha guṇa* create difficulty and discomfort in eliminating flatus, stool, urine and semen. Vāgbhaṭa provides a similar, more condensed explanation in AH Sū.10/37.

Bhāva Prakāśha explains an important exception to the *rasa-doṣha* relationship in BP Pū. 6/172-174. If a *dravya* is expected to calm or decrease *vāta*, yet it is associated with other *guṇas* that typically increase or aggravate vāta, especially *rūkṣha*, *laghu* or *śhīta*, the *dravya* will not calm *vāta* as expected. With *pitta*, the exception includes *dravyas* associated with *tīkṣhṇa*, *uṣhṇa* and *laghu*, and other *pitta*-predominant *guṇas*. With *kapha*, the exception includes *dravyas* associated with *snigdha*, *guru* and *śhīta*, and other *kapha*-predominant *guṇas*.

Rasa and guṇa

Based on the relationship with *rasa* and *pañcha mahābhūtas*, certain *guṇas* can be associated to each *rasa* in a general way. This has been described by Charaka according to the most significant *guṇas* with each *rasa*, in order of least, moderate and maximum influence in Cha. Sū. 26/53-56.

Rasa	*Uttama* Maximum influence	*Madhyama* Moderate influence	*Avara* Least influence
Madhura	*Guru, snigdha, śhīta*		
Amla		*Snigdha, uṣhṇa*	*Laghu*
Lavaṇa	*Uṣhṇa*		*Snigdha, guru (laghu)*
Kaṭu		*Rūkṣha, laghu*	*Uṣhṇa*
Tikta	*Laghu*		*Rūkṣha, śhīta*
Kaṣhāya	*Rūkṣha*	*Guru, śhīta*	

Suśhruta and Vāgbhaṭa provide a more general relationship between *rasas.* In Su. Sū. 42/7 and AH Sū. 10/38, the *rasas* are categorized based on *saumya* and *agneya*, and accordingly, are described as *snigdha* and *guru*, or *rūkṣha* and *laghu*, respectively.

<table>
<tr><th>Rasa</th><th>Saumya</th><th>Agneya</th></tr>
<tr><td>Madhura</td><td rowspan="3">Snigdha
+
Guru</td><td></td></tr>
<tr><td>Amla</td><td></td></tr>
<tr><td>Lavaṇa</td><td></td></tr>
<tr><td>Kaṭu</td><td></td><td rowspan="3">Rūkṣha
+
Laghu</td></tr>
<tr><td>Tikta</td><td></td></tr>
<tr><td>Kaṣhāya</td><td></td></tr>
</table>

The implication of the *rasa-guṇa* relationship can be understood as follows:

- *Guru* → difficult to digest
- *Laghu* → easy to digest
- *Rūkṣha* → causes constipation, discourages elimination of flatus, urine, semen
- *Snigdha* → encourages elimination of stool, urine, flatus, semen
- *Uṣhṇa* → heating *vīrya*
- *Śhīta* → cooling *vīrya*

Rasa and karma

Rasa and *karma* have an extensive relationship. The classics have provided thorough details on the expected actions and outcomes of *rasa* on the human body. These should be reviewed in Cha. Sū. 26/43, Su. Sū. 42/10, AH Sū. 10/7-21, and BP Pū. 6/175-194.

Rasas also impart their own *karmas*, or actions upon contact of the *dravya* within the oral cavity. The descriptions provided in Ca Sū. 26/73-79, Su. Sū. 42/9 and AH Sū. 10/2-6 should be reviewed in detail to understand how to recognize the presence of each *rasa* in a *dravya*.

TEST YOURSELF

Learn, review and memorize key terms from this section.

rasa

anurasa

madhura

svādu

amla

lavaṇa

kaṭu

tikta

kaṣhāya

saumya

agneya

gaṇa

varga

udaka

adho gati

ūrdhva gati

VĪRYA

The term *vīrya* literally means valor, strength, power or energy, and in the context of Āyurveda it is used to describe the final effect of a *dravya* on the body. It is the potency of the *dravya* to produce a primary effect.

Paribhāṣhā

Definition #1:
How it acts

वीर्यं यावदधीवासान्निपाताच्चोपलभ्यते ॥
च. सू. २६।६६

Vīryaṁ yāvadaddhīvāsānnipātāchchopalabyate ||
Cha. Sū. 26/66

Vīryaṁ (The potency of the *dravya*) upalabyate (is known) yāvadaddhīvā (as long as) sānnipātāch-cha (it is in contact [with the body]).

Vīrya is the potency that can be determined while the dravya is in contact with the body between the effects of *rasa* and *vipāka*.

Definition #2:
Cause for all effects

वीर्यं तु क्रियते तेन या क्रिया ।
नावीर्यं कुरुते किंचित् सर्वा वीर्यकृता क्रिया ॥

च. सू. २६।६५

Vīryaṁ tu kriyate tena yā kriyā |
Nāvīryaṁ kurute kiñchit sarvā vīryakṛtā kriyā ||

Cha. Sū. 26/65

Tena (Therefore), vīryaṁ tu (vīrya itself) kriyate (does, is responsible for doing) yā kriya (all actions, outcomes, results, especially therapeutic). Nāvīryaṁ kurute kiñchit (Nothing can be produced without vīrya); sarvā kriya (all actions) vīryakṛtā (are due to vīrya).

Vīrya is that which is responsible for producing all results and effects. No action happens without *vīrya* and all action is because of *vīrya*.

Bheda

The classics state that *vīrya* has two types of accepted classification systems. These two systems actually work together where one is a high-level classification and the other is a more detailed sub-classification. The two types of *vīrya* are the top-level and the eight types of *vīrya* include six which can be classified below the top two.

Classification #1:
Eight and two types

मृदुतीक्ष्णगुरुलघुस्निग्धरूक्षोष्णशीतलम् ।
वीर्यमष्टविधं केचित्,
केचिद्द्विविधमास्थिताः ॥
शीतोष्णमिति,

च. सू. २६।६४

Mṛdutīkṣhṇagurulaghusnigdharūkṣhoṣh ṇaśhītalam |
Vīryamaṣhṭavidhaṁ kecit, kechiddvividhamāsthitāḥ ||
Śhītoṣhṇamiti,

Cha. Sū. 26/64

See also Su. Sū. 40/5

Kechid (According to some), *āsthitāḥ* (there exist) *dvividham* (two types) – *śhīt-oṣhṇam-iti* (cold and hot). *Kecit* (According to others), *vīryam aṣhṭavidhaṁ* (there are eight types of *vīrya*) – *mṛdu* (soft), *tīkṣhṇa* (sharp), *guru* (heavy), *laghu* (light), *snigdha* (oily), *rūkṣha* (dry), *uṣhṇa* (hot and) *śhītalam* (cold).

Suśhruta explains how to recognize the effect of *vīrya* using the sense organs in Su. Sū. 41/11. *Bhāva Prakāśha* explains the *karma*, or general effects, of *vīrya* in BP Pū. 6/239-240.

TEST YOURSELF

Learn, review and memorize key terms from this section.

vīrya

____

VIPĀKA

Vipāka covers the final outputs of digestion. The word is composed of the prefix *vi-*, which expresses distinction, division, change or difference, and *pāka* which indicates cooking, ripening, digestion, assimilation, etc. *Vipāka* is the result of an individual's *agni* on what has been consumed. By understanding *vipāka* and the output, significant information can be inferred about the behavior of *agni* in clinical management.

Paribhāṣhā

Definition #1:
How it acts

विपाकः कर्मनिष्ठया ।

च. सू. २६।६५.५

Vipākaḥ karmaniṣhṭhayā |

Cha. Sū. 26/65.5

Vipākaḥ (*Vipāka* [is that which performs]) *karma niṣhṭhayā* (the complete action or final outcome).

Vipāka is responsible for the final outcome (of digestion). The final outcomes considered for assessing *vipāka* primarily include the *trimala*.

Definition #2:
Role in digestion

जाठरेणाग्निना योगाद्यदुदेति रसान्तरम् ।
रसानां परिणामान्ते स विपाक इति स्मृतः ॥

अ. हृ. सू. ९।२०

Jāṭhareṇāgninā yogādyadudeti rasāntaram |
Rasānāṁ pariṇāmānte sa vipāka iti smṛtaḥ ||

AH Sū. 9/20

Jāṭhareṇāgninā (*Jāṭhara-agni*, the main digestive power which resides in the *grahaṇī* [around the duodenum]) *yogādyad udeti* (coming in contact with and performing its function on) *rasāntaram* (the *rasa* inside [the digestive tract]) *rasānāṁ pariṇāmānte* (is the transformation after [being in contact with] the *rasana*, sense of taste on the tongue) *sa vipāka iti smṛtaḥ* (and so this is remembered as *vipāka*).

Vipāka is the transformation of the *dravya* after its contact with the tongue and conversion by *jāṭhara-agni* to become the taste inside the digestive tract (the post-digestive taste).

Bheda

The major classification method for *vipāka* is the three-type structure described by Vāgbhaṭa which corresponds to the concept of *avasthapāka*. The two-type classification method may be an older classification method, mentioned by Suśhruta.

Classification #1:
Three types (avastha pāka)

स्वादुः पटुश्च मधुरमम्लोऽम्लं पच्यते रसः ।
तिक्तोषणकषायाणां विपाकः प्रायशः कटुः ॥

अ. हृ. सू. ९।२१

Svāduḥ paṭuśhcha madhuramamlo ' mlaṁ pachyate rasaḥ |
Tiktoṣhaṇakaṣhāyāṇāṁ vipākaḥ prāyaśhaḥ kaṭuḥ ||

AH Sū. 9/21

Pachyate rasaḥ (When the *rasas* undergo digestion) *svāduḥ paṭuśhcha madhuram* (sweet and salt [become] sweet), *amlo ' mlaṁ* (sour [becomes] sour), *tikta uṣhaṇa kaṣhāyāṇāṁ* (bitter, pungent and astringent) *kaṭuḥ* ([become] pungent); *vipākaḥ prāyaśhaḥ* (these are the general rules of *vipāka*).

Vipaka is generally:

Rasa Flavor	*Vipāka* Post-digestive effect	Effect on *doṣhas* BP Pū. 6/241-244
Madhura, lavaṇa Sweet, salty	*Madhura* Sweet	Increases *kapha* Relieves *vāta* and *pitta*
Amla Sour	*Amla* Sour	Increases *pitta* Relieves *vāta* and *kapha*
Tikta, kaṭu, kaṣhāya Bitter, pungent, astringent	*Kaṭu* Pungent	Increases *vāta* Relieves *kapha* and *pitta*

Classification #2:
Two types

द्रव्येषु पच्यमानेषु येष्वम्बुपृथ्वीगुणाः ।
निर्वर्तन्तेऽधिकास्तत्र पाको मधुर उच्यते ॥ ११
तेजोऽनिलाकाशगुणाः पच्यमानेषु येषु तु ।
निर्वर्तन्तेऽधिकास्तत्र पाकः कटुक उच्यते ॥

सु. सू. ४०।१२

Dravyeṣhu pachyamāneṣhu yeṣhvambupṛthvīguṇāḥ |
Nirvartante ‘ dhikāstatra pāko madhura uchyate || 11
Tejo ‘ nilākāśhaguṇāḥ pachyamāneṣhu yeṣhu tu |
Nirvartante ‘ dhikāstatra pākaḥ kaṭuka uchyate ||

Su. Sū. 40/12

Dravyeṣhu pachyamāneṣhu (The *dravya* in the process of being digested) *yeṣhv-ambu-pṛthvī-guṇāḥ* (with the *guṇas* of *ambu* [water element] and *pṛthvī* [earth element]) *nirvartante ‘ dhikāstatra* (after completing the digestive processes) *pāko madhura uchyate* (is said to be *madhura pāka* [sweet post-digestive effect]). *Tejo ‘ nil- ākāśha- guṇāḥ pachyamāneṣhu* (*Tejas*, *anila*, and *ākāśha guṇas* present during the process of being digested) *pākaḥ kaṭuka uchyate* (are said to undergo *kaṭu pāka*.

In the two types of *vipāka* classification, *madhura* and *kaṭu* are the primary *vipāka*. When the *dravya* contains a predominance of *ap* and/or *pṛthvi*, the *vipāka* is *madhura*. Or, when the *dravya* contains a predominance of *tejas*, *anila* and/or *ākāśha*, the *vipāka* is *kaṭu*.

TEST YOURSELF

Learn, review and memorize key terms from this section.

vipāka

---

avastha pāka

GENERAL MECHANICS OF *DRAVYA, RASA, VĪRYA* AND *VIPĀKA*

Based on all the information on *dravya* and its components, certain behaviors can be anticipated for a *dravya* having a predominant *rasa*. The following chart summarizes these predictable concepts.

Rasa	*Guṇa*	*Karma*	*Vīrya*	*Vipāka*	*Doṣhas*
Madhura Sweet	*Guru, snigdha, śhīta*	*Adho gati* (strong)	*Śhīta*	*Madhura*	K ↑↑↑ VP ↓↓↓
Amla Sour	*Snigdha, uṣhṇa, laghu*	*Adho gati* (moderate)	*Uṣhṇa*	*Amla*	PK ↑↑ V ↓↓
Lavaṇa Salty	*Uṣhṇa, snigdha, guru (laghu)*	*Ūrdhva gati* (moderate)	*Uṣhṇa*	*Madhura*	PK ↑ V ↓
Kaṭu Pungent	*Rūkṣha, laghu, uṣhṇa*	*Ūrdhva gati* (strong)	*Uṣhṇa*	*Kaṭu*	VP ↑↑↑ K ↓↓↓
Tikta Bitter	*Laghu, rūkṣha, śhīta*	*Ūrdhva gati* (mild)	*Śhīta*	*Kaṭu*	V ↑↑ PK ↓↓
Kaṣhāya Astringent	*Rūkṣha, guru, śhīta*	*Adho gati* (mild)	*Śhīta*	*Kaṭu*	V ↑ PK ↓

Rasa, *vīrya* and *vipāka* all have an effect on the final outcome of the *dravya*. Whichever is more powerful, potent or strong will exert the most effect in the end. If all three are of equal strength, *rasa* will be overcome by *vipāka*, and *vipāka* will be overcome by *vīrya* (see Cha. Sū. 26/72, AH Sū. 9/25 and BP Pū. 6/249).

PRABHĀVA

The effect which wins over all of the other factors in a draya is *prabhāva*. It occurs when *dravya* do not behave as expected according to the standard profiles. This is a special effect that is exerted. It explains contradictory *dravya* that are capable of exerting unanticipated effects even though they have the same profile as similar *dravya*. Specific examples of these exceptions are mentioned in Cha. Sū. 26/48-52 and 26/68-71, AH Sū. 10/33-35 and BP Pū. 6/195-200.

Paribhāṣhā

Definition #1:

How it works

रसवीर्यविपाकानां सामान्यं यत्र लक्ष्यते ।
विशेषः कर्मणा चैव प्रभावस्तस्य स स्मृतः ॥

च. सू. २६।६७

Rasavīryavipākānāṁ sāmānyaṁ yatra lakṣhyate |
Viśheṣhaḥ karmaṇā chaiva prabhāvastasya sa smṛtaḥ ||

Cha. Sū. 26/67

Rasa, *vīrya*, *vipākānāṁ* (*Rasa*, *vīrya*, *vipāka*) *sāmānyaṁ yatra lakṣhyate* (known to be the same in specific ways) *viśheṣhaḥ karmaṇā chaiva* (and still create a different action or result) – *prabhāvastasya sa smṛtaḥ* (this is to be known as due to *prabhāva*).

The concept of *prabhāva* is consistent among classical authors (see AH Sū. 9/26 and BP Pū. 6/245-246). Vāgbhaṭa additionally describes a concept called *vicitra pratyayārabdha dravya* in AH Sū. 9/27-28 which is similar to *prabhāva* and explains special effects of *dravyas* based on their *pañchabhautika* composition along with examples.

TEST YOURSELF

Learn, review and memorize key terms from this section.

prabhāva ____________________

Chapter 3: Review

ADDITIONAL READING

Read and review the references listed below to expand your understanding of the concepts in this chapter. Write down the date that you complete your reading for each. Remember that consistent repetition is the best way to learn. Plan to read each reference at least once now and expect to read it again as you continue your studies.

References marked with (skim) can be read quickly and do not require commentary review.

CLASSICS		1st read	2nd read
Charaka	Cha. Sū. 1/49-67 Cha. Sū. 25/36 Cha. Sū. 26/ Cha. Sū. 27/200 Cha. Vi. 1/6-8 Cha. Vi. 6/139-144 Cha. Vi. 8/138 Cha. Śhā. 1/27-28 Cha. Śhā. 1/72 Cha. Śhā. 6/10		
Suśhruta	Su. Sū. 40-42 Su. Sū. 45/11 Su. Sū. 46/511-530		
Aṣhṭāṅga Hṛdaya	AH Sū. 1/15-18 AH Sū. 9-10/		
Bhāva Prakāśha	BP Pū. 6/169-end		

JOURNALS & CURRENT RESOURCES

Insight of sandra and drava guna, Jyoti Devangamath

QUESTIONS & ANSWERS

Record your questions for this chapter here for further research and discussion.

Question:

Answer:

Question:

Answer:

Question:

Answer:

SELF-ASSESSMENT

1. Which component does not have a *samavāyi* relationship with *dravya*?
   a. *guṇa*
   b. *kāla*
   c. *prabhāva*
   d. *rasa*
   e. *vīrya*

2. *Pārthiva dravya* consists of which *pañcha mahābhūta(s)*?
   a. *ap*
   b. *pṛthvi*
   c. *tejas*
   d. *vāyu*
   e. All of the above

3. *Tejas* is primarily composed of _____ *guṇa* and _____ *karma*
   a. *Laghu guṇa* and *lāghava karma*
   b. *Manda guṇa* and *bandha karma*
   c. *Mṛdu guṇa* and *mārdava karma*
   d. *Śhīta guṇa* and *glāni karma*
   e. *Tīkṣhṇa guṇa* and *prakāśha* karma

4. The *sāmānya guṇas* include which two subcategories?
   a. *Ātma* and *pratnāntā guṇas*
   b. *Gurvādi* and *parādi guṇas*
   c. *Sārtha* and *viśheṣha guṇas*
   d. *Śhlakṣhṇa* and *viśhada guṇas*
   e. None of the above

5. *Vyavāyi* is
   a. Not considered a *guṇa* by Chakrapāṇi
   b. One of the *parādi guṇas*
   c. One of the 20 *gurvādi guṇas*
   d. That which moves slowly and causes stagnation
   e. The opposite of *śhīta*

6. Of the *parādi guṇas,* which is also a *pramāṇa?*
   a. *Abhyāsa*
   b. *Parimāṇa*
   c. *Saṁyoga*
   d. *Saṅkhya*
   e. *Yukti*

7. *Madhura rasa* is composed of what *pañcha mahābhūtas*?
   a. *Ap* and *tejas*
   b. *Pṛthvi* and *ap*
   c. *Tejas* and *vāyu*
   d. *Vāyu* and *pṛthvi*
   e. None of the above

8. Which *rasa* decreases *pitta doṣha* most?
   a. *Amla*
   b. *Kaṭu*
   c. *Kaṣhāya*
   d. *Madhura*
   e. *Tikta*

9. *Prabhāva*
   a. Comes after digestion.
   b. Does not behave as expected according to standard profiles.
   c. Follows standard rules according to *rasa, vīrya, vipāka.*
   d. Is always the most important factor in any dravya.
   e. Is experienced with the eyes.

10. A meal predominant in *kaṭu rasa* would most likely cause an increase of
    a. *Kapha*
    b. *Kaṣhāya*
    c. *Rūkṣha*
    d. *Śhīta*
    e. *Vāta*

CRITICAL THINKING

1. Consider the relationship between *dravya*, *guṇa* and *karma*. Using the correct *siddhānta* terminology, demonstrate the application of *anumāna pramana* in a simple practical example.

2. Which types of *guṇas* are used to describe the *pañcha mahābhūtas*?

3. Looking at the *guṇas* of the *pañcha mahābhūtas*, which are common or opposite among the *bhūtas*? Should these *guṇas* be considered more important? Why?

4. What is special about the *Vaiśheṣhikā guṇas*?

5. Using any concept from this chapter where more than one classification method is listed, can you demonstrate how multiple classifications can all be used together to correctly describe the concept?

6. Take any *dravya* with a predominant single *rasa* and test all of its listed components. Use the scientific method, record your findings and explain them using the information in this chapter.

7. List the components that have a *samavāyi* relationship with *dravya* in order by their power to affect the body. Explain why this relationship is important, what is actually inducing the final effect, and the term used to describe the effect when it does not happen in this standard order.

8. Draw a picture that shows the process of rasa manifestation. Label each step in the process in your picture.

9. Explain the *siddhāntas* responsible for the relationship between the *rasas*, *doṣhas* and *guṇas*.

Chapter 4 : Tridoṣha siddhānta

KEY TERMS

ādāna	dehī	prāṇa	śhleṣhmalā
āgneya	dhātu	puruṣha	soma
agni	doṣha	rañjaka	tarpaka
ālocaka	kapha	sādhaka	udāṇa
apāna	karma puruṣha	samāna	vāta
avalambaka	kāya	saṁsarga	vātalā
avikṛta	kledaka	sannipāta	vāyu
bhrājaka	mala	śharīra	vikṛta
bodhaka	pāchaka	śhārīra	vikṣhepa
chetanā	pañcha mahābhūtas	saumya	visarga
chikitsā puruṣha	pitta	śhleṣhaka	vyāna
deha	pittalā	śhleṣhma	

The *tridoṣha siddhānta* is a core principle unique to Āyurveda. It originated in a rudimentary way in the older Vedic texts, and was then thoroughly developed in the Āyurvedic classics.

The *tridoṣha*, *vāta, pitta* and *kapha*, are the three primary controllers of the human body. In their correct, normal states they maintain health, happiness and life. In improper or abnormal states, the same *doṣhas* are the causes for disease, unhappiness, and eventually death (Ca Vi. 1/5).

The *tridoṣhas* operate within the scope of the human body which is called *karma puruṣha* for the purposes of applying Āyurveda. In order to understand how they work, a review of the human body is required. Classical Āyurveda has always considered the human body to be a single, functioning holistic system which is more than the sum of its parts. Traditionally, this included both anatomy and physiology simultaneously because both are required for the body to function.

The concepts of *deha*, *śharīra, kāya* and *puruṣha* cover this well from an introductory perspective. While all of these terms can be loosely translated as the "human body," they each carry their own distinct meaning and provide deeper insight into the application of the *tridoṣha siddhānta*.

DEHA

The term *deha* refers to the human body as an entity capable of growing. The term is defined as:

Deha दिह् गात्र

Dih gātra

Gātra (The body) *dih* (increases).

Deha is the body which increases, or grows.

Deha is used classically to indicate the body which is capable of growing. This indicates a healthy body which is operating according to standard functions because the natural state of the body is to keep growing to outpace decay. This is similar to the concept of anabolism.

BP Pū. 2/32 states that the person who is focused on sin or good deeds, discomfort or contentment, and attached and bound to the actions of the mind and their outcomes, is called *dehī*. The *dehī* can be considered as one who's attention is focused towards feeding, supplementing or providing for their physical existence. Any normal, healthy individual should have this type of desire in an appropriate form to maintain their own life and being.

TEST YOURSELF

Learn, review and memorize key terms from this section.

deha

____

dehī

____

ŚHARĪRA

The terms *śharīra* and *śhārīra* should be distinguished first. *Śharīra* (with a short first a) refers to the physical body itself, while *śhārīra* (with a long first a) refers to the study of the human body, especially in preparation for clinical practice.

Here, when referring to the body as the object of practice, the term *śharīra* is used. This term carries the implication that *śharīra* is constantly decaying, or dying. This refers to the ongoing processes of the body breaking down on all levels.

Chakrapāṇi provides the definition of *śharīra* in Cha. Sū. 1/6-14. The fact that he placed this commentary at the very beginning of the text is significant. He further states that the object of Āyurveda is the human body because of its nature to decay.

Śharīra शीर्यते इति शरीरम्

Śhīryate iti śharīram

Iti (And so) *śharīram* (the body) *śhīryate* (decays).

And so, *śharīra* constantly decays.

Specific causes for the growth of *śharīra* are mentioned by Charaka in Cha. Śhā. 6/12.

TEST YOURSELF

Learn, review and memorize key terms from this section.

śharīra

____

śhārīra

____

KĀYA

The term kāya is especially valuable in the context of applied Āyurveda because it includes the potential intelligence of the human body to maintain health. The term is defined as:

Kāya चीयते अन्नादिभिः

Chīyate annādibhiḥ

Annādibiḥ (Food, etc) *chīyate* (increases [the body] through proper selection).

Kāya is that which selects the proper food (and nourishment) for growth.

The term '*chīyate*' means:

Chīyate चित् चयन

Chit chayana

Chit (Increase) *chayana* (by selection).

Chit means to increase, collect or grow. *Chayana* means making a selection.

Kāya is the physical body which grows by choosing the right food for the individual. Considering this definition within the context of the classics, it is clear that making the right food choices is one of the key, fundamental means to good health and happiness.

TEST YOURSELF

Learn, review and memorize key terms from this section.

kāya

PURUṢHA

Recall that the term *puruṣha* can broadly refer to a human being, man, or mankind, in a general sense. It is a concept and term which can be found in many branches of Vedic sciences, and within each subject it can convey a meaning appropriate to the context.

Within applied Āyurveda, *puruṣha* has been defined and accepted as the association of the *pañcha mahābhūtas* with *chetanā*, simultaneously. When these six factors are combined, life is present in the human body and this combination of the body activated with life becomes the purpose and scope of applied Āyurveda.

Many additional classifications and explanations exist for *puruṣha*. Even though they are recognized as valid, they are not applicable within the scope of Āyurveda. Chakrapāṇi makes this point clear along with the definition of *puruṣha*, in Cha. Śhā. 1/16. His commentary is extremely relevant to establish the boundaries of the science and practice of Āyurveda.

The following definitions of *puruṣha* clarify the scope, meaning and application of the term.

Charaka's perspective

खादयश्चेतनाषष्ठा धातवः पुरुषः स्मृतः ।
चेतनाधातुरप्येकः स्मृतः पुरुषसंज्ञकः ॥

च. शा. १।१६

Khādayaśhchetanāṣhaṣhṭhā dhātavaḥ puruṣhaḥ smṛtaḥ |
Chetanādhāturapyekaḥ smṛtaḥ puruṣhasaṁjñakaḥ ||

Cha. Śhā. 1/16

Puruṣhaḥ (A human being, or mankind) *smṛtaḥ* (is known as) *kha-ādayaśh* (the five gross elements and) *chetanā* (consciousness) *ṣhaṣhṭhā dhātavaḥ* (as the sixth supportive component). *Chetanā* (Consciousness) *dhāturapyekaḥ* (as the single supportive component) *smṛtaḥ* (should also be remembered) *puruṣhasaṁjñakaḥ* (and known as a human being, or mankind).

Puruṣha is known as *kha*, etc (the *pañcha mahābhūtas*) along with a sixth *dhātu*, *chetanā*. Also, *puruṣha* should be remembered as the single *dhātu, chetanā*.

Chakrapāṇi's comments on this line are key to understanding this concept throughout the classics. He states that although the concept of *puruṣha* as a single *dhātu* (ie, *chetanā*) is valid in other branches of Vedic sciences, their implications do not apply within the context of Āyurveda. For example, some sciences consider *puruṣha* to be the "one who sleeps in the body" implying that *puruṣha* has the ability to detach from the body. This perspective is not accepted by Chakrapāṇi in the scope of Āyurveda. He clearly states that the *puruṣha* who is the purpose of application of the science is not the one who is detached from the body.

When this perspective is applied to the remaining statements about *puruṣha* and its classification methods, it becomes clear that the additional methods have been included for posterity. Chakrapāṇi's view can also be applied to other authors of classical Āyurvedic literature.

Later, in Cha. Śhā. 6/3, Charaka restates the definition of *śharīra* and it is equal to *puruṣha*. He says that *śharīra* is named so because it acts as the location (home, abode) of *chetanā* and the *pañcha mahābhūtas*. The *śharīra*, and all of its constituents, are that which is susceptible to disease.

Suśhruta's perspective

अस्मिञ्छास्त्रे पञ्चमहाभूतशरीरिसमवायः पुरुष इत्युच्यते । तस्मिन् क्रिया, सोऽधिष्ठानं;

सु. सू. १।२२

Asmichchhāstre pañchamahābhūtaśharīrisamavāyaḥ puruṣha ityuchyate | Tasmin kriyā, so ‘ dhiṣhṭhānaṁ;

Su. Sū. 1/22

Asmichchhāstre (Within the scope of this field), pañcha mahābhūta (the five gross elements) śharīrisam avāyaḥ (and their perpetual attachment to the physical body) puruṣha ityuchyate (are explained as a human being, or mankind). Tasmin kriyā (For all therapeutic purposes), so ‘ dhiṣhṭhānaṁ (this is the location of activity).

Within this *śhastra*, the *pañcha mahābhūtas* and their perpetual attachment to śh*arīra (chetanā)* are explained as *puruṣha*. This is the location (house, abode) for which all actions (treatment) are applied.

Suśhruta clearly establishes the same definition and scope for the term *puruṣha* and does so significantly from the first chapter of his treatise. The placement of this line is imperative for setting the scope and boundary of the study and application of the science.

Paryāya

Suśhruta additionally mentions two very significant synonyms for *puruṣha* that are relevant for practical application. He describes the phrases *karma puruṣha* and *chikitsā puruṣha* as more specific for usage within the scope of Āyurveda.

पञ्चमहाभूतशरीरिसमवायः पुरुष इति; स एष कर्मपुरुषः चिकित्साधिकृतः ।

सु. शा. १।१६

Pañchamahābhūtaśharīrisamavāyaḥ puruṣha itiḥ, sa eva karmapuruṣhaḥ chikitsādhikṛtaḥ |

Su. Śhā. 1/16

Pañcha mahābhūta (The five gross elements) śharīrisam avāyaḥ (perpetually attached to the physical body) puruṣha itiḥ (are considered a human being), sa eva (and so these are also considered as) karma puruṣhaḥ chikitsā-adhikṛtaḥ (the human being amenable to therapeutic treatment).

And because *puruṣha* is considered the combination of the *pañcha mahābhūtas* and their perpetual attachment to *śharīra (chetanā)*, *puruṣha* can be called *karma puruṣha*, and *chikitsā puruṣha* as it is the reason for therapeutic action.

TEST YOURSELF

Learn, review and memorize key terms from this section.

puruṣha

dhātu

pañcha mahābhūtas

chetanā	
śharīra	
karma puruṣha	
chikitsā puruṣha	

TRIDOṢHA

The *tridoṣha siddhānta* is applied within the scope of *puruṣha*. It encompasses the three *doṣhas*, *vāta, pitta* and *kapha* and all of their behaviors and activities which ultimately determine health or disease. The *tridoṣha siddhānta* is well-developed in Āyurveda, and much more elaborate than its rudimentary concepts in older, classical Vedic literature.

Origin of tridoṣha siddhānta

The *tridoṣha siddhānta* originated from three key concepts that form the foundation of the natural environment - the sun, moon and air. These external concepts were likened to behaviors and functions seen in the human body and organized into the concepts of the three *doṣhas*. The sun is likened to *pitta*, the moon to *kapha* and air to *vāta*. These similarities provide a major basis for understanding physiological concepts which were otherwise difficult to observe directly.

Cha. Sū. 12/ contains perhaps the most beautiful example of this development of the science. In this chapter, a discussion among scholars of the time demonstrates that the external concepts of *agni*, *soma* and *vāyu*, or the sun, the moon and air, were well-developed at that time, and were utilized to draw comparisons between the external environment and the functioning of the human body. By invoking the *loka-puruṣha sāmya siddhānta*, it is clear that early developers of Āyurveda were able to bridge this knowledge to provide the foundation for Āyurveda and a solid base for methodical, scientific development.

Suśhruta adds to this by stating in Su. Sū. 21/8 that the sun, moon and air provide support to the world just as *pitta, kapha* and *vāta* do through the functions of *visarga, ādāna* and *vikṣhepa*. *Visarga* and *ādāna* are the two halves of the year which behave like waxing and waning periods of the moon, and impart a building or depleting effect on all life. *Visarga*, the building effect, corresponds to *kapha*, while *ādāna*, the depleting effect, corresponds to *pitta*. *Vikṣhepa* refers to movement, which corresponds to *vāta*.

Finally, in Su. Sū. 42/5, *Suṣhruta* explains how *vāta, pitta* and *kapha* are generated from the perspective of the environment. He states that:

Vāta	Vāyorātmaivātmā
Pitta	Pittamagneyaṁ
Śhleṣhmā	Śhleṣhmā saumya

Vāta is *ātma-eva-ātma*, or that which originates from itself. *Pitta* comes from the *āgneya* principle, the same which governs the sun. And *kapha* comes from the *saumya* principle, the same which governs the moon. This connection reinforces the fact that the three *doṣhas*, which operate inside the human body, take their fundamental character, qualities and actions from these principles, while being distinct or separate from them.

Nirukti

The term *doṣha* derives from the Sanskrit *dhātu* √ *duṣh*. The Monier Williams dictionary defines *duṣh* as:

duṣh	to become bad or corrupted, to be defiled or impure, to be

ruined, perish; to sin, commit a fault, be wrong; to spoil or corrupt

The term *doṣha* is most commonly defined within the context of Āyurveda as:

doṣha	दूष्यन्ति इति दोषाः
	Dūṣhyanti iti doṣhāḥ

Iti (And so), *doṣhāḥ* (the *doṣhas*) *dūṣhyanti* (are the ones that do "*dūṣhana*" or become bad, corrupted, vitiated).

Doṣhas are the ones with the potential to vitiate, pollute, or make impure.

It must be noted that while the term *doṣha* specifically means to pollute, the classics are clear about that being only one aspect to them. Vitiation is their main function when they are in their abnormal, or unhealthy state.

Suśhruta explains the specific etymology of the terms *vāta, pitta* and *kapha* in Su. Sū. 21/5 as:

Vāta	'Vā' gati-gandhanayoḥ
Pitta	'Tapa' santāpe
Śhleṣhma	'Śhliṣh' āliṅgane

The term *vāta* derives from '*vā*' which means *gati* or *gandha*, movement or smell. *Vāta* can be known to be present using either of these. *Pitta* derives from '*tapa*' which means *santāpe*, to heat. *Kapha* derives from '*Śhliṣh*' which means to embrace, envelope, wrap around or cover. The prefixes or suffixes added to the ends of these roots create the final form of each word.

Each of the *doṣhas* should be known to be present through their effects indicated by this etymology. Although they may appear to be brief explanations, they have very broad and deep applications, and are implicit in every physiological and pathological process.

Paribhāṣhā

Throughout the classics, definitions for the *tridoṣhas* can be found in nearly every treatise. Because of the fundamental nature of this core principle, some authors choose to abbreviate the most basic explanations as they were considered to be known. Here, references are compiled from various authors to provide a comprehensive explanation for students of all levels.

First, it must be clear that the term '*doṣha*' can be used in several contexts, including those which may seem opposing. In BP Pū. 3/100-101, a key statement provides the basis for understanding how the *tridoṣha* and other essential terms can be used interchangeably. He clarifies that *vāta, pitta* and *kapha* can be called *doṣhas*, *dhātus* or *malas*, based on their behavior:

<u>Vāta, pitta and kapha</u>

As doṣhas	*Dhātu and mala dūṣhyanti*
	They harm or contaminate the *dhātus* and *malas*
As dhātus	*Deha dhāraṇāt*
	They support the body in functions of growth and anabolism
As malas	*Raktādīnāṁ malinīkaraṇānyatā*
	They pollute the body in the form of the waste products of rakta, etc (the seven *dhātus*)

With so many definitions available in the classics, it can seem challenging to get an exact, specific answer about what the *doṣhas* are. One of the most succinct definitions is provided in BP Pū. 3/98:

वायुः पित्तं कफश्चेति त्रयो दोषाः समासतः ।
विकृताविकृता देहं घ्नन्ति ते वर्द्धयन्ति च ॥

भा. प्र. पू. ३।९८

Vāyuḥ pittaṁ kaphaśhcheti trayo doṣhāḥ samāsataḥ | Vikṛtāvikṛtā dehaṁ ghnanti te varddhayanti cha ||

BP Pū. 3/98

Vāyuḥ pittaṁ kaphaśhcheti (*Vāta, pitta* and *kapha*) trayo doṣhāḥ (are the three *doṣhas*) samāsataḥ (in short). Vikṛta-āvikṛtā (In their abnormal or normal states) ghnanti (they destroy) te varddhayanti cha (or improve) dehaṁ (the body).

To sum up, *vāta, pitta* and *kapha* are the three *doṣhas*. When in their *vikṛta* state (abnormal, unhealthy), they destroy the body, and in their *avikṛtā* state (normal, healthy) they strengthen, increase and grow the body.

Also see Cha. Sū. 1/57, AH Sū. 1/6, Cha. Śhā. 4/34 for examples of basic definitions from other authors.

More elaborate definitions go on to explain what the *doṣhas* are capable of and what they actually do in the context of the transformation processes that are constantly happening in the body. In Cha. Śhā. 6/18, the characteristic nature of the *doṣhas* is provided.

तेषां सर्वेषामेव वातपित्तश्लेष्माणो दुष्टा दूषयितारो भवन्ति, दोष स्वभावात् ।

च. शा. ६।१८

Teṣhāṁ sarveṣhāmeva vātapittasleṣhmāṇo duṣhṭā dūṣhayitāro bhavanti, doṣha svabhāvāt |

Cha. Śhā. 6/18

Teṣhāṁ sarveṣhāmeva (And out of all of their particular capabilities), vātapittasleṣhmāṇo (*vāta, pitta* and *kapha*) duṣhṭā dūṣhayitāro bhavanti (are the corruptors that cause pollution, vitiation when abnormal); doṣha svabhāvāt (the doṣhas have such nature).

And out of all of their specific functions, *vāta, pitta* and *śhleṣhma* are the ones which are responsible for vitiating, corrupting, and destroying when they themselves are in a state of being vitiated, impure, not right, or abnormal. That is *doṣha svabhāva* (the nature of the *doṣhas*).

Out of all the impurities or pollutants generated inside the body, *vāta, pitta* and *kapha* are the ones responsible for creating these vitiated products when they are unhealthy. By nature, they themselves are the *doṣhas*.

In AH Sū. 11/1 and Su. Sū. 15/3, two more definitions are provided which further emphasize the *doṣhas*' role in supporting the body in its normal healthy state.

दोषधातुमला मूलं सदा देहस्य ।

अ. हृ. ११।१

Doṣhadhātumalā mūlaṁ sadā dehasya |

AH Sū. 11/1

Doṣha (The *doṣhas*), dhātu (*dhātus*) malā (and *malas*) mūlaṁ ([are] the root) sadā (always) dehasya (of the body).

Doṣha, dhātu and *mala* are always (for the duration of life) the roots (of support, health, existence) of *deha*, the body (healthy growth, anabolism).

दोषधातुमलमूलं हि शरीरं,

सु. सू. १५।३

Doṣhadhātumalamūlaṁ hi śharīraṁ

Su. Sū. 15/3

Doṣha (The *doṣhas*), dhātu (*dhātus*) malā (and *malas*) mūlaṁ ([are] the root) hi (for) śharīraṁ (the body),

Doṣha, dhātu and *mala* are the roots (of support, health, existence) for *śharīra*, the body which is naturally prone to deteriorate, decay and undergo catabolism.

One important additional point should be mentioned under the *tridoṣha*. Suśhruta includes references that support the *tridoṣha siddhānta* while also recognizing the existence of a fourth *doṣha, rakta*, in Su. Sū. 21/3. This is done specifically because of the nature of diseases that Suśhruta typically encountered and managed with surgery. It was clear that in this specialty, *rakta* was a major factor in the progression and spread of disease. Although he makes an important point within the practice of Śhalya-tantra, *rakta* cannot be accepted as a fourth *doṣha* in the overall practice of Āyurveda. In Cha. Sū. 24/9, 24/18, 24/22, *rakta* is recognized as a secondary vitiating cause, but not a formal *doṣha*, as it does not have a role to play in the formation of *prakṛti*.

Paryāya and technical terms

Throughout the classics, several synonyms are regularly used for *vāta, pitta* and *kapha*. These include:

Vāta	*māruta* *vāyu* (Cha. Sū. 12/8) *anila*
Pitta	*agni* (Cha. Sū. 12/11) *uṣhma* (Cha. Śhā. 6/15) *anala* (AH Sū. 12/10-11)
Kapha	*śhleṣhma* *soma* (Cha. Sū. 12/12) *bala*

Additionally, Charaka explains in Cha. Vi. 6/13 that use of the terms *vāta, pitta* and *kapha* may refer to *doṣhas* in their *prākṛta* state or in their *vaikṛta* state acting as *dūṣhyas*. In a state of *prakṛti*, Charaka prefers that predominance of a *doṣha* be referred to using the specific terms of *vātalā*, *pittalā* and *śhleṣhmalā*. For example, an individual with a predominance of *vāta* can be identified as *vātalā prakṛti*.

Suśhruta and other authors do not make a distinction here, and instead refer to each *prakṛti* using its predominant *doṣha(s)*, such as *vātika*, *paittika* or *kaphaja prakṛti*. This indicates that the *prakṛti* is born from the *doṣha(s)* in its name.

When *doṣhas* combine, as they most often do, in various states of disequilibrium, they produce ill-health and disease. These combinations are referred to as *saṁsarga* and *sannipāta* (Cha. Vi. 6/10).

Saṁsarga occurs when two *doṣhas* join forces. This may occur in a normal state of *prakṛti* or in a state of *vikṛti*, a deviation from *prakṛti*. *Sannipāta* occurs when all three *doṣhas* combine in a state of *prakṛti* or *vikṛti*. This can occur due to multiple factors and most often includes combinations in similar *guṇas* and *adhiṣhṭhana* (locations). See Cha. Vi. 6/10 and AH Sū. 1/11.5 for a concise explanation.

Tridoṣha bheda

Each of the three *doṣhas* is also classified into five subtypes. This categorization helps provide a clearer structure for the specific functions and responsibilities of the doṣhas on a more granular level. The details of these functions will be covered in Chapter seven.

The high-level overview of *tridoṣha bheda* (also called *doṣha bheda*) is provided here as an introduction:

Doṣha	*Bheda*	Nearest English equivalent
Vāta	*Prāṇa*	Responsible for continuity of life; brings in what is needed to survive
	Udāṇa	Upward and outward movement of *vāyu*
	Vyāna	Circulation
	Samāna	Aids in digestion and absorption
	Apāna	Downward movement of *vāyu*; all forms of excretion, expulsion
Pitta	*Pāchaka*	Responsible for digestion; "cooks" what is consumed
	Rañjaka	Colors *rakta*
	Sādhaka	Intelligence, consciousness
	Ālocaka	Vision
	Bhrājaka	Complexion
Kapha	*Avalambaka*	Support of the upper body
	Kledaka	Supports digestion by moistening incoming food
	Bodhaka	Perceives taste
	Tarpaka	Nourishes *indriya*
	Śhleṣhaka	Lubricates joints

Tridoṣha and pañcha mahābhūtas

Like every *dravya*, the three *doṣhas* are composed of all five *mahābhūtas* with a predominance of one or two *mahābhūtas*. This predominance is what gives the *doṣha* its main characteristics, qualities and actions. Compare this chart to the *pañchabhautika* compositions of *rasas* for a better understanding of how all three concepts work together.

Doṣha gati is also based on *pañchabhautika* composition. *Vāta* has a strong tendency towards *ūrdhva gati*. *Pitta* is primarily directed upwards as well, but can be influenced by its secondary predominance of *ap mahābhūta* to go downwards when that *mahābhūta* becomes more pronounced. *Kapha* has a strong tendency towards *adho gati*. Movement of *doṣhas* in a sideways manner is termed *tiryak gati* (Cha. Sū. 17/112-114, AH Sū. 13/21-22).

Mahābhūta	*Vāta*	*Pitta*	*Kapha*
Pṛthvi	Minor	Minor	Predominant
Ap	Minor	Secondary	Predominant
Tejas	Minor	Predominant	Minor
Vāyu	Predominant	Minor	Minor
Ākāśha	Predominant	Minor	Minor

Tridoṣha and guṇas

Each *doṣha* is responsible for specific *guṇa* and *karma*. In classical literature, the *guṇas* are generally described along with the introduction to the *tridoṣha siddhānta*. The same approach is followed here. Each *doṣhas' guṇas* are listed in this chapter while the details of their *karma* and additional specifics are covered in Chapter seven.

Each chart below compiles multiple references from classical authors and allows for simplified comparisons. Notice that certain *guṇas* have been mentioned by all authors, while others were not as commonly seen. Consider this in the scope of clinical assessment and application.

Vāta Guṇa Characteristics of *vāta*	Cha. Sū. 1/59, 12/4, 20/12	Su. Sū. 42/8	AH Sū. 1/11	BP Pū. 3/102
Rūkṣha Dry	✓	✓	✓	✓
Śhīta Cold	✓	✓	✓	✓
Laghu Light	✓	✓	✓	✓
Sūkṣhma Minute	✓		✓	✓
Chala Moving	✓		✓	✓
Viśhada Clear	✓	✓		
Khara Rough	✓		✓	✓

Dāruṇa Hard	✓			
Viṣhṭambha Stopped		✓		
Śhīghra Fast				✓
Rajo-guṇa Initiation behavior				✓
Mṛdu Soft				✓
Yogavahi Amplification				✓
Vibhāga Separation				✓
Pradhāna doṣha Primary *doṣha*				✓

Pitta Guṇa Characteristics of *pitta*	Cha. Sū. 1/60, 20/15	Su. Sū. 21/11, 42/8	AH Sū. 1/11	BP Pū. 3/120
Sasneha Slighty oily	✓		✓	✓
Uṣhṇa Hot	✓	✓	✓	✓
Tīkṣhṇa Sharp	✓	✓	✓	✓
Drava Liquid	✓	✓	✓	✓
Amla Sour	✓	*vaikṛta*		after *(vi)pāka*
Sara Flowing	✓		✓	✓
Kaṭu Pungent	✓	✓		✓

Laghu Light		√ (42/8)	√	√
Pūti, visra Bad-smelling		√	√	
Nīla Blue		√		√
Pīta Yellow		√		√
Rūkṣha Dry		√ (42/8)		
Viśhada Clear		√ (42/8)		
Sattva-guṇa Determination behavior				√

Kapha Guṇa Characteristics of *kapha*	Cha. Sū. 1/61, 20/18	Su. Sū. 21/15, 42/8	AH Sū. 1/12	BP Pū. 3/126
Guru Heavy	√	√	√	√
Śhīta Cold	√	√	√	√
Mṛdu Soft	√			
Snigdha Oily	√	√	√	√
Madhura Sweet	√	√		√
Sthira Stable	√		√	
Pichchhila, mṛtsna Cloudy, dusty	√	√	√	√
Manda Slow			√	
Śhlakṣhṇa Smooth			√	

Śhveta White		✓		✓
Lavaṇa Salty		*vaikṛta*		*vidagdha*
Tamo-guṇa Inertia behavior				✓

Tridoṣha and special features

Part of the basic introduction to the *tridoṣhas* in the classics includes their general location in the body and the various time periods when each *doṣha* becomes more active, or pronounced. Vāgbhaṭa explains this as:

वयोहोरात्रिभुक्तानां तेऽन्तमध्याधिगाः क्रमात् ।

अ. हृ. सू. १।७.५

Vayohorātribhuktānāṁ te ' ntamadhyādhigāḥ kramāt |

AH. Sū. 1/7.5

Vaya ([In each stage of] lifespan), ahorātri (day and night) bhuktānāṁ (stages of digestion after eating a meal), te (they [the doṣhas]) kramāt (undergo a cycle [of chaya, prakopa and praśhamā]) anta (in the end), madhya (in the middle) ādhigāḥ (and at the beginning of each).

Similar references can be found in Su. Sū. 21/20, 22, 24; Su. Ni. 1/6-9, AH Sū. 1/7; BP Pū. 3/99. The following chart summarizes these basic points.

Predominance in:	*Vāta*	*Pitta*	*Kapha*
Samśhraya Main abode the body	below the *nābhi* (umbilicus)	between *hṛdaya* and *nābhi* (heart and umbilicus)	above *hṛdaya* (heart)
Vaya Age	End	Middle	Beginning
Ahorātra Day			
Rātri Night			
Bhuktānām After eating a meal			

TEST YOURSELF

Learn, review and memorize key terms from this section.

agni

soma

vāyu

visarga

ādāna

vikṣhepa

āgneya

saumya

doṣha

vāta

pitta

kapha

śhleṣhma

vātalā

pittalā

śhleṣhmalā

dhātu

mala

vikṛta

avikṛta

saṁsarga

sannipāta

prāṇa

udāṇa

vyāna

samāna

apāna

pāchaka

rañjaka

sādhaka

ālocaka

bhrājaka

avalambaka

kledaka

bodhaka

tarpaka

śhleṣhaka

Chapter 4: Review

ADDITIONAL READING

Read and review the references listed below to expand your understanding of the concepts in this chapter. Write down the date that you complete your reading for each. Remember that consistent repetition is the best way to learn. Plan to read each reference at least once now and expect to read it again as you continue your studies.

References marked with (skim) can be read quickly and do not require commentary review.

CLASSICS		1st read	2nd read
Charaka	Cha. Sū. 1/6-14 Cha. Sū. 12/ Cha. Sū. 17/112-114 Cha. Sū. 24/9, 24/18, 24/22 Ca Vi. 1/5 Cha. Vi. 6/10-13 Cha. Śhā. 1/16 Cha. Śhā. 6/3 Cha. Śhā. 6/12 Cha. Śhā. 6/18		
Suśhruta	Su. Sū. 1/22 Su. Sū. 15/3 Su. Sū. 21/3-5 Su. Sū. 42/5 Su. Śhā. 1/16		
Aṣhṭāṅga Hṛdaya	AH Sū. 1/6-8 AH Sū. 1/11-12 AH Sū. 11/1 AH Sū. 13/21-22		
Bhāva Prakāśha	BP Pū. 2/32 BP Pū. 3/98-101		

QUESTIONS & ANSWERS

Record your questions for this chapter here for further research and discussion.

Question:

Answer:

Question:

Answer:

Question:

Answer:

SELF-ASSESSMENT

1. According to Suśhruta which two terms best describe *puruṣha*?
   a. *Deha* and *śhārīra*
   b. *Gātra* and *dehī*
   c. *Karma puruṣha* and *chikitsā puruṣha*
   d. *Kāya* and *śharīra*
   e. *Pañcha mahābhūtas* and *chetanā*

2. *Doṣha* has the natural tendency to act as which of the following?
   a. As a *deha*
   b. As a *dhātu*
   c. As a *dūṣhya*
   d. As a *mala*
   e. As a *srotas*

3. Which of the following is a synonym for *vāta*?
   a. *Anala*
   b. *Anila*
   c. *Rajas*
   d. *Sattva*
   e. *Soma*

4. When two *doṣhas* combine, what are they called?
   a. *Avikṛta*
   b. *Prakṛti*
   c. *Saṁsarga*
   d. *Sannipāta*
   e. *Svabhāva*

5. The natural *doṣha gati* of *vāta* tends toward:
   a. *Adho gati*
   b. *Tiryak gati*
   c. *Ūrdhva gati*
   d. All of the above
   e. None of the above

6. The earliest concepts of the *tridoṣha siddhānta* are found in
   a. *Charaka sampradāya*
   b. Kāśhyapa Saṁhitā
   c. Patañjali
   d. *Śhalya Tantra*
   e. Vedic texts

7. The *tridoṣha siddhānta* originated from which concepts?
   a. *Agni*, *māruta*, *soma*
   b. *Ap, tejas, ākāśha*
   c. *Laṅghana, bṛṁhaṇa, rūkṣhaṇa*
   d. *Ṛg, Yajur, Arthava Vedas*
   e. *Uṣhṇa, śhīta, manda*

8. The term *doṣha* derives from which Sanskrit *dhātu?*
   a. *Dhā*
   b. *Dṛśh*
   c. *Duṣh*
   d. *Sidh*
   e. *Śhliṣh*

9. In Āyurveda, *puruṣha* is defined as
   a. Association of the *pañcha mahābhūtas* with *chetanā*
   b. *Ātma*
   c. One who sleeps in the body
   d. One who detaches from the body
   e. *Sattva*, *rajas*, *tamas*

10. Which *guṇas* of *vāta* are shared among all authors of the *Bṛhat Trayī*?
    a. *Chala, khara, viśhada*
    b. *Laghu, rūkṣha, sūkṣhma*
    c. *Mṛdu, śhīghra, vistambha*
    d. *Rūkṣha, śhīta, laghu*
    e. *Yogavahi, vibhāga, sūkṣhma*

CRITICAL THINKING

1. Among the *doṣhas*, first identify each one's significant *guṇas*. Next, identify the common and opposite *guṇas* between pairs.

2. Define the term *doṣha* in your own words using an example.

3. Draw a picture demonstrating *loka-puruṣha siddhānta* between the *doṣhas* and the external world. Label at least five *guṇas* or *karmas* for each *doṣha* in the image.

4. Identify three definitions or explanations of *doṣhas* that would be most important for an Āyurvedic professional to understand, and three that are most important for a layperson to understand.

5. Why would Suśhruta describe four *doṣhas*? List at least three reasons and explain his perspective. Does *Charaka* agree?

6. What is it the "nature" of *doṣhas* to do? Which of the three "bodies" is most affected?

Chapter 5 : Agni

KEY TERMS

agni
āhāra
āhāra pāka
āhāra parināma bhāvas
āhāra rasa
āmāśhaya
amla pāka
antarāgni
asthāyi dhātu
asthi dhātvagni
avasthā pāka
bhūtāgni
dhātu pariṇāma
dhātu poṣhaṇa nyāya
dhātvagni
jāṭharāgni
kāla
kaṭu pāka
kiṭṭā
kleda
koṣhṭha
krūra koṣhṭha
kṣhut
madhura pāka
madhyama koṣhṭha
majja dhātvagni
māṁsa dhātvagni
mandāgni
medo dhātvagni
mṛdu koṣhṭha
mūtra
niṣhṭha pāka
pāchaka pitta
pāchakāgni
pipāsa
pitta
poṣhaka dhātu
poṣhya dhātu
puriṣha
rakta dhātvagni
rasa dhātvagni
samāgni
samayoga
sāra
sāra-kiṭṭa vibhāga
śharīra
sneha
sthāyi dhātu
sthūla bhāga
śhukra dhātvagni
sūkṣhma bhāga
tīkṣhṇāgni
udgāra
uṣhmā
vāta
vāyu
vegas
viṣhamāgni

Agni includes all of the processes that initiate the conversion and transformation of what is consumed thus rendering it into the body. The term *agni* derives from the Sanskrit *dhātu* √ *aṅg*, meaning to move.

The *dhātu* √ *aṅg* forms the verbal root '*ag*' which produces terms including '*agati*,' '*agnā*' and '*agni*.' *Ag* means to move tortuously or to wind. In general, the term *agni* means fire.

Throughout Vedic history, *agni* has been revered as the god of fire and it still maintains the same status in mythology and continued religious practices.

Within the body, *agni* is responsible for the continuation of life, among its key functions. Cha. Chi. 15/3-5 beautifully explains the importance of *agni* in terms of its actions and effects. In its various states, *agni* is responsible for:

State of *Agni*	*Avikṛta* Normal, healthy		*Vikṛta* Abnormal	*Śhānta* Cessation
Functions	*Āyu*	Vitality, life	*Roga* Disease	*Mṛtyu* Death
	Varṇa	Complexion		
	Bala	Strength		
	Svāsthya	Healthy state		
	Utsāha	Enthusiasm		
	Upachaya	Proper growth		
	Prabhā	Glow, complexion		
	Ojas	*Ojas*		
	Tejas	*Tejas*		
	Agnaya	All other *agnis*		
	Prāṇa	*Prāṇa*		

	Chira jīva *Anāmaya* *Mūla*	Long life Absence of disease Root (of health)		

From the explanation above, it is clear that Charaka intends to convey how important the healthy functioning of *agni* is to an individual's overall state of health. All of these results can be considered to be the effects of *agni*. Knowledge and understanding of these effects can also be utilized via *anumāna pramāṇa* to ascertain the general state of *agni* during assessment.

AGNI AS PITTA

The concept of *agni* is described by all of the significant classical authors in relation to *pitta*. Because the two are very similar in nature, it is understood that they have a connection. The question that each author addresses is "What is this relationship between *agni* and *pitta*, and are they the same?" Charaka, Suśhruta and Vāgbhaṭa each provide consistently similar responses.

In Cha. Sū. 12/, a discussion among scholarly experts is recorded, and one of the participants, Mārlci, states that "अग्निरेव शरीरे पित्तान्तर्गतः" (*Agnireva śharīre pittāntargataḥ*). This means that the *pitta* which is *āntar-gataḥ* (going, moving or residing) *śharīre* (inside the body) is *agni*. Based on its state and condition (normal or abnormal), it is responsible for:

State of *Agni*	*Kupita* and *Śhubha* Increased and strong (healthy)	*Akupita* and *Aśhubha* Decreased and weak (unhealthy)
Functions	Creates normal and healthy: *Pakti* (Digestion) *Darśhana* (Vision) *Mātra ūṣhmaṇa* (Regulated body heat) *Prakṛti varṇa* (Healthy complexion) *Śhaurya* (Courage) *Harṣha* (Pleasure, joy) *Prasāda* (Tranquility)	Creates abnormal and unhealthy: *Apakti* (Indigestion) *Adarśhana* (Visual impairment) *Amātra ūṣhmaṇa* (Impaired bodily heat) *Vikṛti varṇa* (Sickly complexion) *Bhaya* (Fear) *Krodha* (Anger) *Moha* (Confusion)

Chakrapāṇi goes on to add that although a comparison has been drawn between the *agni* found in the external world and that present inside the body, the two are not the same. Nor is the *agni* found inside the body the same as the *pitta* within. The reason he cites to prove this is that certain causative factors can result in one or the other changing its states, but not necessarily both. Specifically, certain *dravya* can affect one but not the other, or both may be affected in different ways.

Suśhruta also addresses the question of whether *agni* and *pitta* are the same in Su. Sū. 21/9-10. He clearly states that *pitta* and *agni* can be considered the same when *pitta* performs the role of *agni* and accomplishes its functions. When this happens, *pitta* can be considered as *antarāgni*, or the main *agni* which resides locally in the digestive tract. Additionally, in the very next line he describes the five types of *pittas*, and mentions *pāchaka pitta* as the specific one responsible for *agni*'s function. This type of *pitta* is also named *pāchakāgni*.

Vāgbhaṭa adds more to this explanation in AH Sū. 12/10-11 by stating that *pāchaka pitta* is called *anala* when it does the job of *agni*. This is possible because *pāchaka pitta* is predominant in *tejo mahābhūta*, and when it loses its *drava guṇa*, it performs *pāka* or *pāchana*. It further separates ingested food into the beneficial, nutrient portion and the unwanted waste.

Chakrapāṇi further clarifies on Cha. Chi. 19/6 that an increase or aggravation of *pitta's drava guṇa* will certainly suppress *agni* because of its inherent *śhīta guṇa*. This naturally counteracts the power of *agni* thus causing a reduction.

These processes will be explained in detail later in this chapter.

TEST YOURSELF

Learn, review and memorize key terms from this section.

agni

---

pitta

śharīra

---

antarāgni

---

pāchaka pitta

---

pāchakāgni

PARIBHĀṢHĀ

Even though the concept of *agni* is included throughout the classics with a wide variety of references, it is something which is indirectly defined by most authors. In BP Pū. 3/, a detailed description is provided about the process of food intake and digestion. In that description, the following statement is provided about *agni*, which can be considered a definition:

' ग्रहण्यां पच्यते कोष्ठे वह्निना जायते कटुः ' इति ॥

भा.प्र. पू. ३।१६८

' Grahaṇyāṁ pachyate koṣhṭhe vahninā jāyate kaṭuḥ ' iti ||

BP Pū. 3/168

Iti (And so), *vahninā* (the digestive fire) *grahaṇyāṁ* (inside the *grahaṇī*) *koṣhṭhe* (in the *koṣhṭha*) *pachyate* (breaks down [that which has been consumed]) *jāyate* (rendering it) *kaṭuḥ* (pungent).

Agni, located in the *koṣhṭha*, cooks [the food] in the *grahaṇī* rendering it into a pungent flavor.

The definitions for *agni* may appear lacking because the term *agni* is so versatile. In order to understand *agni* and define it, it must be analyzed from a more granular level. In the definition above, the *agni* that the author refers to is the main one called *jaṭharāgni*. This is the primary *agni* that performs the initial digestive processes and creates the products which then undergo further processing by other types of *agnis*.

अन्नस्य पक्ता पित्तं तु पाचकाख्यं पुरेरितम्
।
दोषधातुमलादीनामूष्मेत्यात्रेयशासनम् ॥

अ. हृ. शा. ३।४९

Annasya paktā tu pāchakādhyaṁ pureritam |
Doṣhadhātumalādeenāmūṣhmetyātreya śhāsanam ||

AH Śhā. 3/49-76

Pāchakā (pitta) has already been described as that which does *annasya paktā* (digestion of food). *Ātreya* instructs that this *ūṣhma* (*pāchakā*, form of *agni*) is inside the *doṣhas, dhātus, malādeenām* (*mala*, etc).

Interestingly, Vāgbhaṭa is the only author of surviving literature to contain this statement. It may be prudent to interpret the *ūṣhma* mentioned as indicating that the *doṣhas, dhātus, malādeenām* (*mala*, etc) as having undergone the effects of *pākā* rather than containing their own individual *agnis*.

More definitions of *agni* are possible only by looking at its subtypes and contexts.

TEST YOURSELF

Learn, review and memorize key terms from this section.

koṣhṭha

____

BHEDA

The classification of *agni* into three subtypes is explained well in Āyurveda. Each type is responsible for specific functions and activities. All three are interdependent and interrelated. The functions of each are listed below and their roles in the overall process of digestion will be explained in the following sections.

Jaṭharāgni

The primary subtype of all *agnis* is *jāṭharāgni*. It is named for its location in the *koṣhṭha* and is the central, or main *agni* responsible for the health and capacity of all of the other subtypes. Charaka explains this in Cha. Chi. 15/38-41. He notes that the condition of *jāṭharāgni* should be carefully maintained by supplying it with appropriate inputs (food, drinks and consumed items). Very similar statements are given by Vāgbhaṭa in AH Śhā. 3/51-54 and 3/71-72.

Jāṭharāgni has several common synonyms:

Anala	represents the internal fire which digests, transforms and assimilates food
Antarāgni	the primary *agni* due to its location in *antara*, the interior portion, or GIT
Koṣhṭhāgni	agni which is located in the *koṣhṭha*
Audaryāgni	located in the abdominal area

	around the stomach or belly
Dehāgni	supports the growth and increase of the body
Kāyāgni	helps maintain growth and normal health through selective, appropriate nourishment

In addition to being the primary *agni* of the body, Vāgbhaṭa notes in AH Sū. 12/8 that *jāṭharāgni* is also responsible for separating the beneficial fractions of consumed food from the waste materials. *Jāṭharāgni* is the one which can be affected by the *doṣhas* to change its state from healthy to various abnormal types (Cha. Chi. 15/51). Suśhruta equates *jāṭharāgni* mythologically to the cause for creation and states that it digests (literally, cooks) consumed food. It cannot be known (investigated, or observed) directly because of its extremely subtle nature (Su. Sū. 35/27).

Various authors provide detailed anatomical explanations for the location of *jāṭharāgni*, as shown below.

Location of *jāṭharāgni*	Cha. Chi. 15/7	Su. Sū.	AH Śhā. 3/51	BP Pū. 3/167
Grahaṇī			√	√
Pittadharā kalā			√	√
Sthitā pakvāśhayadvāri bhukta-mārga-argaleva			√	
Udara	√			

Bhūtagni

Bhūtāgni refers to the subgroup of five *agnis* which are responsible for processing each of the *pañcha mahābhūtas*, as follows:

Mahābhūta	Corresponding *agni*
Pṛthvi	*Pārthiva agni, bhauma agni*
Ap	*Āpya agni*
Tejas	*Taijas agni, Āgneya agni*
Vāyu	*Vāyavya agni*
Ākāśha	*Ākāśha agni, Nābhasa agni*

The *bhūtāgnis* are responsible for transforming the consumed food in its most basic form of *pañcha mahābhūtas* into the corresponding *mahābhūta* components within the body. Because the external nutrients and internal components are ultimately all composed of the *pañcha mahābhūtas*, they can combine based on their *guṇas* (Cha. Chi. 15/13-14, AH Śhā. 3/59, BP Pū. 3/169-170). These activities take place because of *sāmānya-viśheṣha siddhānta*. For example, the *pārthiva bhūta* components of consumed food are processed by *pārthivāgni* which allows the bodily components of the same *bhūta* to be nourished and increased.

Dhātvagni

Dhātvagni encompasses the subgroup of seven *agnis* which are each responsible for converting one product into its corresponding *dhātu*, *upadhātus* and *dhātu-malas*. The process begins with the first *dhātu-agni* which converts the *anna rasa*, or nutrient fluid produced from consumed food, into the first *dhātu*, *rasa dhātu*. The sequence continues through the remaining six, and its complete process is shown below:

Product	Converted by *dhātvagni*	Into the next *dhātu*
Anna rasa (nutrients from food)	*Rasa dhātvagni*	*Rasa dhātu*
Rasa dhātu	*Rakta dhātvagni*	*Rakta dhātu*
Rakta dhātu	*Māṁsa dhātvagni*	*Māṁsa dhātu*
Māṁsa dhātu	*Medo dhātvagni*	*Medo dhātu*
Medo dhātu	*Asthi dhātvagni*	*Asthi dhātu*
Asthi dhātu	*Majja dhātvagni*	*Majja dhātu*
Majja dhātu	*Śhukra dhātvagni*	*Śhukra dhātu*

See Cha. Chi. 15/15-16, AH Śhā. 3/61.5, BP Pū. 3/179 for detailed explanations.

TEST YOURSELF

Learn, review and memorize key terms from this section.

jāṭharāgni

____

bhūtāgni

____

dhātvagni
rasa dhātvagni
rakta dhātvagni
māṁsa dhātvagni
medo dhātvagni
asthi dhātvagni
majja dhātvagni
śhukra dhātvagni

STATES OF AGNI

Agni may function in various states depending on a variety of factors including the consumed food, general health, influence of *doṣhas*, age, season, etc. The four states include one which is normal and healthy, and three that are abnormal and unhealthy. Each of these three is affected by one of the *doṣhas*.

Normal

The normal, healthy state of *agni* is called *samāgni*. Charaka explains this as:

युक्तं भुक्तवतो युक्तो धातुसाम्यं समं पचन् ।

च. चि. १५।५१.५

Yuktaṁ bhuktavato yukto dhātusāmyaṁ samaṁ pachan |

Cha. Chi. 15/51.5

Samāgni digests or processes (literally, cooks) a properly consumed meal to maintain proper *dhātu sāmya*.

And in Cha. Vi. 6/12, *samāgni* is stated to be impaired by even minor variations in food and meal habits. It can only maintain its normal state if inconsistencies with food and meal habits are avoided.

Suśhruta adds in Su. Sū. 35/24:

तत्र यो यथाकालमुपयुक्तमन्नं सम्यक् पचति स समः, समैर्दोषैः ।

सु. सू. ३५।२४

Tatra yo yathākālamupayuktamannaṁ samyak pachati sa samaḥ, samairdoṣhaiḥ |

Su. Sū. 35/24

Samāgni digests (literally, cooks) proper meals within a proper (appropriate) time period, due to *sama doṣha* (the *doṣhas* being in normal, healthy states).

Vāgbhaṭa makes a similar statement in AH Śhā. 3/74:

यः पचेत्सम्यगेवान्नं भुक्तं सम्यक् समस्त्वसौ ॥

अ. हृ. शा. ३।७४

Yaḥ pachetsamyagevānnaṁ bhuktaṁ samyak samastvasau ||

AH Śhā. 3/74

Samāgni digests or processes (literally, cooks) a meal which is properly prepared and consumed at the correct time.

Samāgni is the healthy and ideal state of

jāṭharāgni. Achieving a state of *samāgni* should be the goal for every individual, with the understanding that it is challenging to constantly maintain. It is one of the most effective preventive measures for avoiding unhealthy states of *doṣhas*. The signs of well-maintained and properly functioning *samāgni* are those listed at the beginning of this chapter.

Abnormal

The abnormal, unhealthy state of *agni* can be classified into three types, each one influenced by a primary *doṣha*. These three are responsible for generating unhealthy *doṣhas* as waste products which can cause various problems and obstacles to maintaining health. The three abnormal states of *agni* are *viṣhamāgni, tīkṣhṇāgni* and *mandāgni*, predominant in *vāta, pitta* and *kapha doṣha*, respectively. Various authors have described each of these states and their cardinal features, listed below.

Viṣhamāgni Abnormal *agni* affected by *vāta*	Cha. Chi. 15/50	Cha. Vi. 6/12	Su. Sū. 35/26	AH Śhā. 3/73-76
Dhātu-vaiṣhamya Abnormal state of *dhātus*	√			
Viṣhama pachan Irregular digestion (cooking)	√			
Sama-lakṣhaṇa-viparīta-lakṣhaṇa Presents with features opposite to *samāgni*		√		
Kadāchit samyak pachati Digests (cooks) food properly sometimes			√	
Kadāchit - ādhmāna, śhūla, udāvarta, atisāra, jaṭhara gaurava, āntra kūjana, pravāhaṇi Sometimes produces distension, colic, upward movement of vāta, diarrhea, heaviness in the abdomen, borborygmus, tenesmus			√	
Samyak-āśhu samyak-chirā pachet Sometimes fast or slow to digest				√

Tīkṣhṇāgni Abnormal *agni* affected by *pitta*	Cha. Chi. 15/50	Cha. Vi. 6/12	Su. Sū. 35/26	AH Śhā. 3/73-76
Dhātu-viśhoṣhana with *manda-indhana* Depletion with insufficient fuel or nutrition	√			
Sarva-apachāra-saha Overcomes all improper habits		√		
Āśhu pachati of prabhūta anna Quickly digests too much food			√	
Śhighra-pachet of samyak, etc *bhojana* Fast digestion of proper food (meals)				√

Mandāgni Abnormal *agni* affected by *kapha*	Cha. Chi. 15/51	Cha. Vi. 6/12	Su. Sū. 35/26	AH Śhā. 3/73-76
Vidahati-anna Incompletely digested meals	√			
Na sarva-apachāra-saha Does not tolerate inconsistent meals		√		
Mahatā kālena pachati of alpa yukta Long time to digest small meals			√	
Udara and śhiro-gaurava, kāsa, śhvāsa, praseka, chhardi, gātra-sadana Heaviness in the abdomen and head, cough, difficulty breathing on exertion, salivation, regurgitation, fatigue			√	
Chirāt-pachet of samyak, upayukta anna Slow digestion of proper food (meals)				√
Asya-śhoṣha, āṭopa, āntra kūjana, ādhmāna, gaurava Dry mouth, bloating, borborygmus, abdominal distension, heaviness				√

The state of *agni* can change in as little as a few minutes, depending on the individual and all of their potential causative factors. In general, healthy individuals will tend to be capable of maintaining *samāgni* more easily than those who are easily prone to dysfunction. In these cases, one or more *doṣhas* may become predominant based on various factors and adversely affect *agni* to produce *viṣhamāgni*, *tīkṣhṇāgni* or *mandāgni*. Only one type can act as the primary influencing factor at any time, although they can change easily and quickly in certain situations to appear otherwise.

TEST YOURSELF

Learn, review and memorize key terms from this section.

samāgni

---

viṣhamāgni

---

tīkṣhṇāgni

---

mandāgni

KEY PRINCIPLES

This section covers the key principles that directly impact how *agni* functions.

Koṣhṭha

The term *koṣhṭha* refers to two distinct concepts in Āyurveda. Anatomically, it is the hollow pathway from mouth to anus which allows that which has been consumed to pass through the body, be digested and assimilated. Physiologically, it is the manner in which the anatomical structures function together to perform their functions in a healthy way and generate output in the form of waste materials. In this section, the physiological aspects of *koṣhṭha* will be covered, while their finer anatomical details are listed in Chapter 19.

Koṣhṭha is most commonly categorized into three types, one which is affected by each of the *doṣhas*. Vāgbhaṭa states these in AH Sū. 1/8.5:

कोष्ठः क्रूरो मृदुर्मध्यो मध्यः स्यत्तैः समैरपि ।

अ. हृ. सू. १।८.५

Koṣhṭhaḥ krūro mṛdurmadhyo madyaḥ syattaiḥ samairapi |

AH Sū. 1/8.5

Koṣhṭha may be *krūra, mṛdu* or *madhyama*. When the individual is in a state of *sama* (*dhātu*), *madhya koṣhṭha* is seen.

Additional details in Cha. Sū. 13/69, Su. Chi. 33/21 and AH Sū. 18/34 explain the nature of each type and its predominance of *doṣha*:

Koṣhṭha	Cha. Sū. 13/69	Su. Chi. 33/21	AH Sū. 18/34
Krūra	*Vāta*	*Vāta* and *kapha*	*Vāta*
Mṛdu	*Pitta*	*Pitta*	*Pitta*
Madhyama	not specified	*Sama doṣha*	not specified

Krūra koṣhṭha experiences bowel movements and purgation with difficulty because of the increased presence of *vāta*. Suśhruta adds that *kapha* is involved here. *Mṛdu koṣhṭha* passes bowels and purges easily because of the increased presence of *pitta*. *Madhyama koṣhṭha* is that which is experienced in a state of *sama doṣha*, where the *doṣhas* are normal and healthy.

Additionally, all authors explain in varying levels of depth a procedure called *koṣhṭha parīkṣha*. This is used as a practical test to determine an individual's type of *koṣhṭha* by providing certain foods and drinks. These items were known to increase bowel quantity and/or frequency, and could be used to gauge the current condition of the *koṣhṭha*. Charaka provides the most comprehensive review of *dravyas* for *koṣhṭha parīkṣha* in Cha. Sū. 13/65-69.

Dhātu poṣhaṇa nyāya

The three *dhātu poṣhaṇa nyāya* are the hypotheses proposed to explain how digested food moves through the body in its nutrient state to provide building blocks for growth of the *dhātus*. Each of these three *nyāyas* uses analogies from simple and well-understood real-world events to explain the subtle and undetectable processes occurring in the human body.

The *nyāyas* are explained in the commentary sections of Cha. Sū. 28/4, Su. Sū. 14/10, AH Śhā. 3/62. They are listed on the following page with simple examples.

Ultimately, all three of these *nyāyas* may be used to explain various *dravyas* and how they undergo *pāka* within the human body. Most commonly, *kedāri-kulyā nyāya* is accepted as the general rule because it can explain most standard processes of *pāka* (BP Pū. 3/176).

Kṣhīra-dadhi nyāya

Sequential transformation

This process is analogous to the sequential transformation of a product like milk through various stages into its final form (curd, butter, ghee).

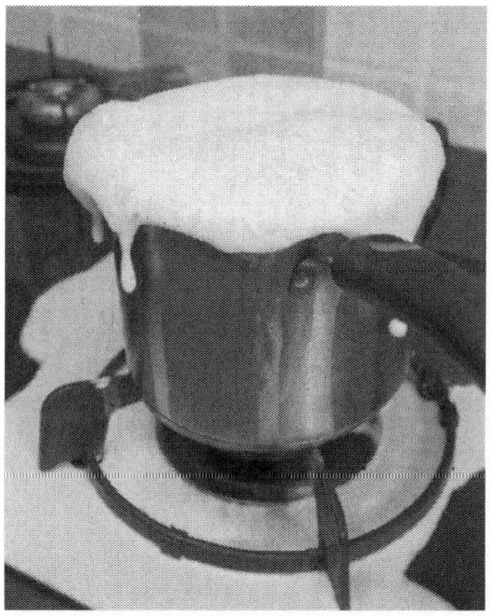

Khale-kapota nyāya

Selective nourishment

This process is analogous to any bird which selects specific, desired food items and carries them to their nest for use.

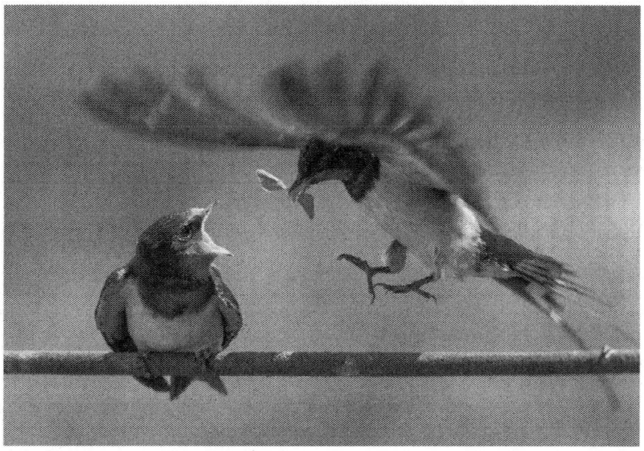

Kedāri-kulyā nyāya

Irrigation

This process is analogous to watering a large field of crops by creating large and small channels to spread the water throughout.

It can also be seen in the structure of plant leaves as shown in this image.

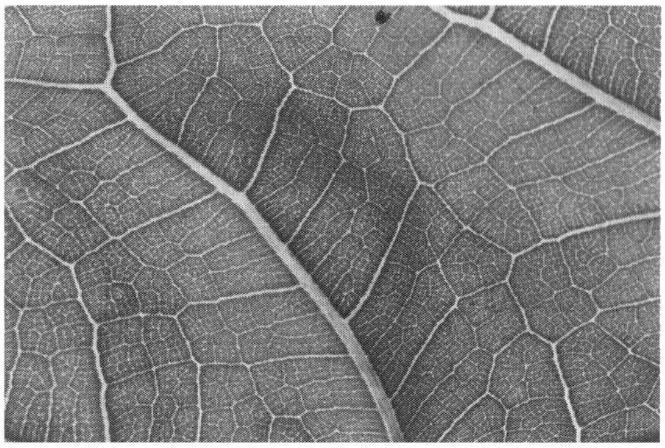

Āhāra parināma bhāvas

The *āhāra parināma bhāvas* are the factors which aid in the process of *pāchana*, or transformation, conversion and assimilation of consumed food items. When these factors are healthy and able to process, they contribute to healthy functioning *agni* at all levels throughout the body. In any other state, *agni* becomes compromised in various ways resulting in an unhealthy aggravation or reduction of the *doṣhas, dhātus* and *malas*.

Charaka describes the *āhāra parināma bhāvas* in Cha. Śhā. 6/14-15 as follows.

Āhāra parināma bhāva Nearest English equivalent	Responsibilities and functions
Uṣhmā Heat (also, *pitta*)	*Pacati* Digests, cooks
Vāyu *Vāta*	*Apakarṣhati* Brings food down by *anulomana* and helps break it down Chakrapāṇi adds that *vāta* brings the food closer to *agni* to promote *pāka* (see also, Cha. Chi. 15/17).
Kleda Moisture	*Śhaithilyam-āpādayati* Produces looseness in the food to help make it smaller
Sneha Unctuousness	*Mardava janayanti* Increases or brings softness into the food
Kāla Time	*Paryāptimabhi-nirvartayati* Allows the processes to complete
Samayoga Proper intake of food	*Pariṇāmā dhātu sāmya karaḥ saṁpadyate* Promotes proper conversion to increase *dhātu sāmya*

Duration for conversion

There are a variety of opinions that propose the length of time required for consumed food to transform into various *dhātus, malas* and other components of the physical body. The specifics of these opinions are discussed in the commentary sections of Cha. Chi. 15/21, Su. Sū. 14/14 and in the verses of AH Śhā. 3/65-66 and BP Pū. 3/178-180. This is a concept which has several plausible theories and one unifying explanation which all authors recognize and accept.

The single, unifying explanation that provides validation to all of the proposed hypotheses and makes them all acceptable under various conditions is the analogy of the process of conversion happening like a wheel. This analogy is significant because it demonstrates constant processing and variability.

Irrespective of how the processes are happening, they are continuously occurring like the passage of time (Cha. Sū. 28/3). This processing works on many levels as well with *jāṭharāgni, bhūtāgni* and *dhātvagni* all functioning simultaneously in their various stages.

It is critical to note here that because these processes are incessant, *agni* will continue to work even in the absence of *āhāra*.

The general consensus is that it can take one day, six days, or one month to complete the full conversion of consumed food into *dhātus*. This variance is based on several factors, including the food consumed, its *dravya prabhāva* and the state of *agni* in the individual. With strong *agni* it is reasonable to assume that the power of conversion can happen more quickly and efficiently. On the other hand, when *agni* is weak, it can take longer to do the same job. The different ways that these transformation processes can occur are explained by the *nyāyas*.

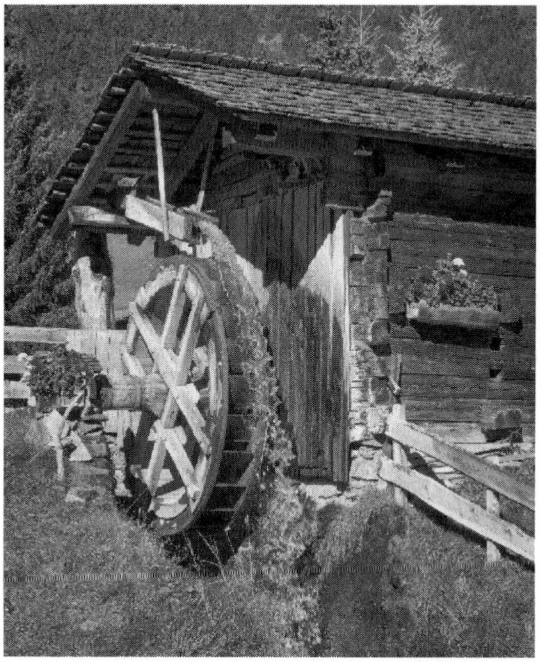

In BP Pū. 5/103, when *āhāra* is not provided in a timely manner, *agni* does *pāchana* of the increased *doṣhas*. Once they have returned to normal or are decreased, *agni* then digests the healthy *dhātus*. When these are diminished, it finally turns to *prāṇa*, resulting in the loss of life.

TEST YOURSELF

Learn, review and memorize key terms from this section.

koṣhṭha

____

krūra koṣhṭha

____

mṛdu koṣhṭha

____

madhyama koṣhṭha

dhātu poṣhaṇa nyāya

āhāra parināma bhāvas

uṣhmā

vāyu

kleda

sneha

kāla

samayoga

DHĀTU PARIṆĀMA

The complete process and mechanics of *agni* are described through the concept of *dhātu pariṇāma*. They explain the complex processes of digestion, metabolism, absorption and excretion in ways which can be understood and managed directly and indirectly through the *pramāṇas* and *jñānendriyas*. Because *dhātu pariṇāma* is constantly happening at many levels, it can be challenging to try to understand which features are being recognized and analyzed at any given point in time. From a practical perspective, the effects of the food most recently consumed and the later final outcomes in terms of *doṣhas, dhātus* and *malas* are generally most readily identifiable in clinical assessments.

Step 1: Intake of *āhāra*

The normal process of *dhātu pariṇāma* begins with the consumption of any type of *āhāra*. Su. Sū. 14/3 defines *āhāra* through several classification methods:

Āhāra	Explanation
Pañcha-bhautika	Composed of the five gross elements, *pṛthvi, ap, tejas, vāyu, ākāśha*
Chatur-vidha	Of four types, that which can be: • *aśhita* → chewed • *peya* → drunk • *lehya* → licked • *bhakṣhya* → eaten (as in a meal)
Ṣhaḍ-rasa	Of six flavors, namely: • *madhura* → sweet • *amla* → sour • *lavaṇa* → salty • *kaṭu* → pungent • *tikta* → bitter • *kaṣhaya* → astringent

Dvi-vidha or *Aṣhṭa-vidha vīrya*	Of two or eight types of potency: • *śhīta* → cold ○ snigdha → unctuous ○ *pichchhila* → slimy ○ *mṛdu* → soft • *uṣhṇa* → hot ○ *rūkṣha* → dry ○ *viṣhada* → clear ○ *tīkṣhṇa* → sharp
Aneka guṇa upayukta	Of many types of qualities when consumed (referring to the twenty *gurvādi guṇas*)

There are many recommendations on how to properly consume food, especially meals, so their beneficial effects can be maximized through efficient *pāka*. These recommendations will be covered in detail in Volume 3.

Āhāra is brought into the body by *prāṇa vāyu* which influences the selection of what to consume (BP Pū. 3/166). Vāgbhaṭa explains this in AH Sū. 12/4 by stating that one of the functions of *prāṇa vāyu* is अन्न प्रवेश कृत् (*Anna praveśha kṛt*), or bringing the food into the body. It should be noted clearly here that eating, especially a meal, was always assumed to be an activity that was done with respect by dedicating proper time, effort and attention. These meal habits are significant in many ways to allow the first stages of digestion to occur well, thus setting the stage for the remaining, dependent processes.

Kapha also plays several important roles in this initial step of *dhātu pariṇama*. First, *bodhaka kapha*, located in the *rasana* allows the *rasas* in the *āhāra* to be perceived and understood (AH Sū. 12/16.5). This provides critical feedback to the rest of the digestive system and the body before the food enters the gut. These brief, but key moments of chewing allow the digestive system to prepare for the incoming food. The sensitivity and response of taste receptors can be seen by the reactions of the body and mind based on an individual's liking or disliking of certain flavors. These responses have been described in depth in Cha. Sū. 26/73-79, Su. Sū. 42/9 and AH Sū. 10/2-6 and can be interpreted as significant diagnostic criteria in clinical practice.

Second, *kledaka kapha* aids the process of bringing *āhāra* into the body by moistening, softening and lubricating each bolus of *āhara* as it enters the *āmāśhaya*, which is most commonly considered the stomach, but here may also include the route from the mouth to the stomach. See AH Sū. 12/16.

Vāgbhaṭa summarizes this step in AH Śhā. 3/55 by stating:

अन्नं कालेऽभ्यवहृतं कोष्ठं प्राणानिलाहृतम्
।
द्रवैर्विभिन्नसङ्घातं नीतं स्नेहेन मार्दवम् ॥

अ. हृ. शा. ३।५५

Annaṁ kāle ' bhyavahṛtaṁ koṣhṭhaṁ prāṇānilāhṛtam |

dravairvibhinnasaṅghātaṁ nītaṁ snehena mārdavam ||

AH Śhā. 3/55

Food (a meal) which is eaten at the correct time is brought down into the *koṣhṭha* by *prāṇa vāta. Drava* (synonymous for *kleda*, ie, *kledaka kapha*) breaks down the larger segments by making them unctuous and soft.

Charaka adds an important statement in Cha. Chi. 15/12. By consuming wholesome meals in the right way at the right time, all of the *indriyas* are nourished.

Step 2: Āhāra pāka

The next step of *āhāra pāka* marks the beginning of the transformation of *āhāra rasa* into *dhātus*. *Āhāra rasa* is the initial juice produced from the consumed food which is then acted upon by *jāṭharāgni* in the *grahaṇī* to initiate and manage the process of *pāka*, or digestion. Additional activities occur during *pāka* which are functions of *bhūtagnis* and various types of *doṣhas*.

The major outcome of this stage of *pāka* is the selective separation of *sāra* (also called *prasāda,* Cha. Sū. 28/4), or the desired nutrient portion, from *kiṭṭā*, the waste materials. This job is done directly by *pāchaka pitta*, which is synonymous for *anala* as Vāgbhaṭa states in AH Sū. 12/11:

... पाकादिकर्मणाऽनलशब्दितम् ।
पचत्यन्नं विभजते सारकिट्टौ पृथक् तथा ॥
अ. हृ. सू. १२।११

... pākādikarmaṇā ' nalaśhabditam |
pachatyannaṁ vibhajate sārakiṭṭau
pṛthak tathā ||

AH Sū. 12/11

(*Pāchaka pitta*) goes by the name of *anala* because it does the *karma* of *pāka*, etc. It does *pāchana* of *anna* (digests, transforms, assimilates meals), and separates the *sāra* (nutrient portion) from the kiṭṭa (waste material).

The process of *sāra-kiṭṭa vibhāga*, or selective separation of nutrients from wastes, happens at the levels of the *bhūtāgnis* and *dhātvagnis* during their active conversion processes. These secondary *agnis* will perform their functions well only when activated and supported by *jaṭharāgni*. As *jaṭharāgni* increases or decreases, so do the *bhūtāgnis* and *dhātvagnis* (Cha. Chi. 15/39-40).

Before the *sāra-kiṭṭa vibhāga* occurs, the *bhūtāgnis* are activated by *jaṭharāgni* to process their appropriate materials. Each *bhūtāgni* is responsible for converting its own related *bhūta* so that it may be utilized by the body to nourish similar substances (BP Pū. 3/169-170). Charaka elaborates on the importance of *bhūtāgni pāka* and explains that it is responsible for activating the various *guṇas* (including *gurvādi, viśhiṣhṭa*, etc) which then go on to nourish all of the *dhātus* and *indriyas* (Cha. Sū. 28/3, Cha. Chi. 15/13-4). This is regulated by *samānya-viśheṣha siddhānta* which allows things of similar nature to increase while things of opposite nature get reduced.

This output of *bhūtāgni* conversion is also called *avasthā pāka*. This occurs in three stages, each of which are responsible for generating one *doṣha*. The progression of these stages lasts for the duration of digestion in the *koṣhṭha*, and their descriptions and outcomes are listed below (Cha. Chi. 15/9-11, Chakrapāṇi; AH Śhā. 3/57-58, BP Pū. 3/171).

Avasthāpāka	1st stage: *Prapāka*	2nd stage: *Pacyamāna*	3rd stage: *Śhoṣhyamāṇa*
Bhāva Result of processing	*Madhura*	*Amla*	*Kaṭu*
Lakṣhaṇas Characteristics	*Phena-bhūta* Foamy	*Vidagdha* Semi-digested, sour *Pittam-accha* Produces clear *pitta*	*Śhoṣhya vahninā* Drying effect by *agni* *Paripiṇḍata* Becomes a bolus
Adhiṣhṭhāna Location	*Ūrdhva āmāśhaya* Upper stomach	*Grahaṇī*	*Pakvāśhaya*
Doṣha Main *doṣha* produced	*Kapha*	*Pitta*	*Vāta*

Each of these stages will only occur properly when the digesting food moves through in a timely manner. This is neither too fast, nor too slow, but at the speed required to produce the appropriate results.

Concurrently, *samāna vāyu* stimulates the main activities of *jaṭharāgni* just as blowing on flames increases their capacity to burn fuel (Cha. Chi. 15/6-8). Vāgbhaṭa states in AH Sū. 12/8 that *samāna vāyu* moves throughout the entire *koṣhṭha*, holds onto the consumed food so it can be digested properly, aids in *pāchana*, stimulates *sāra-kiṭṭa vhibhāga*, and readies the waste materials for their excretion. The functions of *pāchana* and *vibhajana* should be considered in a secondary, supportive role to *jaṭharāgni*. The entire process is analogous to cooking a pot of rice over a wood stove (AH Śhā. 3/56).

The process of *sāra-kiṭṭa vibhajana* results in the *āhāra rasa* being divided into the two portions of *sāra*, nutrient portion, and *kiṭṭa*, the waste materials. The *sāra* is again subdivided into the *sthūla bhāga* (or *sthūla amśha*) and the *sūkṣhma bhāga* (or *sūkṣhma amśha*). Each of these subdivided portions is responsible for:

Sāra-kiṭṭa vibhajana	*Sthūla amśha*	*Sūkṣhma amśha*	*Mala amśha*
Explanation	Major fraction of beneficial nutrients	Minor fraction of beneficial nutrients	Waste products from *vibhajana* process
Nourishes	The immediate *dhātu*	The subsequent *dhātu*	Waste materials
Also called	*Sthāyi dhātu* *Poṣhya dhātu*	*Asthāyi dhātu* *Poṣhaka dhātu*	

This detailed explanation of *sāra-kiṭṭa vibhajana* is provided in the context of *āhāra pāka* (managed by *jaṭharāgni*) as well as all *dhātu pāka* (managed by *dhātvagnis*). The entire process of *vibhajana* goes on at both of the levels of *pāka* continuously. See Cha. Chi. 15/, BP Pū. 3/177.

The *sāra* generated by *jaṭharāgni* from *anna rasa* becomes *rasa dhātu*, the first of the seven supportive systems of the body (BP Pū. 3/172). It comes into the *hṛdaya* by the propulsive action of *samāna vāyu* (BP Pū. 3/175) and then moves throughout the body to support growth of subsequent *dhātus* by the circulatory action of *vyāna vāyu* (AH Sū. 12/6-7). More specifically, the *sthāyi*, or *sthūla amśha* of the newly formed *rasa dhātu* remains in its place while the *asthayi*, or *sūkṣhma amśha* of *rasa dhātu* moves through various *srotases* to nourish the subsequent *dhātus* (Cha. Vi. 5/3).

Suśhruta defines *rasa* in Su. Sū. 14/3 as:

यस्तेजोभूतः सारः परमसूक्ष्मः स रसः ।

सु. सू. १४।३

Yastejobhūtaḥ sāraḥ paramasūkṣhmaḥ sa rasaḥ |

Su. Sū. 14/3

The end of the *āhāra pāka* process is marked by *niṣhṭha pāka*, which is the final result, or *vipāka* as determined by the *āhāra dravya guṇa*. See Chapter three for a complete review of *vipāka*. And finally, the *kiṭṭa bhāga* of the digested food, is brought down by *samāna vāyu*, and then excreted by *apāna vāyu* (AH Sū. 12/9, BP Pū. 3/174).

Āhāra Pāka

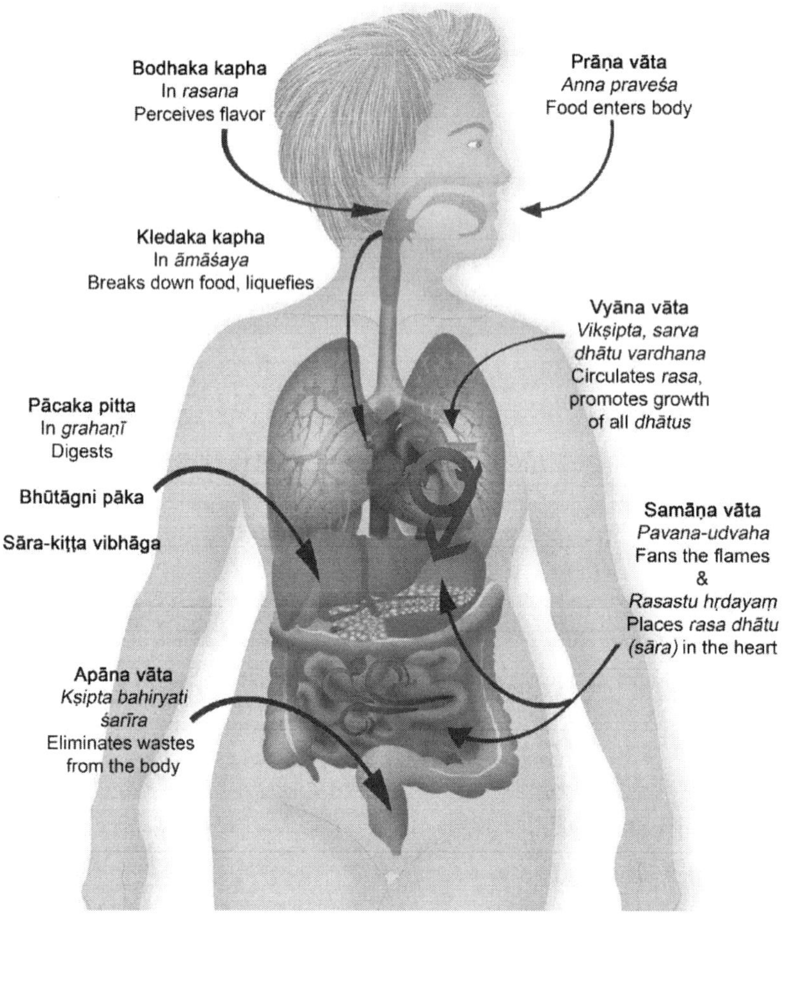

Step 3: Dhātu pariṇāma

The formation of *rasa dhātu* initiates the cycle of *dhātu pariṇāma*. This continues the processes of *sāra-kiṭṭa vibhāga* at the levels of the *dhātus* and is primarily managed by the *dhātvagnis* along with support from the *bhūtagnis*. More so than *jaṭharāgni pāka, dhātu pariṇāma* is constantly ongoing (Chakrapāṇi on Cha. Chi. 15/13) because it can take up to a month to convert any one meal into all of the subsequent *dhātus*. Each one of them requires a certain amount of processing time and all of them are working in their own individual forms concurrently.

It is during these conversion processes that the application of *samānya-viśheṣha* can be predominantly seen. As *āhāra rasa* is broken down and processed, its predominant *guṇas* will naturally be attracted to those *dhātus* having a similar nature, resulting in the increase of those *dhātus* (Cha. Śhā. 6/16-17).

For each of the *saptadhātus*, an individual form of *dhātvagni* exists to manage the conversion of the previous *dhātu's asthayi* (or *poṣhaka*) portion into the next *dhātu*. As part of this conversion process, a certain fraction of the received portion becomes the *kiṭṭa*, or waste material. At each *dhatu* level, one *dhātu* is formed and specific, minor *dhātumalas* are also generated. Additionally, each *dhātu* is capable of creating one or more other, independent tissues, called *upadhātus*. While each *upadhātu* is able to perform certain functions, they are incapable of producing any further *dhātus*. The entire process happens as demonstrated in the following diagram.

TEST YOURSELF

Learn, review and memorize key terms from this section.

dhātu pariṇāma ____________

āmāśhaya ____________

āhāra ____________

āhāra pāka ____________

āhāra rasa ____________

sāra ____________

kiṭṭā ____________

sāra-kiṭṭa vibhāga ____________

avasthā pāka ____________

madhura pāka ____________

amla pāka ____________

kaṭu pāka ____________

sthūla bhāga ____________

sūkṣhma bhāga ____________

sthāyi dhātu ____________

poṣhya dhātu ____________

asthāyi dhātu ____________

poṣhaka dhātu ____________

niṣhṭha pāka ____________

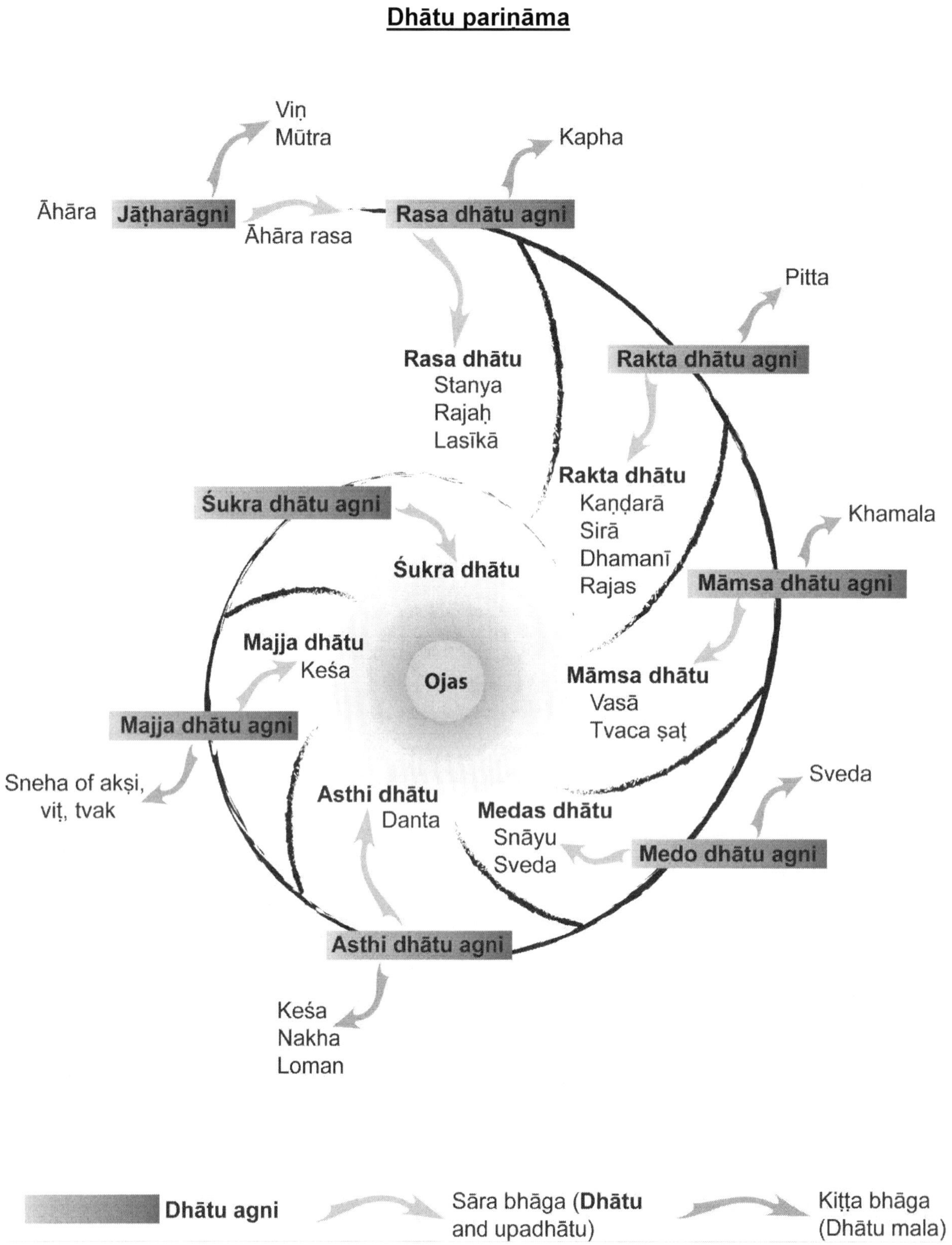
Dhātu pariṇāma
Viṇ
Mūtra
Kapha
Āhāra
Jāṭharāgni
Āhāra rasa
Rasa dhātu agni
Pitta
Rasa dhātu
Stanya
Rajaḥ
Lasīkā
Rakta dhātu agni
Rakta dhātu
Kaṇḍarā
Sirā
Dhamanī
Rajas
Khamala
Māmsa dhātu agni
Śukra dhātu agni
Śukra dhātu
Majja dhātu
Keśa
Ojas
Māmsa dhātu
Vasā
Tvaca ṣaṭ
Majja dhātu agni
Sneha of akṣi,
viṭ, tvak
Sveda
Asthi dhātu
Danta
Medas dhātu
Snāyu
Sveda
Medo dhātu agni
Asthi dhātu agni
Keśa
Nakha
Loman
Dhātu agni
Sāra bhāga (Dhātu and upadhātu)
Kiṭṭa bhāga (Dhātu mala)

OUTPUTS OF CONVERSION

Doṣhas: as dhātus or malas?

The processes that occur during *avasthā pāka* are the main contributors to the generation of all three *doṣhas*. The degree to which the *doṣhas* are generated invariably depends on the many factors which can influence the overall *pāka*. Although the *doṣhas* are by nature inclined to vitiate, they instead can function as *dhātus* and support a state of *sama*, or healthy homeostasis, when *pāka* is well done (Cha. Śhā. 6/18). Charaka reiterates this fact throughout the text that wholesome food is the main cause for *doṣhas* being converted to *dhātus* rather than *malas*.

Dhātus: Supportive tissues

The *saptadhātus* originate from *sāra* (*prasāda*) according to Cha. Sū. 28/4. Their level of health and strength completely depends on their inputs and the powers of conversion at each stage of processing. The *saptadhātus* will be explained in detail in Chapter eight.

Charaka also provides a detailed description of how each *dhātu* converts to the subsequent *dhātu* in Cha. Chi. 15/22-35.

Malas: Waste products

All forms of *malas* (BP Pū. 3/172-174) ultimately originate from *kiṭṭa* according to Cha. Sū. 28/4. The normal functioning of waste products is a sign of healthy digestive processes and is required to maintain normal homeostasis of the *saptadhātus*. Absence, reduction or increase of *malas* from their normal states generally indicate dysfunction and can provide insight into malfunctioning processes of *agni*. *Malas* will be discussed in detail in Chapter nine.

Āma

The term *āma* indicates *apakva*, which is formed by combining the prefix *a-* (not, negation) + *pakva* (ripe). *Āma* is the incompletely or improperly digested remnants that result from faulty *āhāra pāka*. Vāgbhaṭa specifies in AH Śhā. 3/52 that when the *grahaṇī* is weak, it allows incomplete, partially digested *āhāra rasa* to move into the *pakvāśhaya* before it is actually ready for further processing.

भुक्तमामाशये रुध्वा सा विपाच्य नयत्यधः
।
बलवत्यबला त्वन्नमाममेव विमुञ्चति ॥
अ. हृ. शा. ३।५२

Bhuktamāmāśhaye rudhvā sā vipāchya niyatyadhaḥ |
Balavatyabalā tvannamāmameva vimuñchati ||
AH Śhā. 3/52

The consumed food in the *āmāśhaya* undergoes proper *pāka* when *grahaṇī* is strong and able to hold it in place for the appropriate amount of time. However, when *grahaṇī* is weak, it releases the incompletely processed *āhāra pāka* into the *pakvāśhaya* before it is fully ready. This insufficiently or improperly digested material is called *āma*. See also AH Sū. 13/25-27.

Charaka provides another perspective on the formation of *āma* in Cha. Vi. 2/7-8. When a person indulges in specific causative factors listed in the reference, and then they eat too much and drink too much following the meal, it results in all three *doṣhas* becoming excessively aggravated. This disrupts the normal *āhāra pāka* resulting in *āma* that combines with the aggravated *doṣhas* resulting in states called *sāma vāta, sāma pitta and sāma kapha*. This is a more serious situation and its *lakṣhaṇas* will be discussed in later volumes in the context of *chikitsā*.

Vegas: Relieving reflexes

Finally, several of the *vegas* can be considered by-products of normal digestion. These *vegas* fall under the topic of *adhāraṇīya vega*, which are the natural urges of the body, or relieving reflexes which should never be withheld when they manifest. Normally, these are covered within the context of Svastha Vṛtta in all major classical works. In this textbook they are mentioned here in relation to normal digestion and will be covered in detail in Volume three.

Adhāraṇīya vegas that are related to digestion include:

Mūtra	Urine
Purișha	Feces
Vāta	Flatus
Udgāra	Belching
Kșhut	Hunger
Pipāsa	Thirst

The presence of these *vegas* should be understood within normal and abnormal limits and manifestations. Whenever the urge for any of these presents itself, it should be relieved as quickly and appropriately as possible. Withholding these urges, as well as forcefully manifesting them, can result in various unhealthy conditions.

TEST YOURSELF

Learn, review and memorize key terms from this section.

āma

apakva

vega

mūtra

purișha

vāta

udgāra

kșhut

pipāsa

Chapter 5: Review

ADDITIONAL READING

Read and review the references listed below to expand your understanding of the concepts in this chapter. Write down the date that you complete your reading for each. Remember that consistent repetition is the best way to learn. Plan to read each reference at least once now and expect to read it again as you continue your studies.

References marked with (skim) can be read quickly and do not require commentary review.

CLASSICS		1st read	2nd read
Charaka	Cha. Sū. 12/ Cha. Sū. 13/65-69 Cha. Sū. 28/3-4, commentary Cha. Vi. 2/7-8 Cha. Vi. 6/12 Cha. Śhā. 6/14-18 Cha. Chi. 15/3-52		
Suśhruta	Su. Sū. 14/10-14 Su. Sū. 21/9-10 Su. Sū. 35/27		
Aṣhṭāṅga Hṛdaya	AH Sū. 12/3-17 AH Sū. 13/25-27 AH Śhā. 3/51-72		
Bhāva Prakāśha	BP Pū. 3/ BP Pū. 5/103		

JOURNALS & CURRENT RESOURCES

Ayurvedic Concepts of Metabolism – Dhatuparinama, Dr. ABHILASH. M. MD (Ay) (skim)

QUESTIONS & ANSWERS

Record your questions for this chapter here for further research and discussion.

Question:

Answer:

Question:

Answer:

Question:

Answer:

SELF-ASSESSMENT

1. What is the main, primary function of normal *agni*?
   a. Complexion
   b. Cooking food
   c. Eyesight
   d. Life and vitality
   e. Physical strength

2. Suśhruta states that *pitta* and *agni* can be considered the same when
   a. Assimilation and elimination are perfect
   b. *Dravya* affects one but not the other
   c. *Pitta* loses its *drava guṇa* and becomes *rūkṣha*
   d. *Pitta* performs the role of *agni*
   e. None of the above

3. Which *agni* is responsible for the transformation of the gross elements?
   a. *Bhūtāgni*
   b. *Dhātvagni*
   c. *Jāṭharāgni*
   d. *Kāyāgni*
   e. *Koṣhṭhāgni*

4. Which synonym of agni indicates that it is responsible for growth of the body?
   a. *Antarāgni*
   b. *Dehāgni*
   c. *Jāṭharāgni*
   d. *Kāyāgni*
   e. *Koṣhṭhāgni*

5. What is not a function of *Jāṭharāgni*?
   a. Cooking consumed food
   b. Normal and abnormal states of all *agnis*
   c. Production of *āhāra rasa*
   d. Separation of food into each of the *pañcha mahābhūtas*
   e. Separation of *sāra* and *kiṭṭā*

6. Which state indicates healthy or normal *agni*?
   a. *Koṣhṭhāgni*
   b. *Mandāgni*
   c. *Samāgni*
   d. *Tīkṣhṇāgni*
   e. *Viṣhamāgni*

7. Which state of *agni* is capable of cooking food properly only some of the time?
   a. *Koṣhṭhāgni*
   b. *Mandāgni*
   c. *Samāgni*
   d. *Tīkṣhṇāgni*
   e. *Viṣhamāgni*

8. Which of the following is not one of the *āhāra parināma bhāvas*?
   a. *Agni*
   b. *Kāla*
   c. *Kleda*
   d. *Uṣhmā*
   e. *Vāyu*

9. Which analogy classically explains the internal processing of nutrients that ultimately form the body?
   a. A bird that selects specific food items and brings them to its nest for consumption
   b. A wheel constantly turned by a flow of water
   c. The irrigation of a large field of crops by creating large and small channels to spread the water throughout
   d. The transformation of milk through various stages into its final form (curd, butter, ghee)
   e. All of the above

10. Which of the following is a process of *dhātu pariṇāma*?
    a. Consumption of *āhāra*
    b. Initiation of *prāṇa vāyu*, *bodhaka kapha*, *kledaka kapha*
    c. *Sāra-kiṭṭa vibhāga*
    d. Transformation of *āhāra rasa* into *dhātus*
    e. All of the above

CRITICAL THINKING

1. Looking at the *dravyas* mentioned by Charaka for *koṣhṭha parīkṣha*, do you recognize any that you have personally experienced to be effective in yourself or anyone else? If so, describe an experience.

2. Explain how *dravya prabhāva* or *dravya vicitraprabhāva* can have its effect using the information provided in this chapter and any classical references (with citations).

3. Explain and define the concept of *āma* using classical citations.

4. Describe the process of *dhātu pariṇāma* from Charaka's perspective in Chi. 15-22-35. Include *dhātus*, *malas*, *upadhātus* and *dhātumalas*. Which *nyāya(s)* could be involved?

5. What role does the *koṣhṭha* play in *dhātu pariṇāma*? How might different types of *koṣhṭha* influence the final outcomes of *dhātu pariṇāma*?

6. How does normal *āhāra pāka* produce *doṣhas*? How does it produce *dhātus*?

7. Create a chart that shows the relationship between *koṣhṭha bheda*, states of *agni* and *doṣhas*.

8. Using the diagram of *āhāra pāka* in this chapter, identify the roles of the *āhāra pariṇāma bhāvas* in the diagram.

Chapter 6 : Dhātu sāmya

KEY TERMS

agni	dhātu vaiṣhamya	poṣhaṇa	śhamana
āhāra	doṣha prakopa	prakopa	sāmya
ahita	dūṣhya	praśhamana	sañchaya
chaya	hita	rasa	vaiṣhamya
dhāraṇa	kopa	sam	vikāra
dhātu	kṣhaya	sama	vṛddhi
dhātu sāmya	lakṣhaṇa	śhama	

Dhātu sāmya is the purpose and ultimate goal of Āyurveda. It refers to the state of natural homeostasis, or personal, individual equilibrium where a person is in a state of health. Often, this may be referred to as a state of balance, which is partly true at a very simplistic level. It must be understood that balance in this context does not indicate equal measure, but rather an individual's distinct state of being which maintains their normal health and function. The classics refer to this as the *prakṛta* state of the three *doṣhas, vāta, pitta* and *kapha*. The homeostasis achieved by all three operating in their *prakṛta* state is ultimately one's *prakṛti*, or the unique baseline of one's state of being which is standard to themselves only.

Maintaining a permanent, regular state of *dhātu sāmya* is generally difficult from all practical angles. There are a large number of factors which influence *dhātu sāmya* and they may be uncontrollable or controllable, external or internal, etc. Because a certain amount of fluctuation in the *doṣhas* is to be expected, the goal of reaching and maintaining *dhātu sāmya* becomes a constantly moving target.

NIRUKTI & PARIBHĀṢHĀ

To better understand the phrase *dhātu sāmya*, first review the etymology and definitions of each term.

Nirukti

The term *dhātu* derives from the Sanskrit *dhātu* √ *dhā*, which indicates:

√ dhā

dhāraṇa
concentration, the ability to carry, wear or bear

puṣhṭi
growth, increase, comfort, nourishment

'dhāraṇaṁ dharanam' (Śha. Ka.)
'a support, prop or stay which holds, bears, preserves, maintains or protects,' (*Śhabda Kalpa Druma*)

In the scope of Āyurveda, *dhātu* refers to that which supports, nourishes and provides the ability to hold, bear, preserve, maintain, protect and nourish.

Vāgbhaṭa defines *dhātu* in the Hemādri commentary of AH Sū. 1/13 as:

शरीरधारणात् धातवः

अ. हृ. सू. १।१३ (हेमाद्रि)

Śharīra-dhāraṇāt dhātavaḥ

AH Sū. 1/13 (Hemādri)

Dhātu is that which does *dhāraṇa* (provides support, holds up, maintains, etc) to *śharīra* (the body which has the tendency to break down or decay).

When the *tridoṣhas, saptadhātus* and *trimalas* are functioning to provide this type of support to the body, they can be considered as *dhātus*. See Chapter four for an explanation of how the *tridoṣhas* can behave.

The term *sāmya* derives from the Sanskrit *dhātu* √ *sam*, which indicates:

√ sam	*samārtha* (*samā*) same, equal, similar, like, equivalent, having the right measure, regular, normal, right, equally distant from extremes
	prakṛṣhṭa drawn forth, protracted, long (in space and time), superior, distinguished, eminent
	saṅgata consistent, compatible
	śhobhana good, nice, splendid

Sāmya indicates that something is in its right or proper state. Because of this, it will likely experience the beneficial effects of that state, such as extended life span, and generally being good.

Paribhāṣhā

Charaka defines *dhātu sāmya* in several instances:

कार्यं धातुसाम्यमिहोच्यते ।
धातुसाम्यक्रिया चोक्ता तन्त्रस्यास्य प्रयोजनम् ॥

च. सू. १।५३

Kāryaṁ dhātusāmyamihochyate |
Dhātusāmyakriyā choktā tantrasyāsya prayojanam ||

Cha. Sū. 1/53

Dhātu sāmya is the *kārya* (what should be done, the job at hand). The *kriyā* (therapeutic actions) which are applied to achieve *dhātu sāmya* are the purpose (goal) of this science.

कार्यं धातुसाम्यं, तस्य लक्षणं विकारोपशमः ।

च. वि. ८।८९

Kāryaṁ dhātusāmyaṁ, tasya lakṣhaṇaṁ vikāropaśhamaḥ |

Cha. Vi. 8/88-89

The *kārya* (what should be done, the job at hand, responsibility of the Vaidya) is (to achieve) *dhātu sāmya*. This (effect) is to be understood by the *lakṣhaṇas* (signs and symptoms) of *upaśhama* (relief from, absence of) *vikāra* (disease).

In Cha. Sū. 20/9, it is also stated that all three *doṣhas, vāta, pitta* and *kapha*, reside in *sarva śharīra* (the entire body). While in their healthy state, they have the capacity to bring about positive health outcomes such as *upachaya* (growth), *bala* (strength), *varṇa* (complexion), *prasāda* (happiness), etc. Yet when they are not in their healthy state, they themselves are the causes for *vikṛti* (deviation from normal health) and *vikāra* (disease). Notably, this explanation has been provided by Charaka in the main chapter on the full classification of diseases in *Sūtrasthāna*. This explanation prefaces the disorder classification to remind the reader that the source of disease is largely due to internal causes.

Throughout the classics, the concept of *dhātu sāmya* is frequently reiterated to remind the reader that it is the purpose and goal of Āyurveda. Review these additional references as examples: Cha. Sū. 12/8, Cha. Sū. 12/13, Cha. Sū. 18/48, Cha. Vi. 1/5, Cha. Śhā. 6/4, Cha. Śhā. 6/6-7, Cha. Śhā. 6/18, BP Pū. 3/100-101, BP Pū. 4/89.

The same meaning of *sāmya* can also be expressed through the similar terms of *sama, samā* and *samī*. These can be grammatical variants of the same Sanskrit *dhātu*.

TEST YOURSELF

Learn, review and memorize key terms from this section.

dhātu

---

dhāraṇa

---

sam

---

sāmya

---

dhātu sāmya

THE OPPOSITE STATE: DHĀTU VAIṢHAMYA

When *dhātu sāmya* is not in effect, its opposite becomes predominant, in varying degrees. This state of disequilibrium of the *doṣhas, dhātus* and *malas* is termed *dhātu vaiṣhamya*.

In this state, the *doṣhas* behave as they are inclined to, as vitiators (*dūṣhyanti iti doṣhaḥ*). When they attain this state, they have the potential to cause damage to the *saptadhātus* and *malas*, and when that occurs, these normal tissues and waste products take on the role of *dūṣhyas*, or that which is being vitiated. In the early stages of *dhātu vaiṣhamya*, full-fledged disease has usually not yet formed, so it becomes somewhat of a gray zone in between strong, obvious health and clear-cut illness.

Charaka defines *dhātu vaiṣhamya* as:

कार्ययोनिर्धातुवैषम्यं, तस्य लक्षणं
विकारागमः ।

च. वि. ८।८८

Kāryayonirdhātvaiṣhamyaṁ, tasya
lakṣhaṇaṁ vikārāgamaḥ |

Cha. Vi. 8/88

Kārya yoni (the source, cause or reason for what should be done) is *dhātu vaiṣhamya*. It should be known or understood by the *lakṣhaṇas* (signs and symptoms) of *vikāra* (disease) as given throughout this entire treatise.

TEST YOURSELF

Learn, review and memorize key terms from this section.

dhātu vaiṣhamya

---

dūṣhya

---

lakṣhaṇa

---

vikāra

CAUSES FOR DHĀTU SĀMYA

Ultimately, the factors which are primarily responsible for *dhātu sāmya* relate to nourishment by using the right food for the right person at the right time. *Āhāra, agni*, and *rasa* are the top three contributors to *dhātu sāmya* and are repeatedly mentioned in classical literature to remind the reader of their priority and importance.

Āhāra

Āhāra can be considered *hita*, healthy or beneficial, or *ahita*, detrimental to health. *Hita āhāra* is a definite reason for consistent, good health and this point is expressed by Charaka in many instances.

हिताहारोपयोग एकएव पुरुषवृद्धिकरो
भवति, अहिताहारोपयोगः
पुनर्व्याधिनिमित्तमिति ॥

च. सू. २५।३१

Hitāhāropayoga ekaeva
puruṣhavṛddhikaro bhavati,
ahitāhāropayogaḥ
punarvyadhinimittamiti ||

Cha. Sū. 25/31

Hita āhāra upayoga (following the rules of taking wholesome food) is the cause for growth of *puruṣha* (a human being). *Ahita āhāra upayoga* (consuming food which is unwholesome) is the reason for repetitive disease.

समांश्चैव शरीरधातून् प्रकृतौ स्थापयति
विषमांश्च समीकरोतीत्येतद्धितं विद्धि,
विपरीतं त्वहितमिति; ।

च. सू. २५।३३

Samāṁśhchaiva śharīradhātun prakṛtau
sthāpayati viṣhamāṁśhcha
samīkarotītyetaddhitaṁ viddhi,
viparītaṁ tvahitamiti; |

Cha. Sū. 25/33

Hita is that which is capable of producing *sama śharīra, sama dhātu* and *prakṛti sthāpayati* (maintaining an inherent state of health), and can support eliminating the disturbed or abnormal [*doṣhas*] when they are in an unhealthy state. The opposite of this is *ahita*.

The statement above is recorded as coming directly from Punarvasu Ātreya. He also adds that these are the most complete definitions of *hita* and *ahita*.

Additional references reiterating the same point can be found in Cha. Sū. 28/3 (end) and Cha. Sū. 28/5.

Agni

Proper, healthy functioning of *agni* on all levels is required to convert *hita āhāra* to produce *dhātu sāmya*. Review the statements listed at the beginning of Chapter five for Charaka's perspective on how important healthy *agni* is to life. Then compare Vāgbhaṭa's opinion from AH Śhā. 3/54:

यदन्नं देहधात्वोजोबलवर्णादिपोषणम् ।
तत्राग्निर्हेतुराहारान्न ह्यपक्वाद्रसादयः ॥

अ. हृ. शा. ३।५४

Yadānaṁ
dehadhātvojobalavarṇādipoṣhaṣham |
Tatrāgnirheturāhārānna
hyapakvādrasādayaḥ ||

AH Śhā. 3/54

That food, which does *poṣhaṇa* (promotes nourishment) of the *deha* (growing body), *dhātus* (supportive tissues), *ojas* (resistance to disease), *bala* (strength), *varṇa* (complexion), etc, is actually effective because of *agni*. *Apakva* [*āhāra*] (undigested food) cannot do this for *rasa*, etc (*dhātus*).

Rasa

The proper use of the *ṣhaḍ rasa* is one more key to *dhātu sāmya*. This usage must be considered within the context of *āhāra* and *agni* because all three are interrelated. In Cha. Vi. 1/4, the importance of *rasa* is stated as:

ते सम्यगुपयुज्यमानाः शरीरं यापयन्ति,
मिथ्योपयुज्यमानास्तु खलु
दोषप्रकोपायोपकल्पन्ते ॥

च. वि. १।४

Te samyagupayugyamānāḥ śharīraṁ yāpayanti, mithyopayujyamānāstu khalu doṣhaprakopāyopakalpante ||

Cha. Vi. 1/4

These (six flavors) provide the base (ie, maintain) *śharīra* when they are used properly. Incorrect usage results in *doṣha prakopa* (aggravation of the *doṣhas*).

All three of these factors, *āhāra, agni* and *rasa*, are key to supporting *dhātu sāmya*. However, Punarvasu Ātreya reminds Agniveśha in Cha. Sū. 28/7 that just because an individual consumes *hita āhāra* regularly, that will not prevent disease all the time. *Hita āhāra* alone is also not capable of curing every disorder. There are many additional factors which contribute to disease, and often they cannot be controlled. Read the full discussion in Cha. Sū. 28/7 for a thorough explanation.

Additional important factors for the maintenance of *dhātu sāmya* are mentioned in Cha. Śhā. 6/8-11. These will be covered in detail later in separate chapters.

TEST YOURSELF

Learn, review and memorize key terms from this section.

āhāra __________

hita __________

ahita __________

agni __________

poṣhaṇa __________

rasa __________

doṣha prakopa __________

CHANGES IN STATES

The same reasons which have been listed above to help maintain *dhātu sāmya* can also be the cause for *vaiṣhamya* when not used appropriately. The *doṣhas, dhātus* and *malas* can all experience a state of *vaiṣhamya* independently or in combinations. *Vaiṣhamya* refers to disequilibrium, and this may present as any deviation from normal levels. This may manifest as a decrease or an increase in quantity and/or quality. The terms used to describe these states include:

Sama	normal, healthy state
Vaiṣhamya	*vi* (a prefix, meaning deviation from) + *sāmya* (normal, healthy state)
Kṣhaya	decrease in quantity and/or qualities in *doṣha, dhātu* or *mala*

Vṛddhi	increase in quantity and/or qualities in *doṣha, dhātu* or *mala*
Sañchaya	a mild increase in *doṣha* only, also called *chaya*
Prakopa	a great increase in *doṣha* only, also called *kopa*
Praśhamana	return to normal state in *doṣha* only, also called *śhamana*, or *śhama*

The change in state from *dhātu sāmya* to *dhātu vaiṣhamya* is ultimately due to too much or too little nourishment of one or more *dhātus*. *Samānya-viśheṣha siddhānta* is responsible for combining things of similar nature. It also reduces things where they are dissimilar by having the effect of cancelling each other out. This is easiest to understand through the presentation of *guṇa*, although it actually happens at the *mahābhūta* level of the *dravya*.

The unique profile of any individual has certain levels of each *mahābhūta* that are within *dhātu sāmya* range. This can be considered an individual's normal, healthy baseline. Deviation from this baseline, either above or below, results in *dhātu vaiṣhamya.* This is why the classics explain that the very same things (foods, activities, etc) are both the cause for good health and disease, when used correctly or incorrectly.

The instigating cause for *dhātu vaiṣhamya* can come from any source which is capable of fluctuating or destabilizing an individual's state of *dhātu sāmya*. Most often, this initiates with *āhāra, agni* or *rasa* (or a combination). It should be understood that the general rules which promote a healthy state of any *doṣha, dhātu* or *mala* can be broken to create a causative factor for *dhātu vaiṣhamya*. Each of these possibilities will not be listed exhaustively as they can be infinite. Specific factors which support or hamper the *doṣhas, dhātus* and *malas* are listed in various chapters throughout this volume and the other textbooks in this series in the context of understanding each concept.

TEST YOURSELF

Learn, review and memorize key terms from this section.

dhātu sāmya

dhātu vaiṣhamya

sama

vaiṣhamya

kṣhaya

vṛddhi

sañchaya

chaya

prakopa

kopa

praśhamana

śhamana

śhama

Chapter 6: Review

ADDITIONAL READING

Read and review the references listed below to expand your understanding of the concepts in this chapter. Write down the date that you complete your reading for each. Remember that consistent repetition is the best way to learn. Plan to read each reference at least once now and expect to read it again as you continue your studies.

References marked with (skim) can be read quickly and do not require commentary review.

CLASSICS		1st read	2nd read
Charaka	Cha. Sū. 1/53 Cha. Sū. 12/8 Cha. Sū. 12/13 Cha. Sū. 18/48 Cha. Sū. 20/9 Cha. Sū. 25/30-33 Cha. Sū. 28/3-7 Cha. Sū. 28/30 Cha. Vi. 1/4-5 Cha. Vi. 8/88-89 Cha. Śhā. 6/4-18		
Suśhruta			
Aṣhṭāṅga Hṛdaya	AH Sū. 1/13 AH Sa. 3/50-54		
Bhāva Prakāśha	BP Pū. 3/100-101 BP Pū. 4/89		

JOURNALS & CURRENT RESOURCES

QUESTIONS & ANSWERS

Record your questions for this chapter here for further research and discussion.

Question:

Answer:

Question:

Answer:

Question:

Answer:

SELF-ASSESSMENT

1. Which of the following best describes *dhātu sāmya*?
   a. Constantly moving target
   b. Individual state of equilibrium
   c. Personal homeostasis
   d. *Prākṛta*
   e. All of the above

2. Which of the following best describes *dhātu vaiṣhamya*?
   a. *Dhātu* acts as a *dūṣhya*
   b. Individual state of disequilibrium
   c. That which is being vitiated
   d. *Vikṛti*
   e. All of the above

3. Correct nourishment at the correct time for the right person is the main reason for?
   a. *Dhātu sāmya*
   b. *Dhātu vaiṣhamya*
   c. *Prakṛti*
   d. *Vikṛti*
   e. All of the above

4. *Hita āhāra* is responsible for?
   a. *Dhātu sāmya*
   b. Growth of *puruṣha*
   c. *Prakṛti sthāpayati*
   d. *Sama śharīra*
   e. All of the above

5. What are the top three contributors to *dhātu sāmya*?
   a. *Āhāra*, *agni*, and *rasa*
   b. *Doṣha*, *dhātu*, *mala*
   c. *Kārya*, *lakṣhaṇa*, *kriyā*
   d. *Vāta*, *pitta* and *kapha*
   e. None of the above

6. What is *hita āhāra* capable of doing?
   a. Creating consistently good health
   b. *Prakṛti sthāpayati*
   c. *Sama śharīra*
   d. Supporting the elimination of abnormal or vitiated *doṣhas*
   e. All of the above

7. Vāgbhaṭa's opinion on food from AH Śhā. 3/54 states all of the following, except:
   a. *Poṣhaṇa* creates *apakva āhāra*
   b. *Poṣhaṇa* creates *deha*
   c. *Poṣhaṇa* creates *ojas* and *bala*
   d. *Poṣhaṇa* creates the *dhātus*
   e. All of the above

8. The proper use of the *ṣhaḍ rasa* is key to *dhātu sāmya*. Which of the following occurs first with incorrect usage?
   a. *Dhātu vaiṣhamya*
   b. *Doṣha prakopa*
   c. *Dūṣhyas*
   d. *Vikṛti*
   e. All of the above

9. Punarvasu Ātreya reminds Agniveśha in Cha. Sū. 28/7 that just because an individual consumes *hita āhāra* regularly, it will not prevent disease all the time. What are the other causes of disease?
   a. Failure of the intellect
   b. Individual resistance to disease
   c. Seasonal abnormalities
   d. Unwholesome use of the senses
   e. All of the above

10. Punarvasu Ātreya reminds Agniveśha in Cha. Sū. 28/7 that there are individual causes for disease. Which of the following does he state as individual cause?
   a. Excess quantity
   b. Location or environment
   c. Time or potency of the vitiating combination
   d. Weak body and/or mind
   e. All of the above

CRITICAL THINKING

1. Which components of *śharīra* can the concepts of *dhātu sāmya* and *dhātu vaiṣhamya* encompass?

2. In changing state from *dhātu sāmya* to *dhātu vaiṣhamya* what are the most common causes? What is actually responsible for the change in state, and why?

3. Draw a graph (line chart or area chart) showing the interaction between *dhātu sāmya*, *dhātu vaiṣhamya* and the changes of states that can occur (*kṣhaya, vṛddhi*, etc).

4. When changes in state occur in any of the components of *śharīra*, explain how the *guṇa* and *karma* of the components are involved. What is the underlying basis of the change?

5. Why is *samānya-viśheṣha* responsible for *vṛddhi-kṣhaya*?

6. Fill in the blanks:

   Dhātu sāmya is a state of ______________ while *dhātu vaiṣhamya* is ______________.

Chapter 7 : Doṣha

KEY TERMS			
āhāra	kāraṇa	prākṛta doṣha lakṣhaṇas	tarpaka kapha
ālocaka pitta	karma	prākṛta kapha	trividha kāraṇa
apāna vāta	kledaka kapha	prākṛta pitta	udāna vāta
artha	kṣhaya	prākṛta vāta	vaikṛta
avalambaka kapha	kṣhīna doṣha lakṣhaṇas	prāṇa vāta	vaiṣhamya doṣha
bhrājaka pitta	lakṣhaṇa	rañjaka pitta	vāta kṣhaya
bodhaka kapha	pāchaka pitta	rasa	vāta sthāna
doṣha bheda	pañcha kapha	sādhaka pitta	vāta vṛddhi
doṣha sthāna	pañcha pitta	sama doṣha	vihāra
kāla	pañcha vāta	samāṇa vāta	vṛddha doṣha lakṣhaṇas
kapha kṣhaya	pitta kṣhaya	śhleṣhaka kapha	vṛddhi
kapha sthāna	pitta sthāna	sthāna	vyāna vāta
kapha vṛddhi	pitta vṛddhi		
	prākṛta		

The fundamentals of the *tridoṣha siddhānta* have been covered in Chapter four. Here, those basic concepts will be expanded to include specific information on how the *doṣhas* function in the human body. This begins with an overview and is followed by the details for each *doṣha*.

HOW DOṢHAS FUNCTION IN THE BODY

At any given point of time, each *doṣha* will be in one or more of three general states and in certain locations. There are always general and specific causes and reasons for *doṣhas* to be in any given state, and in certain locations. These causes are derived from too much or too little association with *guṇas* which represent the *pañchabhautika* composition of *dravyas*. Ultimately, they influence the physical body through *samānya-viṣhesa*. The outcome of all of the situations and the ability to understand and identify how a *doṣha* is functioning in the body is based on assessing *lakṣhaṇas*. Recall that a *lakṣhaṇa* is a characteristic, quality, sign or symptom. It is the detectable representation of a specific *guṇa* or *karma*, which manifests in the human body and may be assessed through a number of methods.

The classics are replete with *lakṣhaṇas* that thoroughly describe the wide range of functions of the *doṣhas* in the body. In advanced study, *lakṣhaṇas* are also used to describe pathological sequences and processes that may or may not manifest as full-blown disease. The term *lakṣhaṇa* can indicate any feature, characteristic or notable quality or action that is seen in any given individual, presentation or state.

Here, the classical *lakṣhaṇas* are compiled and organized according to each *doṣha*. They are grouped into sections based on how *doṣhas* function in the body. First, the *sthānas*, or specific locations of each *doṣha* are described. Remember that even though *doṣhas* are said to reside in these locations, they actually move all over the body while maintaining a special affinity to these primary "home" areas (AH Sū. 1/7). Next, the general and specific causes for changes in states of *doṣhas* are listed. These include reasons for a *doṣha* to attain a state of *kṣhaya* (decrease) and *vṛddhi* (increase). This is followed by the *doṣha*'s *lakṣhaṇas* in each of those states.

Finally, the *doṣha bheda* are listed along with their *lakṣhaṇas*. These descriptions include specific behaviors, and especially functions and responsibilities of each of the *doṣha bheda*. Review the diagram at the end of this section to understand how the *doṣhas'* functions are organized in this chapter.

To help develop an understanding of the *doṣhas*, their functions in the body, and how to recognize them, Charaka provides wonderful analogies in Cha. Sū. 12/. The entire chapter is dedicated to drawing similarities between the representations of the *doṣhas* in the external world and their internal behavior. These analogies are possible through the application of *loka-samya puruṣha siddhānta*.

States of doṣhas

Cha. Śhā. 6/4-5 provides a good introduction to the states of *doṣhas* and their influence on the state of health. When in their healthy state, the *doṣhas* support the body, but in any other state they are the causes of disease and destruction of the body. The *doṣhas* can be in a state of *vṛddhi* (increased state) or *hrāsa*, better known as *kṣhaya* (decreased state). Both *vṛddhi* and *kṣhaya* fall under *vaiṣhamya*.

The two primary states of *doṣhas* are:

गतिश्च द्विविधा दृष्टा प्राकृती वैकृती च या ॥
च. सू. १७।११५

Gatiśhcha dvividhā dṛṣhṭā prākṛtī vaikṛtī cha yā ||

Cha. Sū. 17/115

Doṣhas can be see in two states - *prākṛta* (normal) and *vaikṛta* (abnormal).

In their *prākṛta* state, *doṣhas* behave in only one way. They act normally and support the healthy functioning of the body. However, in their *vaikṛta* state, they may behave in several different ways. These are described as:

क्षयः स्थानं च वृद्धिश्च दोषाणां त्रिविधा गतिः ।

च. सू. १७।१११.५

Kṣhayaḥ sthānaṁ cha vṛddhiśhcha doṣhāṇāṁ trividhā gatiḥ |

Cha. Sū. 17/111.5

The three ways that *doṣhas* can move, go or be include *kṣhaya* (decrease), *sthāna* (normal, stable) and *vṛddhi* (increase).

In order for a *doṣha* to change its state from *prākṛta* to *vaikṛta*, it must have a specific reason to do so. These reasons are explained in a general way as:

समानगुणाभ्यासो हि धातूनां
वृद्धिकारणमिति ॥

च. सू. १२।५

Samānaguṇābhyāso hi dhātūnāṁ vṛddhikāraṇamiti ||

Cha. Sū. 12/5

Abhyāsa (Regular, continuous usage) of (*dravyas* having) *samāna guṇa* (the same or similar *guṇa*) as the *dhātus* is the *kāraṇa* (cause) for *vṛddhi* (increase).

प्रकोपणविपर्ययो हि धातूनां
प्रशमकरणमिति ॥

च. सू. १२।६

Prakopaṇaviparyayo hi dhātūnāṁ praśhamakaraṇamiti ||

Cha. Sū. 12/6

Viparyaya (the opposite) of *prakopa* (the state of aggravation) is the *kāraṇa* (cause) for *praśhamana* (return to normal state) of the *dhātus*.

Recognizing states of doṣhas

The key to recognizing, assessing and understanding the movement and changes of the *doṣhas* lies in one's ability to identify *lakṣhaṇas* properly and interpret their meanings. The foundations for these skills begin here with the core concepts of the mechanics of the *dosas*. Their mastery can take decades of practice and continued study.

Charaka explains the general rules for recognizing states of *doṣhas* as:

दोषाः प्रवृद्धाः स्वं लिङ्गं दर्शयन्ति यथाबलम् ।
क्षीणा जहति लिङ्गं स्वं, समाः स्वं कर्म कुर्वते ॥

च. सू. १७।६२

Doṣhāḥ pravṛddhāḥ svaṁ liṅgaṁ darśhayanti yathābalam |
Kṣhīṇā jahati liṅgaṁ svaṁ, samāḥ svaṁ karma kurvate ||

Cha. Sū. 17/62

Pravṛddha doṣhas (*doṣhas* in a state of *vṛddhi*) are seen by their own *liṅga*, or *lakṣhaṇas* (characteristics) according to their strength. *Kṣhīṇa doṣhas* (*doṣhas* in a state of *kṣhaya*) give up their own *liṅga*, or *lakṣhaṇas* (their characteristics become absent). And those in a state of *sama* perform their *karma* (actions, behaviors) normally.

Charaka elaborates on this in Cha. Sū. 18/52-53 by stating that *kṣhīṇa doṣhas* can be known in two ways. Their normal behaviors and activities can be reduced, or their opposite behaviors and activities may increase.

Vāgbhaṭa provides additional insight on how to recognize states of *chaya* and *prakopa* by defining them clearly.

Definition of chaya

चयो वृद्धिः स्वधाम्न्येव प्रद्वेषो वृद्धिहेतुषु ॥
विपरीतगुणेच्छा च

अ. हृ. सू. १२।२२

Chayo vṛddhiḥ svadhāmnyeva pradveṣho vṛddhihetuṣhu ||
Viparītaguṇechchhā cha

AH Sū. 12/22

The state of *chaya* (mild increase of *doṣha*) is seen when the *doṣha* undergoes increase in its own (*sthāna, guṇa, karma*) in ways where it would otherwise be normal. It results in a natural disinterest for things which cause the unhealthy, increased state and an inclination towards good (healthy) things of opposite nature.

Definition of kopa

कोपस्तून्मार्गगामिता । लिङ्गानां दर्शनं स्वेषामस्वास्थ्यं रोगसम्भवः ॥

अ. हृ. सू. १२।२३

Kopastūnmārgagāmitā |
Liṅgānāṁ darśhanaṁ sveṣhāmasvāsthyaṁ rogasambhavaḥ ||

AH Sū. 12/23

The state of *kopa* (great increase of *doṣha*) is seen when the *doṣha* moves out of its own normal location and into other places in the body. It makes itself known by displaying its own characteristics, inducing a feeling of *asvasthya* (general ill-health), and presenting early signs and symptoms of disease.

TEST YOURSELF

Learn, review and memorize key terms from this section.

lakṣhaṇa

---

prākṛta

vaikṛta

kṣhaya

sthāna

vṛddhi

DOṢHA VṚDDHI AND KṢHAYA KĀRAṆA

Many *kāraṇa* (general and specific causes) have been listed in the classics as reasons for *doṣhas* to change their state from *sama* to *vṛddhi* (increased), or from *sama* to *kṣhaya* (decreased). These are presented in different ways by various authors, usually within the context of each topic.

Suśhruta provides the general rule for the causes of aggravation for the *doṣhas* in Su. Sū. 15/13. He states that their increase in human beings is the result of *upasevana* (excessive, regular usage) of similar substances. Anything which is similar by its *guṇa, karma*, or *pañchabhautika* composition has the ability to accumulate the same in the body. *Bhāva Prakāśha* elaborates this point to include the influence of seasons on diet and regimens in BP Pū. 5/326.

The specific causes can be categorized into the following, and references can be found as listed below:

Kārana for *doṣha vṛddhi* and *kṣhaya* Causes for increase and decrease of *doṣhas*	Charaka	Suśhruta	Vāgbhaṭa	Bhāvamiśhra
Āhāra Food, meals, dietary preferences		Su. Sū. 21/19, 21, 23, 25		BP Pū. 5/325-326, 7(VII)/41-47
Rasa Predominant flavors and tastes	Cha. Vi. 1/7			
Vihāra Lifestyle activities, habits				
Tri-vidha kāraṇa The three general causes (for disease)	Cha. Sū. 1/54, Sū. 11/43		AH Sū. 12/34-35	
→ *Kāla (ṛtu)* Subtype 1: Time (seasons)	Cha. Sū. 11/42	Su. Sū. 21/20, 22, 24	AH Sū. 12/24	BP Pū. 5/325-326
→ *Artha* Subtype 2: Sense organ activity	Cha. Sū. 11/37-38		AH Sū. 12/36-37	
→ *Karma* Subtype 3: Actions (of 3 types)	Cha. Sū. 11/39-40		AH Sū. 12/40-42	

Charaka lists the specific *prakopa kāraṇa* for *vāta* in Cha. Chi. 28/15-19.

TEST YOURSELF

Learn, review and memorize key terms from this section.

kāraṇa

āhāra

rasa

vihāra

tri-vidha kāraṇa

kāla

artha

karma

SAMA DOṢHA

This section provides a comprehensive review of the *sama lakṣhaṇas* mentioned by major classical authors for each of the *doṣhas*. This state of *sama* indicates that the *doṣha* is operating in its normal, *prākṛta* state. These *lakṣhaṇas* indicate a healthy operating level of each of the *doṣhas*.

Prākṛta doṣha lakṣhaṇas

Prākṛta vāta lakṣhaṇa with nearest English equivalent	Cha. Sū. 17/116, 18/49	Su. Ni. 1/9	AH Sū. 11/1	BP Pū. 3/103
Utsāha Enthusiasm, eagerness	√		√	√
Ucchvāsa Exhalation	√		√	√
Niḥśhvāsa Inhalation	√		√	√
Cheṣhṭa All activities, movements, functions	√		√	√
Vega-pravartana Initiation and execution of all *vegas*			√	√
Samyak-gata of dhātus Proper transportation for healthy *dhātus*	√		√	√
Akṣhāṇā-pāṭava Sharpness and health of *jñānendriyas*			√	√
Hṛdaya-indriya-chitta dhṛk Maintains and supports the heart, sense organs and conscious decision-making				√
Prāṇa Life	√ Sū. 17/116			
Doṣha-dhātu-agni samatā Normal state of *doṣha, dhātu, agni*		√		
Samprāpti viṣhaya Normal process of sense perception		√		
Kriyāṇām-anulomya Normal downward functioning of organs (peristalsis)		√		

Prākṛta pitta lakṣhaṇa with nearest English equivalent	Cha. Sū. 17/116, 18/50	Su. Sū.	AH Sū. 11/1	BP Pū.
Pakti Digestion, breaking down consumed food	√		√	
Ūṣhma Body temperature	√		√	
Darśhana Vision, sight	√		√	
Kṣhut Hunger	√		√	
Tṛṭ Thirst	√		√	
Ruchi Craving, fondness, desire for taste and flavor, having excitement for food			√	
Prabhā Complexion, glow	√		√	
Medhā Intelligence, prudence, wisdom	√		√	
Dhī Thoughts, disposition, discrimination ability			√	
Śhaurya Heroism, valor, prowess, might			√	
Tanu-mārdava Softness, suppleness, delicateness of the body	√		√	
Prasāda Happiness	√			

Prākṛta kapha lakṣhaṇa with nearest English equivalent	Cha. Sū. 17/116, 18/51	Su. Sū. 15/4	AH Sū. 11/1	BP Pū.
Sthiratva Stability	√		√	
Snigdhatva Unctuousness, oiliness, lubrication, friendliness	√		√	
Sandhi-bandha Well-bound joints	√		√	
Kṣhama-adi Tolerance, patience, forbearance, etc	√		√	
Gaurava Heaviness	√			
Vṛṣhata Virility	√			
Bala Strength	√			
Dhṛti Patience	√			
Alobha Absence of greed	√			

VAIṢHAMYA DOṢHA

Vṛddha doṣha lakṣhaṇa

See also AH Sū. 12/49-53 for additional *lakṣhaṇas*.

Vāta vṛddhi lakṣhaṇa with nearest English equivalent	Cha. Sū.	Su. Sū. 15/13	AH Sū. 11/6	BP Pū. 7(VII)/57
Kārśhya Emaciation, excessively thin, weak		√	√	√
Kārśṇya Darkened complexion		√	√	
Uṣhṇa kāmatva Craving for heat		√	√	√
Kampa Tremors			√	
Ānāha Abdominal distention, bloating			√	
Śhakṛt-grahān Constipation		√	√	
Bhramśha of bala, nidra, indriya Loss of strength, sleep, sensory function		√	√	√
Pralāpa Excessive or irrelevant speech			√	
Bhrama Giddiness, dizziness			√	
Dīnata Faint heartedness, weakness			√	
Vāk pāruṣhya Hoarseness of voice		√		
Gātra sphuraṇa Twitching in body parts		√		√
Pārṣhya Roughness (of the skin)				√
Gāḍha mala Hard, compact stools				√

Pitta vṛddhi lakṣhaṇa with nearest English equivalent	Cha. Sū.	Su. Sū. 15/13	AH Sū. 11/6	BP Pū. 7(VII)/57
Pīta of viṇ, mūtra, netra, tvak Yellow discoloration of feces, urine, eyes, skin		✓	✓	✓
Kṣhut Hunger			✓	
Tṛṭ Thirst			✓	
Dāha Burning sensation			✓	
Alpa-nidra Less or little sleep		✓	✓	
Pīta avabhāsa Yellowish complexion		✓		
Santāpa Increase in heat		✓		
Śhīta kāmitva Craving for cold		✓		✓
Mūrchchhā Fainting		✓		✓
Bala hāni Loss of strength		✓		
Indriya daurbalya Weakness of the sense organs		✓		✓
Alpa mūtra Decreased urine				✓

Kapha vṛddhi lakṣhaṇa with nearest English equivalent	Cha. Sū	Su. Sū. 15/13	AH Sū. 11/7	BP Pū. 7(VII)/58
Agni sadana Weak or reduced digestive power			✓	
Praseka Salivation, running or dripping mouth or nose			✓	✓
Ālasya Lassitude, lack of energy			✓	
Gaurava Heaviness		✓	✓	✓
Śhvaitya Whiteness, white coloration		✓	✓	
Śhaitya Coldness		✓	✓	✓
Śhlatha-aṅga Looseness of bodily limbs			✓	
Śhvāsa Difficulty breathing, or catching the breath			✓	
Kāsa Cough			✓	
Ati-nidra Too much sleep		✓	✓	✓
Sthairya Stiffness		✓		
Avasāda Depression		✓		
Tandra Drowsiness		✓		
Sandhi viśhleṣha Looseness of the joints		✓		✓
Viṭ-ādi śhauklya Whitish, pale discoloration of stools, etc				✓
Utkleda Nausea				✓

Kṣhīna doṣha lakṣhaṇa

Vāta kṣhaya lakṣhaṇa with nearest English equivalent	Cha. Sū.	Su. Sū. 15/7	AH Sū. 11/15	BP Pū. 7(VII)/78
Aṅga sāda Exhausted or weary limbs, debility of the body			✓	
Alpa bhāṣhita Speaks very little, diminished speaking		✓	✓	✓
Alpa hita Very little activity, diminished physical activity or interest			✓	
Saṁjña-moha Loss of awareness, distracted or confused perception		✓	✓	✓
Vṛddha śhleṣhma Signs and symptoms of increased kapha			✓	
Manda cheṣhṭa Decreased, reduced activity		✓		✓
Apraharṣha Dissatisfaction, discontent, absence of excitement		✓		

Pitta kṣhaya lakṣhaṇa with nearest English equivalent	Cha. Sū.	Su. Sū. 15/7	AH Sū. 11/15	BP Pū. 7(VII)/78
Manda anala Sluggish digestive power		✓	✓	✓
Śhīta Cold			✓	
Prabhā hāni Loss of radiance, luster		✓	✓	✓
Manda uṣhma Reduced bodily heat		✓		
Ādhika śhleṣhma Increase (excess) of *kapha*				✓

Kapha kṣhaya lakṣhaṇa with nearest English equivalent	Cha. Sū.	Su. Sū. 15/7	AH Sū. 11/16	BP Pū. 7(VII)/79
Bhrama Dizziness, that which is not steady, confusion			✓	
Śhlesṁa-āśhaya-śhūnyatva Emptiness of organs where kapha resides			✓	
Hṛd drava Palpitations of the heart			✓	
Sandhi śhlatha Looseness of joints		✓	✓	✓
Rūkṣhata Dryness		✓		✓
Antardaha Internal heat sensation		✓		✓
Āmāṣhaya-śhleṣhmāśhaya-śhūnyatā Emptiness of organs where *kapha* resides, especially the *āmāśhaya*		✓		
Tṛṣhṇa Thirst		✓		
Daurbalya Weakness		✓		
Prajāgaraṇa Staying awake at night		✓		
Mūrchchha Fainting				✓

DOṢHA STHĀNA

Vāta sthāna with nearest English equivalent	Cha. Sū. 20/8	Su. Sū. 21/6	AH Sū. 12/1	BP Pū. 3/107
Pakvāśhāya (viśheṣha sthāna) Large intestines, large colon	✓		✓	✓
Kaṭi Waist, hips, pelvic girdle	✓		✓	✓
Sakti Thighs	✓		✓	✓
Śhrotra Ears			✓	✓
Asthi Bones			✓	✓
Sparśhana-indriya Sense of touch			✓	✓
Śhroṇi, guda saṁśhraya In the junction of the pelvis and anal sphincter		✓		
Basti Urinary bladder	✓			
Purīṣha dhāna Rectum, receptacle of feces	✓			
Pādāvasthīni Lower legs, calves	✓			

Pitta sthāna with nearest English equivalent	Cha. Sū. 20/8	Su. Sū. 21/6	AH Sū. 12/2	BP Pū.
Nābhi Umbilical area			*(viśheṣh a sthāna)*	
Āmāśhāya (*adho*) Organ that holds undigested food, lower part	(*viśheṣha sthāna*)		✓	
Sveda Sweat	✓		✓	
Lasīkā Lymph	✓		✓	
Rudhira (rakta) The 2nd *dhātu*	✓		✓	
Rasa The 1st *dhātu*	✓		✓	
Dṛk Eyes			✓	
Sparśhana Sense of touch			✓	
Pakva-āmāśhaya madhya In between the *pakvāśhāya* and *āmāśhaya*		✓		

Kapha sthāna with nearest English equivalent	Cha. Sū. 20/8	Su. Sū. 21/6	AH Sū. 12/3	BP Pū.
Uras (viśheṣha sthāna) Chest and lung area	✓		✓	
Kaṇṭha Throat			✓	
Śhira Head	✓		✓	
Kloma The organ that manages kleda			✓	
Parvāṇi Small joints	✓		✓	
Āmāśhāya The organ that holds undigested food	✓	✓	✓	
Rasa The 1st *dhātu*			✓	
Medas The 4th *dhātu*	✓		✓	
Ghrāṇa Nose			✓	
Jihvā Tongue			✓	
Grīva Neck	✓			

DOṢHA BHEDA

The concept of doṣha bheda provides better insight into the detailed functioning of each of the *tridoṣhas*. This can be helpful to explain and understand complex sequences of activities that result in normal and abnormal physiology, as well as pathology. Vāgbhaṭa explains an important point to remember in AH Sū. 12/18:

इति प्रायेण दोषाणां स्थानान्यविकृतात्मनाम् ॥
व्यापिनामपि जानीयात्कर्माणि च पृथक्पृथक् ।

अ. हृ. सू. १२।१८

Iti prāyeṇa doṣhāṇāṁ sthānānyavikṛtāmanām ||
Vyāpināmapi jānīyātkarmāṇi cha pṛthakpṛthak |

AH Sū. 12/18

Even though the *doṣhas* move all over the body, when they are in their normal state, these are their special (specific) functions and locations.

See these additional references for more details - Cha. Sū. 12/8, Su. Sū. 21/10-14, Su. Ni. 1/11.

Pañcha vāta

Prāṇa vāta lakṣhaṇa with nearest English equivalent	Cha. Chi. 28/6	Su. Sū. 15/4, Ni. 1/14	AH Sū. 12/4	BP Pū. 3/109, 111
Mūrdha-gaḥ Located in the head	✓		✓	
Uraḥ-kaṇṭha chara Moves between the chest area and throat	✓		✓	
Buddhi-hṛdaya-indriya-chitta dhṛk Maintains and supports the mind, heart, sense organs and conscious decision-making			✓	
Ṣhṭhīvana Spitting, expectoration	✓		✓	
Kṣhavathu Sneezing	✓		✓	
Udgāra Burping, belching	✓		✓	
Niḥśhvāsa Inhalation, inspiration	✓		✓	
Anna praveśha Bringing food into the body	✓	✓	✓	✓
Pūraṇa To fill (the body with food and air)		✓ Sū. 15/4		
Vaktra sañchārī Moves around the oral cavity		✓		
Deha dhṛk Maintains, supports the body		✓		✓
Prāṇa avalambate Supports life		✓		✓
Jihva, āsya, nāsika Located in the tongue, mouth and nose	✓			
Adha hṛda koṣhṭha Located from below the heart to the abdomen				✓
Mukha gacchati Moves in the mouth				✓

Udāna vāta lakṣhaṇa with nearest English equivalent	Cha. Chi. 28/7	Su. Sū. 15/4, Ni. 1/14	AH Sū. 12/5	BP Pū. 3/109, 110, 116
Uraḥ sthāna Located in the chest area			√	
Nāsa-nābhi-gala charet Moves through the nose, umbilical area and throat			√	
Vāk pravṛtti Initiates speech	√	√	√	√
Prayatna Effort	√		√	
Urjā Enthusiasm	√		√	
Bala Physical strength	√		√	
Varṇa Complexion	√		√	
Smṛti Memory			√	
Udvahana To carry, lift, bring up (air, exhalation)		√ Sū. 15/4c		
Pavana uttama The best of the vāyus		√		√
Nābhi, uraḥ, kaṇṭha Located in (between) the umbilicus, chest and throat	√			
Kaṇṭha Present in the throat				√
Ūrdva Moves in an upwards direction				√
Ūrdva jatru gatān roga Diseases especially above the clavicles				√

Vyāna vāta lakṣhaṇa with nearest English equivalent	Cha. Chi. 28/9	Su. Sū. 15/4, Ni. 1/12	AH Sū. 12/6	BP Pū. 3/109, 116
Hṛdaya sthāna Located in the heart			✓	
Kṛtsna deha chāri mahājavaḥ Moves all over the body with great speed	✓	✓	✓	✓
Gati Movement, walking, going	✓		✓	✓
Apakṣhepaṇa Abduction	✓		✓	✓
Utkṣhepa Adduction			✓	✓
Nimeśha Opening the eyelids	✓		✓	✓
Unmeśha, ādi Closing the eyelids, etc	✓		✓	✓
Sarvā kriyā in śharīra All activities in the body			✓	✓
Praspandana To move, throb, pulse		✓ Sū. 15/4		✓
Udvahana To carry, lift, bring up (air, exhalation)				✓
Pūraṇa Filling				✓
Virechana Expelling				✓
Dhāraṇa Holding up, supporting				✓
Rasa saṁvahana Constantly circulates rasa		✓		✓
Sveda Supports sweat		✓		✓
Asṛk srāvaṇa Circulates rakta		✓		✓

Pañchadhā cheṣhṭa Responsible for five directions of movement (expansion, contraction, up, down, oblique)		√		√
Prasārana Stretch, extend, diffuse	√			

Samāṇa vāta lakṣhaṇa with nearest English equivalent	Cha. Chi. 28/8	Su. Sū. 15/4, Ni. 1/12	AH Sū. 12/8	BP Pū. 3/109, 113
Agni samīpastha Located near agni	√		√	√
Koṣhṭhe charati sarvataḥ Moves throughout the digestive system			√	
Anna ghṛṇāti Holds on to the food			√	
Pachati Breaks down, digests		√	√	√
Vivechayati Separates food into useful and non-useful parts		√	√	
Muñchati Eliminates waste products			√	
Viveka To separate (*sāra* from *kiṭṭa*)		√ Sū. 15/4		
Āma-pakvāśhaya chara Moves between the *āmāśhaya* and *pakvāśhāya*		√		√
Vahni saṅghata Associates with *agni*		√		√
Sveda, doṣha, ambu vaha srotas Present within the channels of sweat, *doṣhas* and fluid (water)	√			
Antaragni, pārśhva stha Located around *jāṭharāgni* and the sides of the thorax and abdomen	√			
Agni bala Promotes strength of *agni*	√			

Apāna vāta lakṣhaṇa with nearest English equivalent	Cha. Chi. 28/10	Su. Sū. 15/4, Ni. 1/12	AH Sū. 12/9	BP Pū. 3/109, 114
Apāna-gaḥ Located in the anal canal			✓	
Śhroṇi-basti-meḍhra-uru chara Moves in the pelvic girdle, bladder, penis, thighs			✓	
Śhukra-ārtava-śhakṛt-mūtra-garbha niśhkramana Eliminates or expels the male reproductive fluid, female reproductive fluid (including menstrual blood), feces, urine and fetus			✓	✓
Dhāraṇa To hold onto, control (the timely release)		✓ Sū. 15/4		
Pakvādhānalaya Located in the lower intestines, bowels		✓		✓
Kāla karśhati - Śhakṛt, mūtra, śhukra, garbha, ārtava Expels feces, urine, semen, fetus and menstrual fluid at the proper time	✓	✓		✓
Vṛṣhaṇa, basti, meḍhra, nābhi, uru, vaṅkṣhaṇa, guda, apāna sthāna Located in the two testicles, urinary bladder, penis, umbilical region, thighs, groin, anal region and pelvis	✓			
Malāśhaya Located in the lower intestines and rectum				✓

Pañcha pitta

Pāchaka pitta lakṣhaṇa with nearest English equivalent	Cha. Sū. 12/11c	Su. Sū. 15/4, 21/10	AH Sū. 12/10	BP Pū. 3/122, 123
Pakva-āmāśhaya-madhyagam Located in between the stomach and large intestine		√	√	
Pañcha-bhūta-ātmaka Composed of five elements			√	
Taijasa-guṇa-udayāt Predominant in the fire element			√	
Tyakta-dravatvam-pakādi-karmaṇā Performs digestive actions after losing its wateriness			√	
Anala-śhabditam Called *"anala"* (a synonym of *agni*)			√	
Anna pachati Cooks the ingested food		√	√	√
Sāra-kiṭṭa pṛthak vibhajate Separates individual components of food essence (useful part) from waste material		√	√	
Tatra-stham-eva pittānām śheṣhāṇām-api-anugraham karoti bala-dānena Located in its own normal place, it gives strength to all the other pittas		√	√	
Pakti, ojas Digestion, vitality	√	√ Sū. 15/4		
Doṣha, rasa, mūtra, purīṣhāṇi vivechayati Separates *doṣha, rasa, mūtra* and *purīṣha* from each other		√		√
Agnyāśhaya Located in the organ where *agni* resides				√
Agni bala vardhana Increases the strength of *agni*				√

Rañjaka pitta lakṣhaṇa with nearest English equivalent	Cha. Sū.	Su. Sū. 15/4, 21/10	AH Sū. 12/12	BP Pū. 3/122, 124
Āmāśhaya-āśhrayam Located in the lower part of the stomach			✓	
Rañjakam-rasa-rañjanāt Colors the *rasa dhātu* red		✓	✓	
Rāga Provides color (to *rasa dhātu*)		✓ Sū. 15/4		
Yakṛt plīha Located in the liver and spleen		✓		✓
Rasa śhoṇitaṁ nayet Converts *rasa dhātu* into *rakta dhātu*				✓

Sādhaka pitta lakṣhaṇa with nearest English equivalent	Cha. Sū. 12/11c	Su. Sū. 15/4, 21/10	AH Sū. 12/13	BP Pū. 3/122, 124
Preta-artha of buddhi, medha, abhi-māna, ādhya Supports the activity of intelligence, knowledge, the mind, etc		✓	✓	
Sādhaka hṛd-gata *Sādhaka pitta* is located in the heart		✓	✓	✓
Medhā Mental grasp, intelligence, ability to know		✓ Sū. 15/4		
Śhaurya Courage	✓			
Harṣha Joy, excitement	✓			
Prasāda Happiness	✓			
Buddhi, dhṛti smṛta Responsible for intelligence, courage, memory				✓

Ālocaka pitta lakṣhaṇa with nearest English equivalent	Cha. Sū. 12/11c	Su. Sū. 15/4, 21/10	AH Sū. 12/14	BP Pū. 3/122, 125
Rūpa Vision	√	√	√	√
Dṛk-stham Located in the eyes		√	√	√
Tejas Illuminate, provide light to see		√ Sū. 15/4		

Bhrājaka pitta lakṣhaṇa with nearest English equivalent	Cha. Sū. 12/11c	Su. Sū. 15/4, 21/10	AH Sū. 12/14	BP Pū. 3/122, 125
Tvak-stham Located in the skin		√	√	√
Bhrājanāt tvacha Makes the skin radiant (gives brightness, luster)		√	√	
Uṣhma To heat (the body), maintain temperature	√	√ Sū. 15/4		
Abhyaṅga, pariṣheka, avagāha, lepa, ādi kriyā dravyāṇāṁ paktā Digests and metabolizes the effects of the *dravyas* (medicaments) used in *abhyaṅga*, *pariṣheka, avagāha*, *lepa*, etc		√		√
Varṇa Complexion	√			√

Pañcha kapha

Avalambaka kapha lakṣhaṇa with nearest English equivalent	Cha. Chi. 28/12c	Su. Sū. 15/4, 21/14	AH Sū. 12/15	BP Pū. 3/127, 130
Uraḥ-sthaḥ sa trikasya Located throughout the chest area and upper back	✓	✓	✓	
Sva-vīrya hṛdayasya-anna-vīrya cha tat-stha eva-ambu-karmaṇa Through its own power and the power of digested food moving through the heart (ie, *rasa dhātu*), it provides support through the actions of *ap mahābhūta*		✓	✓	✓
Kapha-dhāmnām cha śheṣhāṇām yat-karoti-avalambanam Provides strength to all of the other types of *kapha*			✓	
Bala sthairya Supports the strength of the body		✓ Sū. 15/4		
Trika sandhāraṇa Supports (holds up) the chest, shoulders, head		✓		✓
Avalambana Supports the entire body	✓			
Hṛdaya stha Located around the heart				✓

Kledaka kapha lakṣhaṇa with nearest English equivalent	Cha. Chi. 28/12c	Su. Sū. 15/4, 21/14	AH Sū. 12/16	BP Pū. 3/127, 131
Āmāśhaya-saṁsthita Located in the stomach	√	√	√	√
Anna-saṅghata-kledanāt Moistens, liquefies and lubricates the mass of food	√		√	√
Snehana Lubricates		√ Sū. 15/4		
Udaka karmaṇa anugraha Supports the work of fluid in the rest of the body		√		√

Bodhaka kapha lakṣhaṇa with nearest English equivalent	Cha. Chi. 28/12c	Su. Sū. 15/4, 21/12	AH Sū. 12/17	BP Pū. 3/127, 131
Rasa-bodhanāt Responsible for taste perception	√	√	√	√
Rasanā-sthāyī Located in the tongue	√		√	
Ropana Promotes healing		√ Sū. 15/4		
Jihva mūla kaṇṭha stha Located in the root of the tongue and throat		√		
Jihva indriya saumyat Moistens the sense of taste		√		
Kaṇṭhe stha Located in the throat				√
Saumya Having a cooling nature				√

Tarpaka kapha lakṣhaṇa with nearest English equivalent	Cha. Chi. 28/12c	Su. Sū. 15/4, 21/12	AH Sū. 12/17	BP Pū. 3/127, 132
Śhira-saṁstha Located in the head	✓	✓	✓	✓
Akṣhi-tarpaṇāt Nourishes the sense organs (esp. the eyes)	✓		✓	
Pūraṇa Fills (the channels of the sense organs)		✓ Sū. 15/4		
Indriya snehana, santarpaṇa Provides lubrication and strength to the sense organs (in the head)		✓		✓

Śhleṣhaka kapha lakṣhaṇa with nearest English equivalent	Cha. Chi. 2812c	Su. Sū. 15/4, 21/12	AH Sū. 12/18	BP Pū. 3/127, 132
Sandhi-saṁśhleṣhāt Lubricates the joints	✓	✓ Sū. 15/4	✓	✓
Sandhiṣhu-sthita Located in the joints	✓		✓	✓
Sarva sandhi anugraha Supports (movement) of all joints		✓		

Chapter 7: Review

ADDITIONAL READING

Read and review the references listed below to expand your understanding of the concepts in this chapter. Write down the date that you complete your reading for each. Remember that consistent repetition is the best way to learn. Plan to read each reference at least once now and expect to read it again as you continue your studies.

References marked with (skim) can be read quickly and do not require commentary review.

CLASSICS		1st read	2nd read
Charaka	Cha. Sū. 1/54 Cha. Sū. 11/37-43 Cha. Sū. 12/5-6 Cha. Sū. 17/62 Cha. Sū. 17/111-115 Cha. Sū. 18/52-53 Cha. Vi. 1/7 Cha. Śhā. 6/4-5		
Suśhruta	Su. Sū. 15/13 Su. Sū. 21/		
Aṣhṭāṅga Hṛdaya	AH Sū. 11/ AH Sū. 12/		
Bhāva Prakāśha	BP Pū. 3/103-132 BP Pū. 5/325-326 BP Pū. 7/41-79		

JOURNALS & CURRENT RESOURCES

QUESTIONS & ANSWERS

Record your questions for this chapter here for further research and discussion.

Question:

Answer:

Question:

Answer:

Question:

Answer:

SELF-ASSESSMENT

1. Which of the following best describes how *doṣhas* move through the body?
   a. *Abhyāsa guṇa*
   b. *Kṣhaya, sthāna, vṛddhi*
   c. *Samānya-viṣhesa siddhānta*
   d. All of the above
   e. None of the above

2. Which of the following is the best way to determine *prākṛta* from *vaikṛta*?
   a. *Doṣha sthāna*
   b. *Kṣhīṇa doṣha lakṣhaṇa*
   c. *Prākṛta doṣha lakṣhaṇas*
   d. *Vṛddha doṣha lakṣhaṇa*
   e. All of the above

3. When a *doṣha* undergoes *praśhamana*, it is returning to
   a. *Chaya*
   b. *Kṣhaya*
   c. *Prakopa*
   d. *Sthāna*
   e. *Vṛddhi*

4. Which of the following best describes a *doṣha* in the state of *chaya*?
   a. Creates a sense of *asvasthya*
   b. Causes the absence of *lakṣhaṇas*
   c. Displays a mild increase of *lakṣhaṇas* in its own *sthāna*
   d. Displays prominent *lakṣhaṇas*
   e. All of the above

5. Which of the following are the *kārana* for *doṣha vṛddhi* or *kṣhaya*?
   a. *Āhāra*
   b. *Artha, kāla, karma*
   c. *Tri-vidha kāraṇa*
   d. *Vihāra*
   e. All of the above

6. Which of the following indicate *prākṛta vāta lakṣhaṇas*?
   a. Complexion and glow
   b. Enthusiasm and eagerness
   c. Softness and delicateness of the body
   d. Tolerance and patience
   e. Intelligence and discrimination

7. Which of the following indicate *pitta vṛddhi lakṣhaṇas*?
   a. Craving cold and loss of sleep
   b. Giddiness and dizziness
   c. Loss of sleep and bodily heat
   d. Looseness of bodily limbs and joints
   e. Nausea and pale stool

8. Which of the following indicate *kapha kṣhaya lakṣhaṇas?*
   a. Distracted and confused
   b. Dryness and thirst
   c. Loss of luster and digestive power
   d. Dissatisfaction and loss of interest
   e. Sluggish digestion and loss of bodily heat

9. Which of the *pañcha vāta* is responsible for initiating speech and enthusiasm?
   a. *Apāna vāyu*
   b. *Prāṇa vāyu*
   c. *Samāṇa vāyu*
   d. *Udāna vāyu*
   e. *Vyāna vāyu*

10. The function of *pitta* that is responsible for heating the body and maintaining temperature is called
    a. *bhūtāgni*
    b. *Pāchaka pitta*
    c. *pāchana*
    d. *uṣhma*
    e. *uṣhṇa*

CRITICAL THINKING

1. Give examples of how to use the terms *vṛddhi*, *vṛddha*, *kṣhaya* and *kṣhīna*. Explain how they are used as different parts of speech.

2. Could any of the *prākṛta doṣha lakṣhaṇas* be possibly misconstrued as pathological? Which one(s), how and why? Demonstrate through example.

3. Explain the concept of *doṣha sthāna* with references. Does this mean that a *doṣha's sthāna* should always represent characteristics of its own (main) doṣha if *dhātu vaiṣhamya* occurs?

4. Reviewing the *lakṣhaṇas* of *doṣha bheda*, how could each be grouped within the context of *siddhānta*? Hint: consider the structure of *dravya*.

5. Find at least three instances where two or more *doṣhas* within each *doṣha bheda* are involved in the production of a single or similar *lakṣhaṇas*.

6. Which *doṣha* is responsible for the following *lakṣhaṇas*, and in which state?
   a. *Alpa nidra*
   b. *Tṛṣhṇa* or *tṛṭ*
   c. *Mūrchchhā*
   d. Difficulty regulating bodily temperature
   e. Fatigue

Chapter 8 : Dhātu

KEY TERMS

asthi	kāraṇa	medo dhātu vṛddhi	sapta dūṣhya
asthi dhātu kṣhaya	kṣhaya	prākṛta dhātu lakṣhaṇa	śhukra
asthi dhātu vṛddhi	majja	rakta	śhukra dhātu kṣhaya
dhāraṇa	majja dhātu kṣhaya	rakta dhātu kṣhaya	śhukra dhātu vṛddhi
dhātu	majja dhātu vṛddhi	rakta dhātu vṛddhi	upadhātu
dhātumala	māṁsa	rasa	upasevana
kṣhīṇa dhātu lakṣhaṇa	māmsa dhātu kṣhaya	rasa dhātu kṣhaya	vṛddha dhātu lakṣhaṇa
	māmsa dhātu vṛddhi	rasa dhātu vṛddhi	vṛddhi
	medas	saptadhātu	
	medo dhātu kṣhaya		

While *dhātu* may generally refer to any support of the body, it is commonly used to specifically reference the *saptadhātu*. These are the seven supportive systems and products generated as a result of normal, healthy functioning of *agni* at all levels (*jāṭharāgni, bhūtāgni and dhātvagni*). They are capable of growing and generating a healthy body.

PARIBHĀṢHĀ

The definition of *dhātu* is provided by Suśhruta in a clear and concise statement:

त एते शरीरधारणाद्धातव इत्युच्यन्ते ॥

सु. सू. १४।२०

Ta ete śharīradhāraṇāddhātava ityuchyante ||

Su. Sū. 14/20

Ta (Because) *ete* (they) *śharīra-dhāraṇāt* (provide support to the physical body) *dhātava iti uchyante* (they are called *dhātus*).

Suśhruta immediately follows this with an explanation of how the *dhātus* themselves are maintained:

तेषां क्षयवृद्धी शोणितनिमित्ते ... ।

सु. सू. १४।२१

Teṣhāṁ kṣhayavṛddhi śhoṇitanimitte ... |

Su. Sū. 14/21

Their *kṣhaya* (decrease) and *vṛddhi* (increase) is caused by *śhoṇita* (blood) ... |

Chakrapāṇi elaborates on the *dhātus* and their importance in the health of the body. He states in Cha. Śhā. 6/4 that the *dhātus* are composed of the *mahābhūtas* and their existence in a healthy conglomeration is the reason that the body is able to exist.

The *saptadhātus* are also defined by all authors in various instances. Here is Vāgbhaṭa's definition which he includes at the beginning of *Sūtrasthāna*:

रसासृङ्मांसमेदोस्थिमज्जशुक्राणि धातवः ।
सप्त दूष्याः ... ॥

अ. हृ. सू. १।१३

Rasāsṛṅmāṁsamedosthimajjaśhukrāṇi dhātavaḥ | Sapta dūṣhyāḥ ... ||

AH Sū. 1/13

The *sapta dūṣhyas* (meaning the *dhātus*, that which is being vitiated) are *rasa, rakta, māṁsa, medas, asthi, majja*, and *śhukra*.

The relationship between *doṣha* and *dūṣhya* will be discussed in detail in Chapter 12.

Bhāva Prakāśha also provides a similar definition and mentions the purpose of *dhātus* in BP Pū. 3/133:

एते सप्त स्वयं स्थित्वा देहं दधति यन्नृणाम् ।
रसासृङ्मांसमेदोऽस्थिमज्जशुक्राणि धातवः ॥

भा. प्र. पू. ३।१३३

Ete sapta svayaṁ sthitvā dehaṁ dadhati yannṛṇām |
Rasāsṛṅmāṁsamedo ' sthimajjaśhukrāṇi dhātavaḥ ||

BP Pū. 3/133

And so, the seven *dhātus* on their own are *sthitvā* (fixed, firm, stable, in place) and *dadhati* (they stay put) in the *deha* (body) of *nṛṇa* (humans). They are *rasa, rakta, māṁsa, medas, asthi majja* and *śhukra*.

Rakta *dhātu* has several synonyms that are often used. These include *ārtava*, *asṛk*, *rajaḥ* (also, *rajas*), and *śhoṇita*.

TEST YOURSELF

Learn, review and memorize key terms from this section.

dhātu

dhāraṇa

saptadhātu

sapta dūṣhya

rasa

rakta

māṁsa

medas

asthi

majja

śhukra

DHĀTU VṚDDHI AND KṢHAYA KĀRAṆA

Like the *doṣhas*, the *dhātus* have many *kāraṇa* (general and specific causes) for their states of *vṛddhi* and *kṣhaya*. These are listed in many places throughout the classics often as reminders to the reader within the context of a disease or pathological condition.

Suśhruta provides the general rule for the causes of aggravation for the *doṣhas* in Su. Sū. 15/13 which can be readily applied to the *dhātus* as well. He states that their increase in human beings is the result of *upasevana* (excessive, regular usage) of similar substances. Anything which is similar by its *guṇa, karma*, or *pañchabhautika* composition has the ability to accumulate the same in the body. *Bhāva Prakāśha* elaborates this point to include the influence of seasons on diet and regimens in BP Pū. 5/326.

The specific causes can be categorized just

as they are for the *doṣhas*. However, there are fewer references for *kārana* of *dhātu vṛddhi* and *kṣhaya* because they are very similar to the *doṣhas*. Examples can be seen here: Cha. Sū. 17/76-79, Su. Sū. 15/29-33, BP Pū. 7/77.

TEST YOURSELF

Learn, review and memorize key terms from this section.

kāraṇa

---

vṛddhi

---

kṣhaya

---

upasevana

PRĀKṚTA DHĀTU LAKṢHAṆA

When *dhātus* are in their state of *sāmya* they are expected to display certain characteristics and functions. These have been listed in identical form by Vāgbhaṭa and Bhāvamiśhra in AH Sū. 11/4, and BP Pū. 3/134. Suśhruta includes a few more functions in Su. Sū. 15/4.1.

Vāgbhaṭa additionally defines the main purpose of each of the *saptadhātus*. Although only one term is used for the defintion of each *dhātu*, this term elaborately describes extensive functionality when its underlying concept is fully expanded.

प्रीणनं जीवनं लेपः स्नेहो धारणपूरणे ।
गर्भोत्पादश्च धातूनां श्रेष्ठं कर्म क्रमात्स्मृतम् ॥ ४

अ. हृ. सू. ११।४

Prīṇanaṁ jīvanaṁ lepaḥ sneho dhāraṇapūraṇe | Garbhotpādaśhcha dhātūnāṁ śhreṣhṭhaṁ karma kramātsmṛtam ||

AH Sū. 11/4

The concepts of each are described in the following table.

Dhātu	*Prākṛta dhātu lakṣhaṇa* Nearest English equivalent	Su. Sū. 15/4.1	AH Su. 11/4	BP Pū. 3/134
Rasa	*Prīṇana* Satisfies and nourishes (rakta)	✓	✓	✓
	Tuṣhṭi Satisfaction, contentment	✓		
	Rakta puṣhṭi Provides growth, increase, nourishment, plumpness, thriving to rakta	✓		
Rakta	*Jīvana* Enlivens, activates, supports life activities	✓	✓	✓

	Varṇa prasāda Responsible for excellent (easy flowing) complexion	✓		
	Māṁsa puṣhṭi Provides growth, increase, nourishment, plumpness, thriving to *māṁsa*	✓		
Māṁsa	*Lepana* Creates the meat and flesh of the body, covers, spreads and protects		✓	✓
	Śharīra puṣhṭi medasaśhcha Provides growth, increase, nourishment, plumpness, thriving to *śharīra* and *medas*	✓		
Medas	*Snehana* Lubricates		✓	✓
	Sneha-sveda Maintains the unctuousness and sweat	✓		
	Dṛḍhatva Provides steadiness, strength, firmness	✓		
	Asthi puṣhṭi Provides growth, increase, nourishment, plumpness, thriving to *asthi*	✓		
Asthi	*Dhāraṇa* Holds up, supports	✓	✓	✓
	Majja puṣhṭi Provides growth, increase, nourishment, plumpness, thriving to majja	✓		
Majja	*Pūraṇe* (*asthna*, Su.) Fills the spaces (of the bones)	✓	✓	✓
	Sneha bala cha Provides unctuousness and strength	✓		
	Śhukra puṣhṭi Provides growth, increase, nourishment, plumpness, thriving to *śhukra*	✓		
Śhukra	*Garbha-utpāda* Enables reproduction		✓	✓
	Dhairya, chyavana, prīti, deha bala, harṣha, bījārtha Composure, movement (expulsion, ejaculation), satisfaction, bodily strength, excitement, procreation	✓		

VṚDDHA DHĀTU LAKṢHAṆA

Rasa dhātu vṛddhi lakṣhaṇa with nearest English equivalent	Cha. Sū.	Su. Sū. 15/14	AH Sū. 11/8	BP Pū. 7/59
Raso-api śhleṣhmavat Behaves like increased *kapha*			✓	✓
Hṛdaya-utkleda Nausea		✓		
Praseka Salivation		✓		✓
Anna vidveṣha Reluctance, aversion to food (meals)				✓
Gātra gaurava Heaviness of the body, especially limbs				✓
Lālā Salivation				✓
Chhardi Vomiting				✓
Mūrchchhā Fainting				✓
Sāda Weakness, debility				✓
Bhrama Dizziness				✓

Rakta dhātu vṛddhi lakṣhaṇa with nearest English equivalent	Cha. Sū.	Su. Sū. 15/14	AH Sū. 11/9	BP Pū. 7/60
Visarpa A skin disease that spreads quickly			✓	
Plīha Spleen disorders			✓	
Vidradhī Abscesses			✓	
Kuṣhṭha Group of skin diseases			✓	✓
Vātāsra (Syn. for *vātarakta*), a disease characterized by pathological *vāta* and *rakta*			✓	✓
Pittāsra (Syn. for *raktapitta),* a disease characterized by pathological *rakta* and *pitta*			✓	
Gulma A disease characterized by a pathological cluster of *doṣhas* in the abdomen			✓	✓
Upakuśha A disease of the mouth and teeth			✓	
Kāmalā A disease characterized by yellow complexion			✓	✓
Vyaṅga A disease characterized by patches of discoloration on the face			✓	✓
Agni-nāśha Loss or absence of normal agni			✓	✓
Sammoha A state of confusion, disorientation, unconsciousness, etc			✓	✓
Rakta of tvak, netra, mūtra Red discoloration of the skin, eyes, and urine		✓	✓	✓
Raktaṁ sirā pūrayati Blood fills all the veins		✓		✓
Gātra gaurava Heaviness of the bodily limbs				✓

Rakta dhātu vṛddhi lakṣhaṇa with nearest English equivalent	Cha. Sū.	Su. Sū. 15/14	AH Sū. 11/9	BP Pū. 7/60
Nidra, mada, dāha jayate Excessive sleep, intoxication, burning sensation				✓
Guda, meḍhra, āsya pāka Ulceration of the anus, penis and mouth				✓
Arśhas Hemorrhoids				✓
Piṇḍaka Raised eruptions on the skin, ulcerations				✓
Maśhakā Rashes, especially chicken pox				✓
Indralupta Alopecia				✓
Aṅgamarda Generalized body pain				✓
Asṛgdara Menorrhagia				✓
Tāpa Burning sensation, especially in the extremities				✓

Māmsa dhātu vṛddhi lakṣhaṇa with nearest English equivalent	Cha.Sū.	Su. Sū. 15/14	AH Sū. 11/9	BP Pū. 7/64
Gaṇḍa Enlargement of glands (esp. lymph)			✓	✓
Arbuda Abnormal, irregular growths (often malignant)			✓	
Granthi Localized, nodular swelling or growth that is encapsulated (often benign)			✓	
Vṛddhi of gaṇḍa, uru, udara Increased size of cheeks, thighs and abdomen			✓	
Adhi-māmsa of kaṇṭha-adi Excessive growth of muscular tissue of the neck and other areas			✓	
Gaṇḍa, oṣhṭha, sphik, upastha, uru, jaṅgha bahu Enlargement or excessive increase of cheeks, lips, buttocks, genitals, thighs, arms and legs		✓		✓
Gātra gaurava Heaviness of the body limbs		✓		✓

Medo dhātu vṛddhi lakṣhaṇa with nearest English equivalent	Cha. Sū.	Su. Sū. 15/14	AH Sū. 11/10	BP Pū. 7/65
Tadvan-medas Produces similar signs and symptoms as *māmsa*			✓	
Śhrama Exhaustion, fatigue			✓	✓
Śhvāsa from alpa cheṣhṭa Labored breathing even after minimal exertion			✓	✓
Sphik, sthana, udara, grīva lambana Drooping of the buttocks, breasts, neck and abdomen			✓	✓
Udara-parśhva vṛddhi Abdominal enlargement		✓		✓
Kāsa, śhvāsa-ādaya Cough, difficulty breathing, etc		✓		✓
Daurgandhya Bodily odor (bad smell of the body)		✓		✓
Snigdhata Increased unctuousness, oiliness		✓		✓
Tṛṭ, sveda, gala-gaṇḍa, oṣhṭha roga Disorders of thirst, sweat, nodules in the neck, lips				✓
Meha-adi (*prameha*, etc) Disorders of the urinary system, etc				✓
Śhvāsa Difficulty breathing				✓

Asthi dhātu vṛddhi lakṣhaṇa with nearest English equivalent	Cha. Sū.	Su. Sū. 15/14	AH Sū. 11/11	BP Pū. 7/67
Adhi asthi Excessive bone growth		✓	✓	✓
Adhi danta Excessive tooth growth, extra teeth		✓	✓	✓
Danta-anvikaṭān-mahat Teeth that are ugly and big				✓

Majja dhātu vṛddhi lakṣhaṇa with nearest English equivalent	Cha. Sū.	Su. Sū. 15/14	AH Sū. 11/11	BP Pū. 7/68
Netra, aṅga gourava Heaviness of the eyes and limbs		✓	✓	✓
Sthūla parvasu Increased size, thickness, heaviness of body joints (especially smaller joints)			✓	
Kuryāt-kṛcchrāt mūlāni arūṁṣhi Ulcers with deep roots that are difficult to cure			✓	

Śhukra dhātu vṛddhi lakṣhaṇa with nearest English equivalent	Cha. Sū.	Su. Sū. 15/14	AH Sū. 11/12	BP Pū. 7/69
Ati strī kāma Excessive lust, sexual desire (for women)		✓	✓	✓
Śhukra aśhmarī Prostate stones		✓	✓	✓

KṢHĪNA DHĀTU LAKṢHAṆA

Rasa dhātu kṣhaya lakṣhaṇa with nearest English equivalent	Cha. Sū. 17/64	Su. Sū. 15/9	AH Sū. 11/17	BP Pū. 7/79
Ghaṭṭate Restless	✓			
Roukṣhya Dryness			✓	
Śhrama Exhaustion, fatigue	✓		✓	
Śhoṣha Dryness, shriveling, emaciation		✓	✓	✓
Glāni Constant exhaustion even after rest			✓	
Śhabda sahiṣhṇutā Intolerance for sound or noise	✓		✓	
Hṛt pīḍā Squeezing pressure/pain of the heart		✓		✓
Kaṇṭha, tvak śhoṣha Dryness of the throat, skin				✓
Tṛṭ Thirst		✓		✓
Kampa Palpitations, tremors, fine trembles	✓	✓		
Hṛdaya tāmyati svalpa cheṣhṭa Exhaustion of the heart (gasping for breath) with even slight activity (exertion)	✓			

Rakta dhātu kṣhaya lakṣhaṇa with nearest English equivalent	Cha. Sū. 17/65	Su. Sū. 15/9	AH Sū. 11/17	BP Pū. 7/80
Amla-śhiśhira prīti Desire for sour and cool, refreshing things		✓	✓	✓
Sira śhaithilya-rūkṣhata Flaccidity and dryness of the veins		✓	✓	✓
Tvak pāruṣhya Roughness of the skin	✓	✓		✓
Sphuṭitā mlānā tvak-rūkṣhā Cracks, fading (of luster), dryness of the skin	✓			

Māmsa dhātu kṣhaya lakṣhaṇa with nearest English equivalent	Cha. Sū. 17/65	Su. Sū. 15/9	AH Sū. 11/18	BP Pū. 7/80
Akṣha glāni Exhaustion of the senses even after rest			✓	
Gaṇḍa, sphik śhuṣhkata Emaciated and dried up looking cheeks, buttocks, etc	✓ and *udara*	✓	✓	✓
Sandhi vedana Pain in the joints			✓	
Gaṇḍa, oṣhṭha, kandharā, skandha, vakṣha, jaṭhara, sandhi, piṇḍīṣhu śhuṣhkatā Wasting (drying up) of the cheeks, lips, neck, shoulders, chest, abdomen, joints, calves		✓		✓
Upastha śhotha Swelling (inflammation) of the genitals		*śhoṣha*		✓
Gātra rūkṣhatā Dryness of the body		✓		✓
Toda Pricking pain		✓		✓
Dhamanya śhaithilā Flaccidity of the arteries		✓		✓
Gātra sadana Fatigue		✓		

Medo dhātu kṣhaya lakṣhaṇa with nearest English equivalent	Cā. Sū. 17/66	Su. Sū. 15/9	AH Sū. 11/18	BP Pū. 7/82
Kati svapana Loss of sensation in the waist			✓	
Pliha vṛddhi Increase of the spleen		✓	✓	✓
Kṛśha-aṅga Emaciation, thinness of the limbs			✓	
Sandhi śhūnyatā Emptiness, dryness, wasting of the joints		✓		✓
Rūkṣhatā Dryness		✓		✓
Prārthanā snigdha-māṁsa Craving for fatty meat		✓		✓
Sandhīnā sphuṭana Cracking of the joints	✓			
Akṣhi glāni, āyāsa Appearance of exhaustion, stress around the eyes	✓			
Tanutva udara Thinness of the abdomen	✓			

Asthi dhātu kṣhaya lakṣhaṇa with nearest English equivalent	Cha. Sū. 17/67	Su. Sū. 15/9	AH Sū. 11/19	BP Pū. 7/83
Asthi toda Pricking or stabbing pain in the bones			✓	
Danta-keśha-nakha-adi śhadana Falling (prematurely) of teeth, hair on the head, nails, etc			✓	
Asthi śhūla Pain in the bones		✓		✓
Raukṣhya Dryness		✓		✓
Nakha-danta truṭi Breaking, splitting, chipping of nails, teeth		✓		✓
Keśha, loma, nakha, śhmaśhru, dvija prapatana Falling of hair on the head, hair on the body, nails, beard and adult teeth	✓			
Śhrama Exhaustion	✓			
Sandhi śhaithilya Flaccidity of the joints	✓			

Majja dhātu kṣhaya lakṣhaṇa with nearest English equivalent	Cha. Sū. 17/68	Su. Sū. 15/9	AH Sū. 11/19	BP Pū. 7/84
Asthnām majjani souṣhiryam Feeling of hollowness in the filling of the bones		✓	✓	✓
Bhrama Dizziness, feeling of instability			✓	
Timira darśhana Darkness around the eyes, darkened vision			✓	
Alpa śhukra Decrease in *śhukra (dhātu)*		✓		✓
Parva bheda toda Cracking (splitting) pain and pricking pain in the smaller joints		✓		✓
Śhīrya, durbala, laghu of asthi Thin, weak and light bones	✓			
Pratata vāta-roga *Vāta* disorders tend to easily afflict the bones	✓			

Śhukra dhātu kṣhaya lakṣhaṇa with nearest English equivalent	Cha. Sū. 17/69	Su. Sū. 15/9	AH Sū. 11/20	BP Pū. 7/85
Chirāta śhukra Delayed ejaculation		✓	✓	✓
Prasichyeta śhukra śhoṇita Ejaculation with blood		✓	✓	✓
Vṛṣhaṇa toda Pricking pain in the testicles			✓	
Meḍhra dhūmayatī Feeling of smoke, heat coming out of the urethral opening			✓	
Aśhakti maithuna Inability to engage in sexual intercourse		✓		✓
Śhepha-muṣhka vyathā Pain in the penis and scrotum		✓		✓
Daurbalya Weakness	✓			
Mukha śhoṣha Dryness of mouth	✓			
Pāṇḍu Pallor	✓			
Sadana Weakness, tiredness	✓			
Śhrama Exhaustion	✓			
Klaibya Impotency	✓			
Śhukra avisarga Inability to release *śhukra*	✓			

DHĀTUS AND PAÑCHA MAHĀBHŪTAS

Bhāva Prakāśha explains the relationship between the *dhātus* and their predominant *mahābhūtas* in BP Pū. 3/207-8, as follows:

Dhātu	Predominant *mahābhūta(s)*
Rasa	*Ap*
Rakta	*Tejas*
Māṁsa	*Pṛthvi*
Medas	*Ap*
Asthi	*Pṛthvi, vāyu, tejas*
Majja	*Ap*
Śhukra	*Ap*

UPADHĀTU AND DHĀTUMALA

Part of the normal processes of *agni* involve an additional conversion from each *dhātu* into one or more *upadhātus* and *dhātumalas*. Chakrapāṇi explains the difference between *dhātus* and *upadhātus* in the commentary of Cha. Chi. 15/17. *Dhātus* are the primary supportive systems of the body because they help sustain a healthy body and provide nourishment to subsequent *dhātus*. This is what distinguishes them from *upadhātus* which help sustain the body but do not nourish any subsequent *dhātus* or *upadhātus*.

Dhātu	*Upadhātu* with nearest English equivalent	Cha. Chi. 15/17	Su. Sū.	AH Sū. 11/1c	BP Pū. 3/210
Rasa	*Stanya* Breast milk	✓		✓	✓
	Rajaḥ Menstrual blood	✓			
	Lasīkā Watery fluid between *māṁsa* and *tvak*			✓	
Rakta	*Kaṇḍarā* Tendons	✓		✓	
	Sirā Veins	✓		✓	
	Dhamanī Arteries			✓	
	Rajas Menstrual blood				✓
Māṁsa	*Vasā* Muscle fat	✓		✓	✓
	Tvacha ṣhaṭ 6 layers of skin	✓		✓ *(tvak)*	
Medas	*Snāyu* Sinews	✓			
	Sveda Sweat				✓
Asthi	*Danta* Teeth				✓
Majja	*Keśha* Hair (on the head)				✓
Śhukra	*Ojas**				✓

During the processes of *dhātu pariṇāma*, several *malas*, or waste products are formed in addition to the two main *malas* of *purīṣha* and *mūtra*. These additional *malas* are generated from the process of *sāra-kiṭṭa vibhāga*, the splitting of nutrient material (for *dhātu poṣhaṇa*) from the wastes to be excreted. The *kiṭṭa* that are separated are the *dhātumala* and at each level of *dhātu pariṇāma*, one or more specific wastes are produced.

Dhātu	*Dhātumala* with nearest English equivalent	Cha. Chi. 15/18-19	Su. Sū. 46/529	AH Śhā. 3/63	BP Pū. 3/209
*Anna rasa**	*Viṇ* (feces), *mūtra* (urine)	√	√		
Rasa	*Kapha*	√	√	√	√
Rakta	*Pitta*	√	√	√	√
Māmsa	*Khamala* Waste products excreted from the eyes, ears, nose, mouth, genitals	√	√	√	√
Medas	*Sveda* Sweat	√	√	√	√
Asthi	*Keśha* Hair (on the head)	√			
	Nakha Nails		√	√	√
	Loman (*roman*) Hair (on the body)	√	√	√	√
Majja	*Sneha of akṣhi, viṭ, tvak* Oily secretions of eyes, feces, skin	√	√	√	√
Śhukra	None	√	√		√
	Ojas			√	

*Although *anna rasa* is not a fully formed *dhātu*, it is the precursor to the formation of all the *dhātus* and so Charaka and Suśhruta have included its *kiṭṭā* in this list within the context of *dhātu pariṇāma*.

Chapter 8: Review

ADDITIONAL READING

Read and review the references listed below to expand your understanding of the concepts in this chapter. Write down the date that you complete your reading for each. Remember that consistent repetition is the best way to learn. Plan to read each reference at least once now and expect to read it again as you continue your studies.

References marked with (skim) can be read quickly and do not require commentary review.

CLASSICS		1st read	2nd read
Charaka	Cha. Sū. 17/76-79 Cha. Chi. 15/17-20		
Suśhruta	Su. Sū. 14/20-21 Su. Sū. 15/ Su. Sū. 46/525-529		
Aṣhṭāṅga Hṛdaya	AH Sū. 1/13 AH Sū. 11/		
Bhāva Prakāśha	BP Pū. 3/133-165 BP Pū. 3/207-210 BP Pū. 5/326 BP Pū. 7/59-85		

JOURNALS & CURRENT RESOURCES

QUESTIONS & ANSWERS

Record your questions for this chapter here for further research and discussion.

Question:

Answer:

Question:

Answer:

Question:

Answer:

SELF-ASSESSMENT

1. Which of the following describes the *dhātus* and/or their functions?
   a. Composed of a healthy conglomeration of the *mahābhūtas*
   b. *Kṣhaya* and *vṛddhi* is affected by *śhoṇita*
   c. They provide *dhāraṇa* to *śharīra*
   d. The *saptadhātu* on their own are *sthitvā* and *dadhati* in the human body
   e. All of the above

2. Suśhruta states the main *kāraṇa* of *dhātu vṛddhi* and *kṣhaya* is
   a. *Āhāra*
   b. *Jāṭharāgni*
   c. *Sapta dūṣhyas*
   d. *Upasevana*
   e. All of the above

3. Which of the following *prākṛta dhātu lakṣhaṇas* are a function of *medas*?
   a. Provides lubrication
   b. Provides growth, nourishment to *māṁsa*
   c. Provides growth, nourishment to *śhukra*
   d. Promotes reproductive capacity and a long life
   e. Satisfaction and contentment

4. Which of the following is a *lakṣhaṇa of rasa dhātu vṛddhi*?
   a. Behaves like increased *kapha*
   b. Dizziness and fainting
   c. Heaviness of the body and limbs
   d. Weakness and debility
   e. All of the above

5. Which of the following is a *lakṣhaṇa* of *majja dhātu kṣhaya*?
   a. Cracking and pricking pain in the smaller joints
   b. Darkness around the eyes and darkened vision
   c. Dizziness and feeling of instability
   d. Thin, weak and light bones
   e. All of the above

6. Which of the following is a *lakṣhaṇa* of *rasa dhātu kṣhaya*?
   a. Constant exhaustion even after rest
   b. Intolerance for sound or noise
   c. Restlessness
   d. Squeezing pressure or pain around the heart
   e. All of the above

7. Which of the following is a *lakṣhaṇa* of *majja dhātu kṣhaya*?
   a. Cracking and pricking pain in the smaller joints
   b. Darkness around the eyes and darkened vision
   c. Dizziness and feeling of instability
   d. Thin, weak and light bones
   e. All of the above

8. *Ap* is predominant in which *dhātu*(s)?
   a. *Rasa, medas, majja* and *śhukra*
   b. *Rasa, rakta, mamsa* and *śhukra*
   c. *Rakta, mamsa, medas, and śhukra*
   d. *Rakta, medas, majja* and *śhukra*
   e. None of the above

9. What supports *dhātus* but does not provide nourishment to subsequent *dhātus*?
   a. *Dhātumala*
   b. *Dhātu poṣhaṇa*
   c. *Rasadhātu*
   d. *Śhukradhātu*
   e. *Upadhātu*

10. What is the *dhātumala* of *rasadhātu*?
   a. Feces
   b. *Kapha*
   c. Oily secretions of eyes, feces, skin
   d. Sweat
   e. Urine

CRITICAL THINKING

1. Create a chart or diagram starting with the term *dhātu* and identify and explain its possible classifications and perspectives together.

2. Identify at least one *kāraṇa* for *dhātu vṛddhi* and *dhātu kṣhaya* directly from the classical texts and cite the references.

3. Explain how *samānya-viśheṣha* causes *vṛddhi-kṣhaya* to influence the generation of *upadhātus* and *dhātumalas*. Demonstrate the process and important steps using a theoretical example.

4. Using the relationship between *dhātus* and *pañcha mahābhūtas*, classify at least three *dhātu vṛddhi* and *dhātu kṣhaya lakṣhaṇas* for any single *dhātu* and explain how each is generated by the related *pañcha mahābhūta*. Justify this relationship using the appropriate *guṇa(s)*.

5. Using the tables provided in this chapter, how would you identify which *dhātu vṛddhi* and *dhātu kṣhaya lakṣhaṇas* might be more important to memorize than others? Create your own short list where you can reference these priority *lakṣhaṇas* on a single page.

Chapter 9 : Mala

KEY TERMS

kṣhīṇa mala lakṣhaṇa	prākṛta mala lakṣhaṇa	purīṣha	svedo kṣhaya
mūtra	prākṛta mūtra	purīṣha kṣhaya	svedo vṛddhi
mūtra kṣhaya	prākṛta purīṣha	purīṣha vṛddhi	trimala
mūtra vṛddhi	prākṛta svedo	sveda	vṛddha mala lakṣhaṇa

The *trimala* are the three main waste products of the body – *mūtra*, *purīṣha* and *sveda*. They are generated as outcomes of ongoing *dhātu pariṇāma* and must be expelled on a regular basis. All authors have included passing stool and urine under the concept of *adhāraṇīya vegas* because they should never be withheld when the urge arises.

Excessive loss or accumulation of *malas* can be detrimental as Vāgbhaṭa states in AH Sū. 11/25:

मलोचितत्वाद्देहस्य क्षयो वृद्धेस्तु पीडनः ॥
अ. हृ. सू. ११।२५

Malochitatvāddehasya kṣhayo
vṛddhestu pīḍanaḥ ||

AH Sū. 11/25

Mala (waste products) are *uchitatva* (appropriate, suitable, fitting) for *deha* (the body), so *kṣhaya* (decrease, of *malas*) and/or *vṛddhi* (increase, of *malas*) result in *pīḍana* (affliction).

Chakrapāṇi states this even more clearly in the commentary of Cha. Sū. 28/4. He says that even the *malas* can be considered as *dhātus* because they help maintain and sustain the normal, healthy state of the body when they themselves are normal.

Purīṣha (stool) also commonly goes by the synonyms *śhakṛt* or *viṭ*.

PRĀKṚTA MALA LAKṢHAṆA

Prākṛta purīṣha lakṣhaṇa with nearest English equivalent	Cha. Sū.	Su. Sū. 15/4.2	AH Sū. 11/5	BP
Avaṣhṭambha Support or give strength to hold up the body		√	√	
Vāyu-agni dhāraṇa Supports *vāta* and *agni*		√		

Prākṛta mūtra lakṣhaṇa with nearest English equivalent	Cha. Sū.	Su. Sū. 15/4.2	AH Sū. 11/5	BP
Kleda vahāna Elimination of *kleda* (a watery constituent)			√	
Basti pūraṇa Fills the urinary bladder		√		
Vikleda kṛt Manages fluid balance		√		

Prākṛta sveda lakṣhaṇa with nearest English equivalent	Cha. Sū.	Su. Sū. 15/4.2	AH Sū. 11/5	BP
Kleda vidhṛti Retention of *kleda* (a watery constituent)			√	
Kleda tvak Regulates fluid balance through the skin		√		
Saukumārya kṛt Promotes youthfulness (of the skin)		√		

VṚDDHA MALA LAKṢHAṆA

Purīṣha vṛddhi lakṣhaṇa with nearest English equivalent	Cha. Sū.	Su. Sū. 15/15	AH Sū. 11/13	BP Pū. 7/69
Kukṣhi ādhmana-āṭopa Distension of abdomen with gas and gurgling			✓	
Gaurava Heaviness			✓	
Vedana Pain			✓	
Āṭopa kukṣhau śhūla cha Distension and gurgling with abdominal pain		✓		✓

Mūtra vṛddhi lakṣhaṇa with nearest English equivalent	Cha. Sū.	Su. Sū. 15/15	AH Sū. 11/13	BP Pū. 7/69
Basti toda Pricking pain in the bladder		✓	✓	✓ (*vedana*)
Kṛte akṛte saṁjñata Feeling of dissatisfaction after urination			✓	
Mūtra vṛddhi Increase in urine		✓		
Muhuḥ muhuḥ pravṛtti Increased attempts to pass urine, little by little		✓		✓
Ādhmāna Distension (of the urinary bladder)		✓		✓

Svedo vṛddhi lakṣhaṇa with nearest English equivalent	Cha. Sū.	Su. Sū. 15/15	AH Sū. 11/14	BP Pū. 7/69
Ati sveda Excessive sweat, sweating			✓	
Daurgandya Foul body odor		✓ (in *tvak*)	✓	✓
Kaṇḍū Itchiness		✓	✓	✓

KṢHĪNA MALA LAKṢHAṆA

Purīṣha kṣhaya lakṣhaṇa with nearest English equivalent	Cha. Sū. 17/70	Su. Sū. 15/11	AH Sū. 11/21	BP Pū. 7/88
Vāyu antrāṇi Movement of *vāyu* in the intestines	✓		✓	
Sa-śhabdo veṣhṭayanniva kukṣhi bhramati Sound (gurgling) in the abdominal cavity		✓	✓	✓
Ūrdva hṛt *Upward movement toward the heart*			✓	
Pārśhva pīḍayan-bhṛśham Severe discomfort, squeezing sensation of the sides of the abdomen	✓ (abdominal swelling)		✓	
Hṛdaya pārśhva pīḍā Squeezing pain around the heart and sides		✓		✓
Vāyu ūrdva gamana Upward movement of *vāta*	✓ (and *tiryak*)	✓		✓
Kukṣhau sañcharaṇa Movement (gurgling) in the abdomen		✓		

Mūtra kṣhaya lakṣhaṇa with nearest English equivalent	Cha. Sū. 17/71	Su. Sū. 15/11	AH Sū. 11/21	BP Pū. 7/89
Alpa mūtra Reduced quantity of urine		✓	✓	✓
Mūtrayet kṛchchhrā Difficulty in urination	✓		✓	
Vivarṇa sa-asram vā Urine is discolored or mixed with blood	✓		✓	
Basti toda Pricking pain around the bladder		✓		✓
Pippāsā Thirst	✓			
Asya-mukha pariśhuṣhyati Dryness of the mouth and face	✓			

Svedo kṣhaya lakṣhaṇa with nearest English equivalent	Cha. Sū.	Su. Sū. 15/11	AH Sū. 11/22	BP Pū. 7/90
Roma chyuti Falling of bodily hair			✓	
Stabdha romakūpa Stiffness, blockage of the body hair pores		✓	✓	✓
Sphuṭana tvacha Cracking of the skin			✓	
Tvak śhoṣha Dryness of the skin		✓		✓
Sparśha vaigunya Altered, defective sensation of touch		✓		
Sveda nāśha Complete loss or absence of sweat		✓		✓
Chakṣhu rūkṣhatā Dryness of the eyes				✓

Chapter 9: Review

ADDITIONAL READING

Read and review the references listed below to expand your understanding of the concepts in this chapter. Write down the date that you complete your reading for each. Remember that consistent repetition is the best way to learn. Plan to read each reference at least once now and expect to read it again as you continue your studies.

References marked with (skim) can be read quickly and do not require commentary review.

CLASSICS		1st read	2nd read
Charaka	Cha. Sū. 17/70-71 Cha. Sū. 28/4		
Suśhruta	Su. Sū. 15/		
Aṣhṭāṅga Hṛdaya	AH Sū. 11/		
Bhāva Prakāśha	BP Pū. 7/70-90		

JOURNALS & CURRENT RESOURCES

QUESTIONS & ANSWERS

Record your questions for this chapter here for further research and discussion.

Question:

Answer:

Question:

Answer:

Question:

Answer:

SELF-ASSESSMENT

1. Which of the following is directly related to the *malas*?
   a. *Adhāraṇīya vegas*
   b. *Malas as dhātus*
   c. *Mala kṣhaya* and/or *vṛddhi* cause *vaikṛta doṣha*
   d. *Malas* are created by *dhātu pariṇāma*
   e. All of the above

2. Which *prākṛta mala* offers strength and support to the body?
   a. *Mūtra*
   b. *Purīṣha*
   c. *Sveda*
   d. Both A and B
   e. All of the above

3. Which *prākṛta mala* regulates the fluids of the body?
   a. *Mūtra*
   b. *Purīṣha*
   c. *Sveda*
   d. Both A and C
   e. All of the above

4. Which author states *sveda* promotes youthfulness?
   a. *Bhāvamiśhra*
   b. *Chakrapāṇi*
   c. *Charaka*
   d. *Suśhruta*
   e. *Vāgbhaṭa*

5. Which of the following is a *lakṣhaṇa of mūtra vṛddhi*?
   a. Difficulty in urination
   b. Foul body odor
   c. Increased frequency to pass urine, with little satisfaction
   d. Passing loose stools with urine
   e. Urine is discolored or mixed with blood

6. Which of the following is a *lakṣhaṇa of purīṣha kṣhaya*?
   a. Alternating constipation and loose stools
   b. Foul body odor
   c. Movement and sound (gurgling) in the abdomen
   d. Pain
   e. Thirst

7. Which of the following is a *lakṣhaṇa of svedo vṛddhi?*
   a. Altered, defective sense of touch
   b. Falling of bodily hair
   c. Itchiness
   d. Stiffness and blockage of of body hair pores
   e. Thirst

8. Which state of *mala* is associated with thirst?
   a. *Mūtra kṣhaya*
   b. *Mūtra vṛddhi*
   c. *Purīṣha kṣhaya*
   d. *Svedo kṣhaya*
   e. *Svedo vṛddhi*

9. Which state of *mala* is associated with abdominal distention and pain?
   a. *Mūtra kṣhaya*
   b. *Mūtra vṛddhi*
   c. *Purīṣha kṣhaya*
   d. *Purīṣha vṛddhi*
   e. *Svedo kṣhaya*

10. Which state of *mala* is associated with dryness of the face, mouth and eyes?
    a. *Mūtra kṣhaya*
    b. *Purīṣha kṣhaya*
    c. *Svedo kṣhaya*
    d. Both A and C
    e. All of the above

CRITICAL THINKING

1. Do any of the malas share common *prākṛta*, *vṛddhi*, or *kṣhaya lakṣhaṇas*?
2. Using the tables provided in this chapter, how would you identify which *mala vṛddhi* and *mala kṣhaya lakṣhaṇas* might be more important to memorize than others? Create your own short list where you can reference these priority *lakṣhaṇas* on a single page.
3. Demonstrate how the *prākṛta mala lakṣhaṇas* indicate that the malas are functioning as *dhātus* using an example for each.
4. What relationship can be inferred between the *vṛddhi* and *kṣhaya* of *doṣhas* and the *vṛddhi* and *kṣhaya* of *malas*? Does a change in the state of the malas affect the *doṣhas*, and vice versa? If so, how?

Chapter 10 : Ojas

KEY TERMS

apara ojas	kāraṇa	ojo-vaha	Suśhruta sampradāya
bala	kṣhaya	para ojas	tuṣhṭi
cheṣhṭa	lakṣhaṇas	pramāṇa	vṛddhi
chetanā	mahā-mūlā	puṣhṭi	
deha	ojas	srotas	
hṛdaya	ojo-nāśha	sthāna	

At the end of *dhātu pariṇāma*, the culmination is the formation of *ojas*. This is considered to be the best, final result of all of the internal processing, conversion and uptake from consumed food. For the most part, classical descriptions of *ojas* are similar. And in certain cases, authors provide additional insight and unique perspectives.

PARIBHĀṢHĀ: DEFINITIONS

Ojas is defined by each of the classical authors as:

हृदि तिष्ठति यच्छुद्धं रक्तमीषत्सपीतकम् ।
ओजः शरीरे संख्यातं तन्नाशान्ना विनश्यति ॥

च. सू. १७।७४

Hṛdi tiṣhṭhati yachchhuddhaṁ raktamīṣhatsapītakam |
Ojaḥ śharīre saṅkhyātaṁ ṭannaśhānnā vinaśhyati ||

Cha. Sū. 17/74

Ojas is *hṛdi tiṣhṭhati* (situated or located in the heart), *śhuddha* (white, clean, pure), *rakta īṣhat* (slightly reddish, like blood) and *pītaka* (slightly yellowish). *Ojas* in the *śharīra* (body) is *saṅkhyāt* (measurable). When it gets destroyed, so does the body.

ओजस्तु तेजो धातूनां शुक्रान्तानां परं स्मृतम् ।
हृदयस्थमपि व्यापि देहस्थितिनिबन्धनम् ॥

अ. हृ. सू. ११।३७

Ojostu tejo dhātūnāṁ śhukrāntānāṁ param smṛtam |
Hṛdayasthamapi vyāpi dehasthitinibandhanam ||

AH Sū. 11/37

Ojas smṛta (Ojas is known as) *tejo dhātūnāṁ* (the processed outcome of all the *dhātus*), *śhukrāntānāṁ* (ending with *śhukra*), and *paraṁ* (the best, final product). It is *hṛdaya-stha* (located in the heart), *api vyāpi* (and also moves throughout) *deha-sthiti* (the body, where it is also located), which it *nibandhanam* (supports, constructs, binds together, regulates).

तत्र रसादीनां शुक्रान्तानां धातूनां यत् परं तेजस्तत् खल्वोजस्तदेव बलमित्युच्यते, स्वशास्त्रसिद्धान्तात् ॥

सु. सू. १५।१९

Tatra rasādīnāṁ śhukrāntānāṁ dhātūnāṁ yat paraṁ tejastat khalvojastadeva balamityuchyate, svaśhāstrasiddhāntāt ||

Su. Sū. 15/19

And so, from *rasādi* to *śhukrānta dhātus* (*rasa* through *śhukra*), the *paraṁ* (the best, final product) *tejastat* (is created through processing and conversion) *khalu* (and is definitely) *tad eva ojas* (known as *ojas*). *Iti uchyate* (And it is also known as) *bala, svaśhāstra* (in our *śhāstra*) *siddhāntāt* (as a core principle).

In the commentary of Cha. Sū. 28/4, Chakrapāṇi echoes Suśhruta's definition to better explain the main text.

TEST YOURSELF

Learn, review and memorize key terms from this section.

ojas

---

hṛdaya

---

bala

ARE *OJAS* AND *BALA* THE SAME?

According to the *Suśhruta sampradāya*, *ojas* and *bala* are two terms used to explain the same concept. They may be used interchangeably as synonyms in the context of this *sampradāya*. Suśhruta follows his definition with an explanation of terminology in Su. Sū. 15/20 by providing a description of the normal functions and responsibilities of *bala*:

तत्र बलेन स्थिरोपचितमांसता
सर्वचेष्टास्वप्रतिघातः स्वरवर्णप्रसादो
बाह्यानामाभ्यन्तराणां च
करणानामात्मकार्यप्रतिपत्तिर्भवति ॥
सु. सू. १५।२०

Tatra balena sthiropachitamāṁsatā
sarvacheṣhṭāsvapratighātaḥ
svaravarṇaprasādo
bāhgyānāmābhyantarāṇāṁ cha
karaṇānāmātmakāryapratipattirbhavati ||
Su. Sū. 15/20

And so, *bala* is responsible for *sthira-upachita-māṁsa* (stable or strong, well-developed *māṁsa*), *sarva cheṣhṭa pratighāta* (proper functioning, execution of all activities), *svara-varṇa-prasāda* (clearness and brightness of voice and complexion), *bāhya* and *abhyantara karaṇām* (all external and internal causes) for *ātma-kārya pratipatti* (everything which should be done and everything which is done by *ātma*).

Bhāvamiśhra quotes Suśhruta's perspective on the concept of *bala* in BP Pū. 7/114-118. He adds that *bala* is that which allows one to perform *cheṣhṭa* (all types of actions and activities) quickly, immediately or directly (without delay).

TEST YOURSELF

Learn, review and memorize key terms from this section.

Suśhruta sampradāya

---

ojas

---

bala

---

cheṣhṭa

OJO GUṆA AND KARMA

The effects of *ojas* are felt on all aspects of life and health through their *guṇa* and *karma*. Charaka likens this in Cha. Sū. 17/75(1) to the way bees collect honey from fruits and flowers. They carefully select their sources of nourishment according to what they most enjoy (for their health) and then process and refine it through digestion, turning it into honey which is the best final product. Likewise, *ojas* chooses from the available nourishment to create the best essence of the body and accordingly displays its characteristics and actions based on the quality of inputs.

Most authors have provided similar information on *ojas*. Use the table below to compare their perspectives.

Ojo guṇa and karma Characteristics and actions of *ojas*	Cha. Sū. 17/74-75	Su. Sū. 15/21-22	AH Sū. 11/38-41	BP Pū. 3/181-187
Hṛdi tiṣhṭhati Primarily based (located) in the heart	✓		✓	
Śhuddha Clean, pure, white	✓	✓ (*śhukla*, white)	✓	
Īṣhat rakta Slightly reddish in color (like blood)	✓		✓	
Sa-pītaka Slightly yellowish in color	✓		✓	
Sarpi varṇa Ghee-colored (when initially produced)	✓			
Madhu rasa Honey-flavored	✓			
Laja gandhi Aroma of *laja* (puffed rice)	✓			
Somātmaka Predominant in *soma guṇa*		✓	✓	✓
Snighdha Unctuous		✓	✓	✓
Śhīta Cold, cool		✓		✓
Sthira Stable		✓		✓
Sara Flowing		✓		
Vivikta Clear		✓		
Mṛdu Soft		✓		✓
Mṛtsna Fragrant		✓		
Prāṇa-āyatana uttama One of the best (most important) locations or seats for *prāṇa* (life)		✓		

Deha-avayava vyāpta Pervades all limbs of the body		✓	✓	✓
Deha nibandhana Regulates all functions of the body			✓	
Sita White-colored, like natural sugar				✓
Bala puṣhṭi kara Increases strength and nourishment			✓	✓
Guru Heavy				✓
Sāndra Thick, dense				✓
Svadu Sweet				✓
Prasanna Bright, pure, clear				✓
Pichchhila Slimy				✓
Sūkṣhma Subtle				✓

Vāgbhaṭa adds in AH Sū. 11/41 that when *ojas* is specifically increased or strong, it is also responsible for *deha tuṣhṭi, puṣhṭi* and *bala* (contentment or satisfaction, nourishment and strength of the body).

In Cha. Sū. 30/9-11, Charaka also provides a detailed explanation of *ojas*' importance and functions from the moment of conception. It is responsible for life itself, including conception.

Bhāva Prakāśha includes a useful summary of the perspectives of several authorities, including Charaka, Vāgbhaṭa and Suśhruta in BP Pū. 3/182-187.

TEST YOURSELF

Learn, review and memorize key terms from this section.

deha

____

tuṣhṭi

____

puṣhṭi

____

bala

____

OJO BHEDA

Charaka describes two subtypes of *ojas* - *para ojas* and *apara ojas* in Cha. Sū. 30/6-7. He directly states that *para ojas* has its *sthāna* in *caitanya-saṅgraha*, or the place where *chetanā* gathers, ie the heart. This implies that *apara ojas* moves throughout the entire body.

Chakrapāṇi comments on these statements and Cha. Sū. 17/73-75 to clarify these points, as follows:

	Para ojas	*Apara ojas*
Sthāna Location	*Chaitanya-saṅgraha* Heart	*Mahatā mahāmūlā daśha* 10 major vessels rooted in the heart
Pramāṇa Quantity	*Aṣhṭa bindu* 8 drops	*Ardha añjali** One-half volume of cupped hands
Ojo-nāśha Loss of ojas	*Nāśha dhāri* Loss of life (immediate)	*Ojo-vikāra* Disorders due to loss of ojas

*See Cha. Śhā. 7/15.

TEST YOURSELF

Learn, review and memorize key terms from this section.

para ojas

apara ojas

sthāna

chetanā

pramāṇa

ojo-nāśha

OJO STHĀNA

Charaka states that the heart is the main *sthāna*, or location for *para ojas*:

तत् परस्यौजसः स्थानं तत्र चैतन्यसंग्रहः ।

च. सू. ३०।६.५

Tat parasyaujasaḥ sthānaṁ tatra chaitanyasaṅgrahaḥ |

Cha. Sū. 30/6.5

That (which is) *parasyaujasaḥ* (*para ojas*) *sthānaṁ* (is located) *tatra* (in that place) *chaitanya saṅgrahaḥ* (where *chetanā* gathers or is collected, ie, the heart).

Vāgbhaṭa also notes in AH Sū. 11/37 that the *sthāna* of *ojas* is the *hṛdaya*. Additionally, it is *deha-sthiti-nibandhanam*, or located throughout the body, which is its entire receptacle. Essentially, he is stating that *ojas* pervades throughout the body while having its main location in the heart. This can also be understood in reference to the two types of *ojas*.

TEST YOURSELF

Learn, review and memorize key terms from this section.

sthāna

para ojas

chetanā

hṛdaya

CHANNELS CARRYING OJAS

Charaka describes ten channels which are responsible for carrying *ojas* throughout the body. These are described as:

तेन मूलेन महता महामूला मता दश ।
ओजोवहाः शरीरेऽस्मिन् विधम्यन्ते समन्ततः ॥

च. सू. ३०।८

Tena mūlena mahatā mahāmūlā matā daśha |
Ojovahāḥ śharīre ' smin vidhamyante samantataḥ ||

Cha. Sū. 30/8

Thus, at the *mūlena mahatā* (root of the heart) *mahā-mūlā* (the major root channels) *matā* (are considered to be) *daśha* (ten). *Ojo-vahaḥ* (These are the channels of *ojas*) and *vidhamyante* (they pulsate, move *ojas*) *samantataḥ* (through the entire) *śharīre* (body).

A more detailed explanation of the concept of *srotas* which are considered the main channels of the body will be covered in Chapter 11.

TEST YOURSELF

Learn, review and memorize key terms from this section.

mahā-mūlā

ojo-vaha

srotas

FACTORS RESPONSIBLE FOR OJAS AND BALA

Increasing *ojas* and *bala* is key to maintaining a healthy state for every individual. These classical recommendations include both general and a few specific instructions. The general rules are preferred because the specific requirements for each application must be considered based on many factors.

Ojo vṛddhi kāraṇa Factors to increase *ojas* (and *bala*)	Cha. Sū. 30/13-14	Su. Sū. 15/29-30	AH Sū. 11/42	BP Pū.
Duḥkha-hetavaḥ Avoid anything which causes unhappiness	✓			
Prasādana for *hṛdaya, ojas, srotas* Soothing, appeasing, gratifying for heart, ojas, channels of circulation	✓			
Sevyaṁ prayatnena praśhamo jñāna Regular effort to calm the mind (higher knowledge)	✓			
Svayoni vardhana anna-pāna Food and drinks of the same sources (similar properties) to that which is decreased (among *doṣhas, dhātus, malas*)		✓	✓	
Prārthayate Fulling cravings (for specific types of foods that will correct a deficiency)		✓	✓	

TEST YOURSELF

Learn, review and memorize key terms from this section.

ojas

vṛddhi

kāraṇa

OJO KṢHAYA KĀRAṆA

Because *ojas* is responsible for so many positive health outcomes, it should be clear that its maintenance and promotion are a constant priority. One of the most effective ways to increase *ojas* is to not allow it to be decreased. The classics have listed several specific causes for the decrease of *ojas* and these should be avoided as much as possible.

Ojo kṣhaya kāraṇa Causes for decrease of *ojas*	Cha. Sū.	Su. Sū. 15/24	AH Sū. 11/39-40	BP Pū. 7/86
Abhitghāta External trauma or injury		✓		
Kṣhaya Decrease (of dhātus)		✓		
Kopa Anger		✓	✓	✓
Śhoka Sadness		✓	✓	✓
Bhayāna Anxiety		✓	✓	
Śhrama Exhaustion		✓	✓ (*ādi*, etc)	✓ (*ādi*, etc)
Kṣhut Hunger		✓	✓	
Chinta Worry				✓
Rūkṣha, tīkṣhṇa, uṣhṇa, kaṭu Excessive use of dry, sharp, hot and pungent (foods)				✓
Karśhaṇa para Effecting too much reduction in any form (therapeutically, physically, etc)				✓

Rather than listing both causes of increase and decrease for *ojas*, Charaka focused on the increasing factors where other authors identified decreasing causes. The inverse of each can serve as a guide to understanding each state through its opposite.

TEST YOURSELF

Learn, review and memorize key terms from this section.

ojas

kṣhaya

kāraṇa

OJO KṢHAYA LAKṢHAṆAS

When *ojas* is decreased, specific *lakṣhaṇas* can help identify this state.

Ojo kṣhaya lakṣhaṇas Characteristics of decreased *ojas*	Cha. Sū. 17/73	Su. Sū. 15/24	AH Sū. 11/39-40	BP Pū. 7/87
Bibheti Constant fear	✓		✓	✓
Durbala Weakness	✓		✓	✓
Abhīkṣhṇa Worry	✓		✓	✓
Dhyāyati vyathitendriya Sense organs being afflicted with pain	✓		✓	✓
Duśhchhāya Poor complexion	✓		✓	
Durmanā Sad, bad disposition, low spirits	✓		✓	✓
Rūkṣha Dryness	✓		✓	✓
Kṣhāma Thin, wasted, sickly	✓		✓	✓
Mūrchchhā Fainting		✓		
Māṁsa kṣhaya Reduction, wasting of māṁsa		✓		
Moha Delerium		✓		
Pralāpa Excessive, irrelevant speech		✓		
Maraṇa Death		✓		
Chinta Worry				✓

Suśhruta has provided a description of disorders of *ojas* using three clinical presentations. This is described in Su. Sū. 15/23-31 and includes the management of each.

TEST YOURSELF

Learn, review and memorize key terms from this section.

ojas

kṣhaya

lakṣhaṇas

Chapter 10: Review

ADDITIONAL READING

Read and review the references listed below to expand your understanding of the concepts in this chapter. Write down the date that you complete your reading for each. Remember that consistent repetition is the best way to learn. Plan to read each reference at least once now and expect to read it again as you continue your studies.

References marked with (skim) can be read quickly and do not require commentary review.

CLASSICS		1st read	2nd read
Charaka	Cha. Sū. 17/73-75 Cha. Sū. 28/4 Cha. Sū. 30/9-11 Cha. Sū. 30/6-8 Cha. Sū. 30/13-14		
Suśhruta	Su. Sū. 15/19-31		
Aṣhṭāṅga Hṛdaya	AH Sū. 11/37-42		
Bhāva Prakāśha	BP Pū. 3/181-187 BP Pū. 7/86-87 BP Pū. 7/114-118		

JOURNALS & CURRENT RESOURCES

Journal article: *Ojas: The Vital Nectar of Life*

QUESTIONS & ANSWERS

Record your questions for this chapter here for further research and discussion.

Question:

Answer:

Question:

Answer:

Question:

Answer:

SELF-ASSESSMENT

1. Which of the following describes *ojas*?
   a. Color is white, slightly red and yellow
   b. Located in the heart
   c. Located throughout the body
   d. The best, final result of *dhātu pariṇāma*
   e. All of the above

2. Which of the following describes *bala*?
   a. Ability to perform actions without delay
   b. All which is done by *ātma*
   c. Bright clear voice and complexion
   d. Stable, strong, developed *māṁsa*
   e. All of the above

3. Which of the following is a *guṇa* and/or *karma* of *ojas*?
   a. Color of ghee, taste of honey, smell of puffed rice
   b. Heavy, dense and salty
   c. Located in the heart, seat of *prāṇa* and *śhukra*
   d. Sweet, slimy and cloudy
   e. Warm, clear and fragrant

4. Vāgbhaṭa states that *ojas* is strong due to
   a. Being ghee-colored
   b. Being collected like bees collect honey
   c. Capable of deha *tuṣhṭi, puṣhṭi* and *bala*
   d. Providing the seat for *prāṇa*
   e. All of the above

5. According to Charaka, the *sthāna* of *para ojas* is where *chetanā* gathers, which is
   a. The seat of *prāṇa*
   b. The ten major vessels rooted in the heart
   c. The heart
   d. The entire body
   e. All of the above

6. The *pramāṇa* of *apara ojas* is
   a. Disorders due to loss of *ojas*
   b. Eight drops
   c. Loss of life
   d. One-half volume of cupped hands
   e. All of the above

7. *Apara ojas* is found
   a. Throughout the entire body
   b. In the brain
   c. Rooted in the ten major vessels emanating from the heart
   d. A and C only
   e. All of the above

8. Which of the following is not a key factor for *ojo vṛddhi*?
   a. Avoiding *āhāra* which causes *kṣhaya* of *doṣhas, dhātus, malas*
   b. Excessive use of *tīkṣhṇa, uṣhṇa, kaṭu*
   c. Fulfilling food cravings
   d. Regular effort to calm the mind
   e. All of the above

9. Which of the following is not a key factor for *ojo kṣhaya?*
   a. Lack of appetite
   b. Anxiety, worry, anger
   c. Avoiding unhappy situations
   d. Too much work or exercise
   e. All of the above

10. Which of the following describes *ojo kṣhaya*?
    a. Dull dry complexion
    b. Excessive speech, worry, fear
    c. Fainting and delirium
    d. Thin body with wasting of *māṁsa*
    e. All of the above

CRITICAL THINKING

1. In the explanations of normal functioning of *ojas* and *bala*, *cheṣhṭa* is commonly cited as one of the *lakṣhaṇas*. How could this be interpreted? Provide at least five examples of voluntary and involuntary physiological functions that can be supported by healthy *ojas* and *bala*.

2. Looking at the *lakṣhaṇas* of *ojo kṣhaya*, what conclusions can be drawn from the descriptions provided by different authors? How could these present clinically?

3. Analyze the *ojo kṣhaya kāraṇa* along with the *doṣha* and *dhātu kṣhaya kāraṇa*. What is similar? What is different?

4. Can any other analogies accurately describe the concept of *oja*s?

5. Consider the *prākṛta* and *vaikṛta lakṣhaṇas* of *doṣha, dhātu, mala* and *ojas*. Describe at least three examples based on assessable *lakṣhaṇas* that could be due to more than one cause (*doṣha, dhātu, mala, ojas*).

Chapter 11 : Srotas

KEY TERMS

abhiṣhyandi
anabhiṣhyandi
annavahā srotas
asthivahā srotas
atipravṛtti
dhamani
majjavahā srotas
māṁsavahā srotas
medovahā srotas
mūtravahā srotas
prāṇavahā srotas
purīṣhavahā srotas
raktavahā srotas
rasavahā srotas
samānya nidāna
saṅga
sirā
sirā granthi
srotas
sroto duṣhṭi
sroto duṣhṭi lakṣhaṇa
sroto duṣhṭi nidāna
sroto mūla
sroto mūla sthāna
śhukravahā srotas
svedavahā srotas
udakavahā srotas
vimārga gamana
viśheṣha nidāna

The systems of *srotases* are one of the main methods of transportation within the body. Within the *Charaka sampradāya*, these networks of *srotases* would likely be considered the most important of several types of transportation systems. Unlike other networks of channels, such as *dhamani* (arterial networks) and *sirā* (venous networks), the concept of *srotas* has an entire chapter dedicated to it in Cha. Vi. 5/.

Suśhruta provides his perspective on the concept of *srotas* with the specification that they are meant for use in surgical contexts. Vāgbhaṭa and later authors follow either of the main *sampradāya* in their works.

While *srotas* is often translated as "channel" it should be noted that there are many other anatomical components in Āyurveda which perform similar functions and can be translated the same way. What makes *srotases* different? Charaka provides perhaps the most rational explanation for practical application in a general clinical setting.

In this chapter and throughout this series, the technical term *srotas* will be used to refer to a complete network of exudative channels, as a whole system. The usage of *srotases* will refer to the innumerable, individual exudative channels within the network. For more details on rules for Anglicization of Sanskrit terms, review the preface at the beginning of this volume.

As a broad translation, "channels" may refer to any or all of the *sirā*, *dhamani* and *srotas*.

PARIBHĀṢHĀ AND PARYĀYA

Charaka and Suśhruta provide key statements to understand *srotas* and differentiate their specialized functions.

Definition #1: General overview

Suśhruta's definition of srotas is the most comprehensive as a general overview.

मूलात् खादन्तरं देहे प्रसृतं त्वभिवाहि यत् ।
स्रोतोस्तदिति विज्ञेयं सिराधमनिविर्जितम् ॥ १३

सु. शा. ९।१३

Mūlāt khādantaraṁ dehe prasṛtaṁ tvabhivāhi yat | Srotostaditi vijñeyaṁ sirādhamanivirjitam || 13

Su. Śhā. 9/13

Mūlāt (Having their root) khād-antaraṁ (in the central portion [ie, the heart]) dehe (in the body) prasṛtaṁ tvabhivāhi yat (and spreading out carrying the major channels such as rasa, etc) srotostaditi vijñeyaṁ (are the *srotases*), sirā-dhamani-virjitam (which are distinct from *sirā* and *dhamani*).

Suśhruta clearly states that *srotases* are different from both *sirā* and *dhamani* even though they perform similar functions. This definition is similar to Charaka's descriptions.

Definition #2: Primary function

In Cha. Sū. 30/12, three types of anatomical structures are succinctly defined based on their primary actions.

ध्मानाद्धमन्यः स्रवणात् स्रोतांसि
सरणात्सिराः || १२

च. सू. ३०।१२

Dhmānāddhamanyaḥ sravaṇāt srotāṁsi saraṇātsirāḥ || 12

Cha. Sū. 30/12

Dhmānād (That which flows out [from the heart] in pulsations) dhamanyaḥ (is [carried by] *dhamanis*); sravaṇāt (that which oozes or exudes) srotāṁsi (is [carried by] *srotases*) saraṇāt (that which is [constantly] moving) sirāḥ (is [carried by] *sirās*).

This reference provides three key definitions:

Dhamani	*Dhmānāt dhamanyaḥ* *Dhamanis* pulsate
Srotas	*Sravaṇāt srotāṁsi* *Srotases* ooze or exude
Sirā	*Saraṇāt sirāḥ* *Sirās* constantly move

Each definition specifies the distinguishing characteristics based on their function.

Structure	Primary function
Dhamani Artery	*Dhmānāt* Flows with pulsation
Srotas Exudative channel	*Sravaṇāt* Oozes, exudes
Sirā Vein	*Saraṇāt* Constantly moving

Dhamani and *sirā* will be covered in Chapter 19.

Definition #3: Detailed functions

In Cha. Vi. 5/3, the functions of the *srotases* are described in more detail.

स्रोतांसि खलु परिणाममापद्यमानानां
धातूनामभिवाहीनि भवन्त्ययनार्थेन || ३

च. वि. ५।३

Srotāṁsi khalu
pariṇāmamāpadyamānānāṁ
dhātūnāmabhivāhīni
bhavantyayanārthena || 3

Cha. Vi. 5/3

Srotāṁsi (The srotases) khalu (are then) pariṇāmamāpadyamānānāṁ (responsible for the conversion processes) dhātūnām (of the *dhātus*) abhivāhīni (by carrying near to them [the *dhātus*]) bhavanti ayana ārthena (all the necessary nutrients via circuation).

The main function of the *srotases* is described here. They are responsible for supplying nutrition to the *dhātus* during the ongoing processes of *dhātu pariṇāma*. Each *dhātu* is supplied by its own *srotas* which provides its specific nourishment.

Charaka reiterates this point in Cha. Vi. 5/8. While the primary function of the *srotases* is to supply selective, required nutrition, they may also serve as transportation networks for vitiated *doṣhas*. In this capacity, the *doṣhas* are able to spread and infect multiple *srotases* under the right conditions.

तेषां प्रकोपात् स्थानस्थाश्चैव मार्गगाश्च शरीरधातवःप्रकोपमापद्यन्ते, इतरेषां प्रकोपादितराणि च | स्रोतांसि स्रोतांस्येव, धातवश्च धातूनेव प्रदूषयन्ति प्रदुष्टाः | तेषां सर्वेषामेव वातपित्तश्लेष्माणः प्रदुष्टा दूषयितारो भवन्ति, दोषस्वभावादिति || ९

च. वि. ५|९

Teṣhāṁ prakopāt sthānasthāśhchaiva mārgagāśhcha śharīradhātavaḥ prakopamāpadyante, itareṣhāṁ prakopāditarāṇicha | Srotāṁsi srotāṁsyeva, dhātavaśhcha dhātūneva pradūṣhayanti praduṣhṭāḥ | Teṣhāṁ sarveṣhāmeva vātapittaśhleṣhmāṇaḥ praduṣhṭā dūṣhayitāro bhavanti, doṣhasvabhāvāditi || 9

Cha. Vi. 5/9

Teṣhāṁ (With their) prakopāt (great aggravation), sthānasthāśhchaiva (the location in which they reside) mārgagāśhcha (and the pathway) śharīra-dhātavaḥ (of the *dhātus* of the body) prakopamāpadyante (becomes completely involved in the great aggravation), itareṣhāṁ ([this is] one of their) prakopāditarāṇicha (modes of great aggravation, also leading to another). Srotaṁsi (The *srotases*) srotāṁsyeva (and even their contents), pradūṣhayanti (vitiate) dhātavaśhcha (their own *dhātus*) praduṣhṭāḥ dhātūneva (and even vitiate other *dhātus*). Teṣhāṁ sarveṣhāmeva (With all of these), vāta (*vāta*), pitta (*pitta*) śhleṣhmāṇaḥ (and *kapha*) praduṣhṭā (vitiate) dūṣhayitāro bhavanti (all of these), doṣhasvabhāvāditi (as it is their nature to do).

The complex possible outcomes of vitiated *doṣhas* and *dhātus* can be seen here. An almost infinite number of permutations, combinations and sequences can occur depending on each individual scenario.

Definition #4: Anatomical features

Charaka provides a description of the characteristic appearance of *srotases*. This is largely influenced by their function.

स्वधातुसमवर्णानि वृत्तस्थूलान्यणूनि च | स्रोतांसि दीर्घाण्याकृत्या प्रतानसदृशानि च || २५

च. वि. ५|२५

Svadhātusamavarṇāni vṛttasthūlānyaṇūni cha | Srotāṁsi dīrghāṇyākṛtyā pratānasadṛśhāni cha || 25

Cha. Vi. 5/25

Sva-dhātu (Just like their own *dhātu*), sama (the same) varṇāni (color), vṛtta (round shape), sthūla (thickness), ānyaṇūni cha (or thinness), dīrghāṇ (length), yākṛtyā pratāna cha (and tendril-like shape) sadṛśhāni (are seen) srotāṁsi (in the *srotases*).

The main characteristic features described here help to visually identify the *srotases*. Each *srotas* should be noted for its similarity to its own *dhātu* as well as its shape, thickness, size and growth pattern.

Lakṣhaṇa	Characteristic features
Sva-dhātu	Just like their own *dhātu*
Sama varṇāni	Same or similar color, as well as other characteristics
Vṛtta	Round shape
Sthūla-ānyaṇūni cha	Thickness or thinness
Dīrgha	Length
Yākṛtyā pratāna cha	Tendril-like shape

Synonyms

स्रोतांसि, सिराः, धमन्यः, रसायन्यः, रसवाहिन्यः, नाड्यः, पन्थानः, मार्गाः, शरीरच्छिद्राणि, संवृतासंवृतानि, स्थानानि, आशयाः, निकेताश्चेति शरीरधात्ववकाशानां लक्ष्यालक्ष्याणां नामानि भवन्ति | ... ९

च. वि. ५|९

Srotāṁsi, sirāḥ, dhamanyaḥ, rasāyanyaḥ, rasavāhinyaḥ, nāḍyaḥ, panthānaḥ, mārgāḥ, śharīrachchhidrāṇi, saṁvṛtāsaṁvṛtāni, sthānāni, āśhayāḥ, niketāśhcheti śharīradhātvavakāśhānāṁ lakṣhyālakṣhyāṇāṁ nāmāni bhavanti | ... 9

Cha. Vi. 5/9

Srotāṁsi (*Srotases*), sirāḥ (*sirās*), dhamanyaḥ (*dhamanis*), rasāyanyaḥ (*rasāyanis*), rasavāhinyaḥ (*rasavāhinis*), nāḍyaḥ (*nāḍis*), panthānaḥ (*panthas*), mārgāḥ (*mārgas*), śharīrachchhidrāṇi (*śharīrachchhidras*), saṁvṛtāsaṁvṛtāni (*saṁvṛtāsaṁvṛtas*), sthānāni (*sthānas*), āśhayāḥ (*āśhayas*), niketāśhceti (*niketas*) nāmāni bhavanti (are the names) śharīra-dhātvavakāśhānāṁ (of the visible spaces in the *dhātus*) lakṣhyālakṣhyāṇāṁ (that display characteristic features, and those that do not).

Many of the synonyms provided for *srotas* refer to other networks of channels, transportation systems and primary locations. *Srotas* networks are not literally equivalent to these other channels and structures, but are capable of performing similar functions. *Srotas* networks behave like the other transportation systems listed.

These synonyms are defined as:

Srotas	*Sravaṇāt srotāṁsi* *Srotases* ooze or exude
Sirā	*Saraṇāt sirāḥ* *Sirās* constantly move
Dhamani	*Dhmānāt dhamanyaḥ* *Dhamanis* pulsate
Rasāyani	Canal or channel for fluids; implies those channels that carry fluids to regenerate the body
Rasavāhini	The *rasavahā srotas* which carry nutritive fluid
Nāḍi	Any tubular channel
Pantha	A channel through which substances move or flow
Mārga	A pathway
Śharīrachchhidra	Perforations that act as passages through the body
Saṁvṛtāsaṁvṛta	Concealed (minute, hidden) and visible
Sthāna	Location, especially of primary importance
Āśhaya	A receptacle, seat of specific functions and activities, an organ
Niketa	House, habitation; a seat for a constituent component of the body

TEST YOURSELF

Learn, review and memorize key terms from this section.

srotas

dhamani

sirā

BHEDA

There are several perspectives on the classification of *srotases*. While all authors agree that there are an infinite number of potential *srotases* existing in the body on a minute, physical level, they also state that there are a fixed number of primary *srotas* networks as main systems of channels. These two perspectives are not contradictory. Each author identifies the set number and names of the *srotas* networks that are most significant within their scope of practice.

Potential for infinite srotases

Charaka explains the reasoning for the possibility of an infinite number of *srotases* by considering the manner in which the physical body is constructed.

यावन्तः पुरुषे मूर्तिमन्तो
भावविशेषास्तावन्त एवास्मिन् स्रोतसां
प्रकारविशेषाः| सर्वे हि भावा पुरुषे
नान्तरेण स्रोतांस्यभिनिर्वर्तन्ते, क्षयं
वाऽप्यभिगच्छन्ति ... || ३

च. वि. ५।३

Yāvantaḥ puruṣhe mūrtimanto
bhāvaviśheṣhāstāvanta evāsmin
srotasāṁprakāraviśheṣhāḥ | Sarve hi
bhāvā puruṣhe
nāntareṇasrotāṁsyabhinirvartante,
kṣhayaṁ vā ' pyabhigachchhanti ... ||3

Cha. Vi. 5/3

Yāvantaḥ puruṣhe mūrtimanto (For all the types of manifested human beings), bhāva-viśheṣhāstāvanta evāsmin (there are even specific types) srotasāṁ (of *srotases*) prakāra-viśheṣhāḥ (that are individually identifiable). Sarve hi bhāvā puruṣhe (All of these types of human beings) apyabhigachchhanti (advance their growth) nāntareṇa (only by) srotāṁsyabhinirvartante (build up due to *srotases*), kṣhayaṁ vā (reduction due to their withering away).

The key concept is that *srotases* are an absolute necessity for proper functioning of the human body. Their variety is infinite in the sense that each individual is a product of their unique factors which creates their particular physical structure.

Although this may lead one to infer that the human body is a conglomeration of different *srotases*, that is not completely true. Networks of *srotases* are distinct structures and they are identifiable. From this perspective, the most important *srotas* networks are enumerated systematically and detailed for practical application.

अपि चैके स्रोतसामेव
समुदयंपुरुषमिच्छन्ति, सर्वगतत्वात्
सर्वसरत्वाच्च दोषप्रकोपणप्रशमनानाम् | न
त्वेतदेवं, यस्य हि स्रोतांसि, यच्च वहन्ति,
यच्चावहन्ति, यत्र चावस्थितानि, सर्वं
तदन्यत्तेभ्यः || ४
अतिबहुत्वात् खलु
केचिदपरिसङ्ख्येयान्याचक्षते स्रोतांसि,
परिसङ्ख्येयानि पुनरन्ये || ५

च. वि. ५।५

Api chaike srotasāmeva samudayaṁ puruṣhamichchhanti, sarvagatatvāt sarvasaratvāchcha doṣhaprakopaṇapraśhamanānām | Na tvetadevaṁ, yasya hi srotāṁsi, yachchavahanti, yachchāvahanti, yatra chāvasthitāni, sarvaṁ tadanyattebhyaḥ || 4
Atibahutvāt khalu kechidaparisaṅkhyeyānyāchakṣhate srotāṁsi, parisaṅkhyeyāni punaranye || 5

Cha. Vi. 5/4-5

Api chaike (According to some), srotasāmeva samudayaṁ (the aggregation of *srotases*) puruṣhamichchhanti (is believed to produce a human being) sarvagatatvāt (due to their ability to move through everything [in the body]) sarvasaratvāchcha (and effuse nutritive supplies to all) doṣha (the *doṣhas*) prakopaṇa (resulting in *prakopa*) praśhamanānām (and *praśhamana*). Na tvetadevaṁ (But that is not entirely true), yasya hi srotāṁsi (as the *srotases* themselves), yachchavahanti (are under the control of), yachchāvahanti (and provide the nutritive supply for) yatra chāvasthitāni (the very places in which they reside [ie, the *dhātus*]), sarvaṁ (all of which) tadanyattebhyaḥ (are their own separate structures).

Atibahutvāt khalu (Isn't it that there are so many) kechidaparisaṅkhyeyānyāchakṣhate (which have been told as innumerable) srotāṁsi (srotases)? Parisaṅkhyeyāni punaranye (Then again, others say that they can be identified and numbered).

13 systems of srotases

Charaka classifies 13 systems of specific *srotases*, while maintaining that other types of networks may exist.

Note Charaka's method of introducing the specific systems of *srotases*. Rather than specify a particular number, he states that he will list them and leave the reader to infer any remaining.

तेषां तु खलु स्रोतसां यथास्थूलं कतिचित्प्रकारान्मूलतश्च प्रकोपविज्ञानतश्चानुव्याख्यास्यामः; ये भविष्यन्त्यलमनुक्तार्थज्ञानाय ज्ञानवतां, विज्ञानाय चाज्ञानवताम् || ६

च. वि. ५।६

Teṣhāṁ tu khalu srotasāṁ yathāsthūlaṁ katichitprakārānmūlataśhcha prakopavijñānataśhchānuvyākhyāsyāmaḥ; ye bhaviṣhyantyalamanuktārthajñānāya jñānavatāṁ, vijñānāya chājñānavatām || 6

Cha. Vi. 5/6

Teṣhāṁ tu khalu (So then, these) srotasāṁ (srotases) yathā-sthūlaṁ (being the gross, discernable type) katichit-prakārān (and being numerable) mūlataśhcha (with specific, primary root sources) prakopa-vijñānataśhchānu (and known through measurable features of aggravation) vyākhyāsyāmaḥ (will now be described by me, [says Punarvasu Ātreya]). Ye (These) bhaviṣhyantyalamanukt-ārtha-jñānāya (provide sufficient knowledge about the mechanics of operation) jñānavatāṁ (for those who understand the science [to infer more]), vijñānāya (and for those who can understand these alone) chājñānavatām (this information is sufficient).

तद्यथा – प्राणोदकान्न रसरुधिरमांसमेदोस्थिमज्जशुक्र मूत्रपुरीषस्वेदवहानीति वातपित्तश्लेष्मणां पुनः सर्वशरीरचराणां सर्वाणि स्रोतांस्ययनभूतानि, तद्वदतीन्द्रियाणां पुनः सत्त्वादीनां केवलं चेतनावच्छरीरमयनभूतमधिष्ठानभूतं च | तदेतत् स्रोतसां प्रकृतिभूतत्वान्न विकारैरुपसृज्यते शरीरम् || ७

च. वि. ५।७

Tadyathā – prāṇodakānna rasarudhiramāṁsamedosthimajjaśhukra mūtrapurīṣhasvedavahānīti; vātapittaśhleṣhmaṇāṁ punaḥ sarvaśharīracharāṇāṁ sarvāṇi srotāṁsyayanabhūtāni, tadvadatīndriyāṇāṁ punaḥ sattvādīnāṁ kevalaṁ chetanāvachchharīramayanabhūtamadhiṣhṭhānabhūtaṁ cha | Tadetat srotasāṁ prakṛtibhūtatvānna vikārairupasṛjyate śharīram || 7

Cha. Vi. 5/7

Tadyathā (And the systems of *srotases* are) – prāṇa (*prāṇa*), udaka (*udaka*), anna (*anna*), rasa (*rasa*), rudhira (*rakta*), māṁsa (*māṁsa*), medo (*medas*), asthi (*asthi*), majja (*majja*), śhukra (*śhukra*), mūtra (*mūtra*), purīṣha (*purīṣha*), sveda (*sveda*) vahānīti. Vāta (*Vāta*), pitta (*pitta*) śhleṣhmaṇāṁ (and *kapha*) punaḥ (as mentioned previously), sarva-śharīra-charāṇāṁ (move throughout the entire body) sarvāṇi (and all) srotāṁsya (of the networks of *srotases*) yana-bhūtāni (act as their channels of passage). Tad (Likewise), vadatīndriyāṇāṁ (the expressions of the indriyas) punaḥ (and even) sattvādīnāṁ (the mind and all of its components) adhiṣhṭhānabhūtaṁ cha (are located and can move) kevalaṁ (only) chetanāvach (where *chetanā*) chharīramayanabhūtam (is present throughout the body). Tadetat srotasāṁ (When these *srotases*) prakṛti-bhūtatvānna (are in a normal, healthy state of *prakṛti*), upasṛjyate (they build up) śharīram (the body) vikārair ([to prevent] disease).

Other classifications of srotases

Suśhruta provides a description of nine systems of *srotases* that are to be considered in the practice of Śhalya Tantra. The remaining later authors follow either Charaka's or Suśhruta's original classifications.

Review Su. Sā. 9/ and AH Sā. 3/41-48 for a comparison of perspectives. Note that other types of *srotases* are mentioned outside of these classifications when required. For example, while discussing the physiology of normal sleep, Suśhruta refers to *saṁjñāvahāni srotāṁsi* in Su. Śhā. 4/33.

TEST YOURSELF

Learn, review and memorize key terms from this section.

---

prāṇavahā srotas

---

udakavahā srotas

---

annavahā srotas

---

rasavahā srotas

---

raktavahā srotas

---

māṁsavahā srotas	
medovahā srotas	
asthivahā srotas	
majjavahā srotas	
śhukravahā srotas	
mūtravahā srotas	
purīṣhavahā srotas	
svedavahā srotas	

SROTO MŪLA AND DUṢHṬI

The specific features of each network of *srotases* are described through two major concepts. First, each *srotas* has two *mūla sthānas*, or two primary root sources. These root sources are the main locations that provide the generative source and strength for the *srotas* and ultimately their respective *dhātus*.

Second, each *srotas* has specific *lakṣhaṇas* that indicate its normal or abnormal function. These are called *sroto duṣhṭi lakṣhaṇas*. By ascertaining the presence or absence of these *lakṣhaṇas*, a clinical assessment can determine the current state of the particular *srotas*.

While describing the *sroto duṣhṭi lakṣhaṇas*, Charaka notes that for the *srotases* of each *dhātu*, their specific features are listed earlier in the text, in Cha. Sū. 28/.

प्रदुष्टानां तु खल्वेषां रसादिवहस्रोतसां विज्ञानान्युक्तानि विविधाशितपीतीये; यान्येव हि धातूनां प्रदोषविज्ञानानि तान्येव यथास्वं प्रदुष्टानां धातुस्रोतसाम् |

च. वि. ५।८

Praduṣhṭānāṁ tu khalveṣhāṁ rasādivahasrotasāṁ vijñānānyuktāni vividhāśhitapītīye; yānyeva hi dhātūnāṁ pradoṣhavijñānāni tānyeva yathāsvaṁ praduṣhṭānāṁ dhātusrotasām |

Cha. Vi. 5/8

Praduṣhṭānāṁ tu khalveṣhāṁ (In regards to their state of vitiation) rasādi-vaha srotasāṁ (the *rasa*, etc *srotases*) vijñānānyuktāni (are to be known from) vividhāśhitapītīye (the chapter titled "Vividhāśhitapītīyam adhyāya" [Cha. Sū. 28/]). Yānyeva hi dhātūnāṁ pradoṣhavijñānāni (Specific knowledge about the vitiation of the *dhātus*) tānyeva yathāsvaṁ praduṣhṭānāṁ dhātusrotasām (should be considered in context of the vitiation of the *srotases*).

Each *dhātu* and its respective *srotas* are so intimately linked that their features of normal and abnormal functioning can be understood in context of both. If one is dysfunctional, it should be understood that the other is likely to be abnormal as well. From a clinical perspective, this approach helps to streamline the assessment of the body and potentially simplify management protocols.

Next, each *srotas* will be reviewed through its original reference. Its *mūla sthānas* and *sroto duṣhṭi lakṣhaṇas* are identified in context of the *śhloka*. At the end of this section, a complete review of all *srotas* networks with their details is provided.

Prāṇavahā srotas

Air network

तत्र प्राणवहानां स्रोतसां हृदयं मूलं महास्रोतश्च, प्रदुष्टानां तु खल्वेषामिदं विशेषविज्ञानं भवति; तद्यथा - अतिसृष्टमतिबद्धं कुपितमल्पाल्पमभीक्ष्णं वा सशब्दशूलमुच्छ्वसन्तं दृष्ट्वा प्राणवहान्यस्य स्रोतांसि प्रदुष्टानीति विद्यात् ।

च. वि. ५।८

Tatra prāṇavahānāṁ srotasāṁ hṛdayaṁ mūlaṁ mahāsrotaśhcha, praduṣhṭānāṁ tu khalveṣhāmidae viśheṣhavijñānaṁ bhavati; tadyathā - atisṛṣhṭamatibaddhaṁ kupitamalpālpamabhīkṣhṇaṁ vā saśhabdaśhūlamuchchhvasantaṁ dṛṣhṭvā prāṇavahānyasya srotāṁsi praduṣhṭānītividyāt |

Cha. Vi. 5/8

Tatra (And so), prāṇavahānāṁ srotasāṁ (*prāṇavahā srotas*) mūlaṁ (are rooted in) hṛdayaṁ (the heart) mahā-srotaśhcha (and the *mahā-srotas*, or gastrointestinal tract). Praduṣhṭānāṁ (When vitiated) tu (then), khalveṣhāmidae (they are definitely) viśheṣhavijñānaṁ bhavati (known by the specific features) tadyathā (as follows) – ati-sṛṣhṭam (too much) ati-baddhaṁ (too constricted), kupitam (aggravated), alpa-alpam (too little, shallow) abhīkṣhṇaṁ vā (or too frequent [breaths]) sa-śhabda (accompanied with sound), śhūlam (gastrointestinal pain), uchchhvasantaṁ (accompanying inhalation). Dṛṣhṭvā (These are [the signs and symptoms] seen) prāṇavahānyasya srotāṁsi (in *prāṇavahā srotases*) praduṣhṭānītividyāt (when they are known to be vitiated).

Udakavahā srotas

Fluid network

उदकवहानां स्रोतसां तालुमूलं क्लोम च, प्रदुष्टानां तु खल्वेषामिदं विशेषविज्ञानं भवति; तद्यथा - जिह्वाताल्वोष्ठकण्ठक्लोमशोषं पिपासां चातिप्रवृद्धां दृष्ट्वोदकवहान्यस्य स्रोतांसि प्रदुष्टानीति विद्यात् |

च. वि. ५।८

Udakavahānāṁ srotasāṁ tālumūlaṁ kloma cha, praduṣhṭānāṁ tu khalveṣhāmidaṁ viśhēṣhavijñānaṁ bhavati; tadyathā - jihvātālvoṣhṭhakaṇṭhaklomaśhoṣhaṁ pipāsāṁ chātipravṛddhāṁ dṛṣhṭvodakavahānyasya srotāṁsi praduṣhṭānīti vidyāt

Cha. Vi. 5/8

Udakavahānāṁ srotasāṁ (*Udakavahā srotas*) mūlaṁ (are rooted in) tālu (the palate) kloma cha (and thirst center). Praduṣhṭānāṁ (When vitiated) tu (then), khalveṣhāmidaṁ (they are definitely) viśhēṣhavijñānaṁ bhavati (known by the specific features) tadyathā (as follows) – jihvā (the tongue), tālu (the palate), oṣhṭha (the lips), kaṇṭha (the throat), kloma (and the thirst center) śhoṣhaṁ (dry up and waste away) pipāsāṁ cha (and thirst) ati-pravṛddhāṁ (is excessively increased). Dṛṣhṭva (These are [the signs and symptoms] seen) udakavahānyasya srotāṁsi (in *udakavahā srotases*) praduṣhṭānīti vidyāt (when they are known to be vitiated).

Annavahā srotas

Food network

अन्नवहानां स्रोतसामामाशयो मूलं वामं च पार्श्वं, प्रदुष्टानां तु खल्वेषामिदं विशेषविज्ञानं भवति; तद्यथा - अनन्नाभिलषणमरोचकविपाकौ छर्दिं च दृष्ट्वाऽन्नवहान्यस्य स्रोतांसि प्रदुष्टानीति विद्यात् |

च. वि. ५।८

Annavahānā srotasāmāmāśhayo mūlaṁ vāmaṁcha pārśhvaṁ, pradușhțānāṁ tu khalveșhāmidaṁ viśheșhavijñānaṁ bhavati; tadyathā - anannābhilașhaṇamarochakavipākau chhardiṁ cha dṛshṭvā ' nnavahānyasya srotāṁsi pradușhțānīti vidyāt |

Cha. Vi. 5/8

Annavahānā srotasām (*Annavahā srotas*) mūlaṁ (are rooted in) āmāśhayo (the upper portion of the stomach) cha (and) vāmaṁ (the left) pārśhvaṁ (side of the torso). Pradușhțānāṁ (When vitiated) tu (then), khalveșhāmidaṁ (they are definitely) viśheșhavijñānaṁ bhavati (known by the specific features) tadyathā (as follows) – anannābhilașhaṇam (lack of cravings for any type of food), arochaka (a digestive disorder characterized by loss of appetite, abnormal taste sensation and indigestion), vipākau (improper digestion of consumed items), chhardiṁ cha (and vomiting). Dṛșhțvā (These are [the signs and symptoms] seen) annavahānyasya srotāṁsi (in *annavahā srotases*) pradușhțānīti vidyāt (when they are known to be vitiated).

Rasavahā srotas

Rasa dhātu network

रसवहानां स्रोतसां हृदयं मूलं दश च धमन्यः |

च. वि. ५।८

Rasavahānāṁ srotasāṁ hṛdayaṁ mūlaṁ daśha cha dhamanyaḥ |

Cha. Vi. 5/8

Rasavahānāṁ srotasāṁ (*Rasavahā srotas*) mūlaṁ (are rooted in) hṛdayaṁ (the heart) daśha cha dhamanyaḥ (and its ten major *dhamanis* that emerge from it).

Raktavahā srotas

Rakta dhātu network

शोणितवहानां स्रोतसां यकृन्मूलं प्लीहा च |

च. वि. ५।८

Śhōṇitavahānāṁ srotasāṁ yakṛnmūlaṁ plīhā cha |

Cha. Vi. 5/8

Śhōṇitavahānāṁ srotasāṁ (*Raktavahā srotas*) mūlaṁ (are rooted in) yakṛt (the liver) plīhā cha (and spleen).

Māṁsavahā srotas

Māṁsa dhātu network

मांसवहानां च स्रोतसां स्नायुर्मूलं त्वक् च |

च. वि. ५।८

Māṁsavahānāṁ cha srotasāṁ snāyurmūlaṁ tvak cha |

Cha. Vi. 5/8

Māṁsavahānāṁ cha srotasāṁ (And *māṁsavahā srotas*) mūlaṁ (are rooted in) snāyu (the sinews and tendons) tvak cha (and the skin).

Medovahā srotas

Medo dhātu network

मेदोवहानां स्रोतसां वृक्कौ मूलं वपावहनं च
|

च. वि. ५।८

Medovahānāṁ srotasāṁ vṛkkaumūlaṁ vapāvahanaṁ cha |

Cha. Vi. 5/8

Medovahānāṁ srotasāṁ (*Medovahā srotas*) mūlaṁ (are rooted in) vṛkkau (the two kidneys) vapāvahanaṁ cha (and the channels of the omentum).

Asthivahā srotas

Asthi dhātu network

अस्थिवहानां स्रोतसां मेदो मूलं जघनं च |

च. वि. ५।८

Asthivahānāṁ srotasāṁ medo mūlaṁ jaghanaṁ cha |

Cha. Vi. 5/8

Asthivahānāṁ srotasāṁ (*Asthivahā srotas*) mūlaṁ (are rooted in) medo (*medas* and *medo dhātu*) jaghanaṁ cha (and the buttocks).

Majjavahā srotas

Majja dhātu network

मज्जवहानां स्रोतसामस्थीनि मूलं सन्धयश्च |

च. वि. ५।८

Majjavahānāṁ srotasāmasthīni mūlaṁ sandhayaśhcha |

Cha. Vi. 5/8

Majjavahānāṁ srotasām (*Majjavahā srotas*) mūlaṁ (are rooted in) asthīni (the bones) sandhayaśhcha (and joints).

Śhukravahā srotas

Śhukra dhātu network

शुक्रवहानां स्रोतसां वृषणौ मूलं शेफश्च |

च. वि. ५।८

Śhukravahānāṁ srotasāṁ vṛṣhaṇau mūlaṁ śhephaśhcha |

Cha. Vi. 5/8

Śhukravahānāṁ srotasāṁ (*Śhukravahā srotas*) mūlaṁ (are rooted in) vṛṣhaṇau (both testicles) śhephaśhcha (and the penis).

Mūtravahā srotas

Urinary excretion network

मूत्रवहानां स्रोतसां बस्तिर्मूलं वङ्क्षणौ च,
प्रदुष्टानां तु खल्वेषामिदं विशेषविज्ञानं
भवति; तद्यथा - अतिसृष्टमतिबद्धं
प्रकुपितमल्पाल्पमभीक्ष्णं वा बहलं सशूलं
मूत्रयन्तं दृष्ट्वा मूत्रवहान्यस्य स्रोतांसि
प्रदुष्टानीति विद्यात् |

च. वि. ५।८

Mūtravahānāṁ srotasāṁ bastirmūlaṁ vaṅkṣhaṇau cha, praduṣhṭānāṁ tu khalveṣhāmidaṁ viśheṣhavijñānaṁbhavati; tadyathā - atisṛṣhṭamatibaddhaṁ prakupitamalpālpamabhīkṣhṇaṁ vā bahalaṁ saśhūlaṁ mūtrayantaṁ dṛṣhṭvā mūtravahānyasya srotāṁsi praduṣhṭānīti vidyāt |

Cha. Vi. 5/8

Mūtravahānāṁ srotasāṁ (*Mūtravahā srotas*) mūlaṁ (are rooted in) bastir (the urinary bladder) vaṅkṣhaṇau cha (and both sides of the pelvis). Praduṣhṭānāṁ (When vitiated) tu (then), khalveṣhāmidaṁ (they are definitely) viśheṣhavijñānaṁbhavati (known by the specific features) tadyathā (as follows) – ati-sṛṣhṭam (too much), ati-baddhaṁ (too constricted), prakupitam (aggravated) alpa-

alpam (too little, shallow, dribbling) abhīkṣhṇaṁ vā (or too frequent [urination]), bahalaṁ saśhūlaṁ (along with great, sharp pain), mūtrayantaṁ (and a sense of blockage when passing urine). Dṛṣhṭvā (These are [the signs and symptoms] seen) mūtravahānyasya srotāṁsi (in *udakavahā srotases*) praduṣhṭānīti vidyāt (when they are known to be vitiated).

Purīṣhavahā srotas

Fecal excretion network

पुरीषवहानां स्रोतसां पक्वाशयो मूलं स्थूलगुदं च, प्रदुष्टानां तु खल्वेषामिदं विशेषविज्ञानं भवति; तद्यथा - कृच्छ्रेणाल्पाल्पं सशब्दशूलमतिद्रवमतिग्रथितमतिबहु चोपविशन्तं दृष्ट्वा पुरीषवहान्यस्य स्रोतांसि प्रदुष्टानीति विद्यात् |

च. वि. ५।८

Purīṣhavahānāṁ srotasāṁ pakvāśhayo mūlaṁ sthūlagudaṁ cha, praduṣhṭānāṁ tu khalveṣhāmidaṁ viśheṣhavijñānaṁ bhavati; tadyathā - kṛchchhreṇālpālpaṁ saśhabdaśhūlamatidravamatigrathitama tibahu chopaviśhantaṁ dṛṣhṭvā purīṣhavahānyasya srotāṁsi praduṣhṭānīti vidyāt |

Cha. Vi. 5/8

Purīṣhavahānāṁ srotasāṁ (*Purīṣhavahā srotas*) mūlaṁ (are rooted in) pakvāśhayo (the lower intestines housing digested food) sthūlagudaṁ cha (and the large portion of the anal canal). Praduṣhṭānāṁ (When vitiated) tu (then), khalveṣhāmidaṁ (they are definitely) viśheṣhavijñānaṁ (known by the specific features) bhavati tadyathā (as follows) – kṛchchhreṇa (difficulty [passing stools]), alpa-alpaṁ ([stools pass] little by little, in small quantity), sa-śhabda (associated with sound) śhūlam (and sharp pain), ati-dravam (too liquidy), ati-grathitam (too lumpy, knotty, hardened), ati-bahu cha (and too much) upaviśhantaṁ (sitting required to pass stools). Dṛṣhṭvā (These are [the signs and symptoms] seen) purīṣhavahānyasya srotāṁsi (in *purīṣhavahā srotases*) praduṣhṭānīti vidyāt (when they are known to be vitiated).

Svedavahā srotas

Sweat excretion network

स्वेदवहानां स्रोतसां मेदो मूलं लोमकूपाश्च, प्रदुष्टानां तु खल्वेषामिदं विशेषविज्ञानं भवति; तद्यथा -अस्वेदनमतिस्वेदनं पारुष्यमतिश्लक्ष्णतामङ्गस्य परिदाहं लोमहर्षं च दृष्ट्वा स्वेदवहान्यस्य स्रोतांसि प्रदुष्टानीति विद्यात् || ८

च. वि. ५।८

Svedavahānāṁ srotasāṁ medo mūlaṁ lomakūpāśhcha, praduṣhṭānāṁ tu khalveṣhāmidaṁ viśheṣhavijñānaṁ bhavati; tadyathā - asvedanamatisvedanaṁ pāruṣhyamatiśhlakṣhṇatāmaṅgasya paridāhaṁ lomaharṣhaṁ cha dṛṣhṭvā svedavahānyasya srotāṁsi praduṣhṭānīti vidyāt || 8

Cha. Vi. 5/8

Svedavahānāṁ srotasāṁ (*Svedavahā srotas*) mūlaṁ (are rooted in) *medo* (*medas*, or *medo dhātu*) lomakūpāśhcha (and the follicles of the body hair). Praduṣhṭānāṁ (When vitiated) tu (then), khalveṣhāmidaṁ (they are definitely) viśheṣhavijñānaṁ (known by the specific features) bhavati tadyathā (as follows) – asvedanam (absence of sweat), ati-svedanaṁ (excessive sweat), pāruṣhyam (roughness [of the skin]), ati-śhlakṣhṇatām-aṅgasya (excessive smoothness of the limbs of the body), paridāhaṁ (a sensation of heat or burning), lomaharṣhaṁ ca (and horripilation). Dṛṣhṭvā

(These are [the signs and symptoms] seen) svedavahānyasya srotāmsi (in *svedavahā srotases*) praduṣhṭānīti vidyāt (when they are known to be vitiated).

Sroto mūla and duṣhṭi (Input networks)

Srotas Exudative network of channels	*Mūla sthāna* Primary root sources	*Sroto duṣhṭi lakṣhaṇa*	Specific features of dysfunction
Prāṇavahā srotas Air network	• *Hṛdaya* Heart • *Mahā-srotas* Gastro-intestinal tract	• Ati-sṛṣhṭa • Ati-baddha • Kupita • Alpa-alpa • Abhīkṣhṇa vā • Sa-śhabda • Śhūla • Uchchhvasanta	• Too much • Too constricted • Aggravated • Too little, shallow • Or too frequent • Accompanied with sound • Gastrointestinal pain • Accompanying inhalation
Udakavahā srotas Fluid network	• *Tālu* Palate • *Kloma* Thirst center	• Jihvā • Tālu • Oṣhṭha • Kaṇṭha • Kloma • Śhoṣha • Pipāsā cha • Ati-pravṛddhā	• Tongue • Palate • Lips • Throat • Thirst center • Dry up and waste away • And thirst • Excessively increased
Annavahā srotas Food network	• *Āmāśhaya* Upper portion of the stomach • *Vāma pārśhva* Left side of the torso	• Anannābhilaṣhaṇa • Arochaka • Vipākau • Chhardi cha	• Lack of cravings for any type of food • A digestive disorder characterized by loss of appetite, abnormal taste sensation and indigestion • Improper digestion of consumed items • And vomiting

Sroto mūla and dușhți (Transformation networks)

Srotas Exudative network of channels	*Mūla sthāna* Primary root sources	*Sroto dușhți lakșhaṇa*	Specific features of dysfunction
Rasavahā srotas Rasa dhātu network	• *Hṛdaya* Heart • *Daśha dhamani* Ten major *dhamanis* that emerge from the heart	• Aśhraddha • Aruchi • Āsya vairasya arasajñatā • Hṛllāsa • Gaurava • Tandrā • Sa-aṅga-marda • Jvara • Tamaḥ • Pāṇḍu • Sroto-rodha • Klaibya • Sāda • Kṛśhāṅgatā • Nāśho anerayathākāla • Valaya • Palitāni	• Disinterested in food • Lacking taste, appetite • Abnormal sense of taste, unable to taste • Regurgitating hiccup • Heaviness of the body • Exhaustion • Squeezing pain of the limbs • Fever • Overcome by darkness • Paleness complex • Obstruction of exudative channels • Impotence • Weariness, weakness • Emaciation of the limbs • Cessation of normal biological activites at their normal time, such as agni • Premature wrinkles • Premature greying, etc
Raktavahā srotas Rakta dhātu network	• *Yakṛt* Liver • *Plīhā* Spleen	• Kușhțha • Vīsarpa • Piḍakā • Raktapitta • Asṛgdara • Guda, meḍhra, āsya pāka • Plīhā • Gulma • Vidradhi • Nīlikā • Kāmalā • Vyaṅga • Piplu • Tila-kālakāḥ	• Complex skin disorders • Spreading skin pathology • Pustules, boils • Bleeding disorder • Menorrhagia • Suppuration of the anus, penis, mouth • Splenic disorders • Abdominal lump or tumor • Abscess • Dark mole • Jaundice • Freckles, blemishes • Portwine mark • Black mole like a sesame seed

		• Dadru • Charmadala • Śhvitra • Pāmā • Koṭha • Āsramaṇḍala	• Ringworm • Dermatitis • Leucoderma • Scabies • Urticaria • Circular erythema
Māṁsavahā srotas Māṁsa dhātu network	• *Snāyu* Sinews and tendons • *Tvak* Skin	• Adhi-māṁsa • Arbuda • Kīla • Gala-śhālūka • Gala-śhuṇḍike • Pūtimāṁsa • Alajī • Gaṇḍa • Gaṇḍa-māla • Upajihvikā	• Muscular overgrowth • Myoma • Hemorrhoids • Uvulitis • Tonsillitis • Putrid, decayed muscle • Boils • Goiter • Cervical lymphadenitis • Epiglottal overgrowth
Medovahā srotas Medo dhātu network	• *Vṛkkau* Two kidneys • *Vapāvahana* Channels of the omentum	• Ninditāni • Pramehāṇāṁ pūrvarūpāṇi	• Any of the eight types of physical presentations that are most challenging to manage (Cha. Sū. 21/) • Premonitory symptoms of complex urinary disorders including diabetes mellitus
Asthivahā srotas Asthi dhātu network	• *Medo* Medas and medo dhātu • *Jaghana* Buttocks	• Adhi-asthi • Adhi-danta • Danta, asthi bheda, śhūlaṁ • Vivarṇatā • Keśha, loma, nakha, śhmaśhru doṣha	• Excessive bone growth • Supernumary teeth • Splitting, sharp pain in the teeth and bones • Discoloration • Body hair, nails and beard prone to disease
Majjavahā srotas Majja dhātu network	• *Asthīni* Bones • *Sandhi* Joints	• Ruk parvaṇa • Bhrama • Mūrchchhā • Darśhanaṁ tamas astathā • Aruṣhāṁ sthūlamūlānāṁ parvajānā	• Pain in the small joints • Dizziness • Loss of consciousness • Overcome visually by complete darkness • Reddish (hot, angry), deeply set nodules growing from the same location

Śhukravahā srotas Śhukra dhātu network	• *Vṛṣhaṇau* Both testicles • *Śhepha* Penis	• Klaibya • Aharṣhaṇa rogi • Klība, alpa, āyurvirūpaṁ vā prajāyate • Na chāsya jāyate garbha • Patati prasravati	• Impotency • Afflicted with the inability to penetrate even with an erection • Produces impotent, few or short-lived, defective offspring • No conception is produced • Miscarriage

Sroto mūla and dușhți (Output networks)

Srotas Exudative network of channels	*Mūla sthāna* Primary root sources	*Sroto dușhți lakșhaṇa*	Specific features of dysfunction
Mūtravahā srotas Urinary excretion network	• *Basti* Urinary bladder • *Vaṅkșhaṇau* • Both sides of the pelvis	• Ati-sṛșhța • Ati-baddha • Prakupitam • Alpa-alpa • Abhīkșhṇaṁ vā • Bahalaṁ sa-śhūlaṁ • Mūtrayantaṁ	• Too much • Too constricted • Aggravated • Too little, shallow, dribbling • Or too frequent urination • Associated with great, sharp pain • A sense of blockage when passing urine
Purīșhavahā srotas Fecal excretion network	• *Pakvāśhaya* Lower intestines housing digested food • *Sthūla guda* Large portion of the anal canal	• Kṛchchhreṇa • Alpa-alpa • Sa-śhabda śhūla • Ati-drava • Ati-grathita • Ati-bahu cha upaviśhanta	• Difficulty passing stools • Stools pass little by little, in small quantity • Associated with sound and sharp pain • Too liquidy • Too lumpy, knotty, hardened • And too much sitting required to pass stools
Svedovahā srotas Sweat excretion network	• *Medo* • *Medas*, or *medo dhātu* • *Loma kūpa* • Follicles of the body hair	• Asvedana • Ati-svedana • Pārușhya • Ati-śhlakșhṇatā aṅgasya • Paridāha • Lomaharșha	• Absence of sweat • Excessive sweat • Roughness of the skin • Excessive smoothness of the limbs of the body • A sensation of heat or burning • Horripilation

TEST YOURSELF

Learn, review and memorize key terms from this section.

sroto mūla

sroto mūla sthāna

sroto duṣhṭi

sroto duṣhṭi lakṣhaṇa

SROTO DUṢHṬI BHEDA

Four types of *sroto duṣhṭi lakṣhaṇas* describe the mechanisms by which the *srotases* can become dysfunctional. These mechanisms often combine as one can produce another. One or more is always seen when a *srotas* or its respective *dhātus* reach a *vaikṛta* state.

अतिप्रवृत्तिः सङ्गो वा सिराणां ग्रन्थयोऽपि वा | विमार्गगमनं चापि स्रोतसां दुष्टिलक्षणम् || २४

च. वि. ५।२४

Atipravṛttiḥ saṅgo vā sirāṇāṁ granthayo ' pi vā | Vimārgagamanaṁ chāpi srotasāṁ duṣhṭilakṣhaṇam || 24

Cha. Vi. 5/24

Atipravṛttiḥ (Increased flow), saṅgo (accumulation causing obstruction), vā (or) sirāṇāṁ granthayo (obstruction like a knot in the sirā) api vā (or even) vimārga-gamanaṁ (moving the wrong way in a pathway) chāpi (and these are) srotasāṁ duṣhṭi-lakṣhaṇam (the ways in which the *srotases* may present their signs and symptoms of vitiation).

The four mechanisms are:

Sroto duṣhṭi	Lakṣhaṇa
Atipravṛtti	Increased flow
Saṅga	Accumulation causing obstruction
Sirā granthi	Obstruction like a knot in the *sirā*
Vimārga gamana	Moving the wrong way in any pathway

The manner in which these four present can vary widely because of different possible root causes. For example, *saṅga* may eventually lead to *sirā granthi*, causing *atipravṛtti* in the process and later *vimārga gamana*. *Sroto duṣhṭi lakṣhaṇa* may present singly or in any combination.

TEST YOURSELF

Learn, review and memorize key terms from this section.

atipravṛtti

saṅga

sirā granthi

vimārga gamana

SROTO DUṢHṬI NIDĀNA

Nidāna are any causative factors that contribute to a state of abnormality of any bodily structure or function. The details of *nidāna* and its related concepts will be covered later in this series.

In the context of *srotas*, *nidāna* contribute to *sroto duṣhṭi* on all levels. *Nidāna* are classified as *samānya* (general causative factors) and *viśheṣha* (specific causative factors for each *srotas*). Each are reviewed separately below and are summarized at the end of this section.

Samānya nidāna

The general causative factors for *sroto duṣhṭi* include generic factors that are commonly cited as potential causes for disease.

आहारश्च विहारश्च यः स्याद्दोषगुणैः समः |
धातुभिर्विगुणश्चापि स्रोतसां स प्रदूषकः ||
२३

च. वि. ५।२३

Āhāraśhcha vihāraśhcha yaḥ
syāddoṣhaguṇaiḥ samaḥ |
Dhātubhirviguṇaśhchāpi srotasāṁ sa
pradūṣhakaḥ || 23

Cha. Vi. 5/23

Āhāra (Food) śhcha (and) vihāraśhcha (activities) yaḥ syād (which themselves are) doṣha guṇaiḥ samaḥ (similar to the characteristics of the *doṣhas*) dhātubhir-viguṇa-śhchāpi (yet contrary to the characteristics of the *dhātus*), srotasāṁ sa pradūṣhakaḥ (vitiate the very same *srotas* networks).

Charaka states that virtually any type of food or activity has the potential to cause *sroto duṣhṭi*. The ability to determine the potential risk of any of these lies in the application of the foundational *siddhānta*. When any food or activity is similar to the *doṣha*'s *guṇas*, it will cause an increase in those *guṇas*, thus producing an increase of the *doṣha* as well. This directly raises the risk of the *doṣha*'s tendency to behave in its natural state of *dūṣhaṇa*.

Additionally, if the food and activities are *viguṇa* to the *dhātus*, they will have an antagonistic effect to the increase of the normal strength and health of the *dhātus*. The result is the increase of the *doṣha*(s) having the potential to vitiate, and the decrease of the *dhātus*, which are supposed to support the strength and health of the body.

The outcome of this combination of events may be realized over short or long durations of time. The continuation of this process largely depends on the individual's ability to recognize discomfort and change their food and activities accordingly.

Abhiṣhyandi and anabhiṣhyandi

A major factor that is seen across most *samānya nidāna* for *sroto duṣhṭi* is a specific *karma* called *abhiṣhyandi*. This action has the effect of promoting obstruction and blocking whatever is passing or moving through any type of network, channel or transportation system. Its opposite effect is *anabhiṣhyandi*, which deters obstruction and encourages normal movement and flow.

Bhāva Prakāśha provides a clear definition for *abhiṣhyandi*:

पैच्छिल्याद्गौरवाद् द्रव्यं रुद्ध्वा रसवहाः
शिराः । धत्ते यद्गौरवं तत्स्यादभिष्यन्दि
यथादधि ॥ २३५

भा. प्र. पू. ५।२३५

Paichchhilyādgauravād dravyaṁ ruddhvā rasavahāḥ śhirāḥ | Dhatte yadgauravaṁ tatsyādabhiṣhyandi yathādadhi || 235

BP Pū. 5/235

Paichchhilyād (Cloudy), gauravād (and heavy) dravyaṁ (substances) ruddhvā (which block) rasavahāḥ (the *rasavahā*) śhirāḥ (*sirā*, or *srotas*) dhatte (produce) yadgauravaṁ (the very same heaviness) tatsyād (in those locations, ie, *srotases*). Abhiṣhyandi (This is known as *abhiṣhyandi*), yathā ([which has an effect] just like) dadhi (curd).

The primary *guṇas* required to produce the effect of *abhiṣhyandi* are *pichchhila* and *guru*. When these are imparted to the body either through direct consumption as food or drink, or through activities, they have the potential to cause obstruction of the *srotases*, especially in *rasavahā srotas*. *Agni* is directly responsible for supplying the power needed to convert these effects into a lighter form.

Anabhiṣhyandi, or the opposite of *abhiṣhyandi*, can be considered as any *dravya* with the potential to exert the opposite effects. Logically, these *dravya* would be assumed to have primary *guṇas* such as *viśhada* and *laghu*.

Based on the definition above, *abhiṣhyandi* will be translated as blockage of the exudative channels, specifically referring to *srotas*.

Viśheṣha nidāna

The specific causative factors for *sroto duṣhṭi* are described by Charaka for each *srotas*. They are detailed here in their original format and summarized at the end of this section.

Prāṇavahā srotas

Air network

भवन्ति चात्र - क्षयात्
सन्धारणाद्रौक्ष्याद्व्यायामात् क्षुधितस्य च |
प्राणवाहीनि दुष्यन्ति स्रोतांस्यन्यैश्च दारुणैः
|| १०

च. वि. ५|१०

Bhavanti cātra - Kṣhayāt sandhāraṇādraukṣhyādvyāyāmāt kṣhudhitasya cha | Prāṇavāhīni duṣhyanti srotāṁsyanyaiśhca dāruṇaiḥ || 10

Cha. Vi. 5/10

Bhavanti cātra (And so it is said that) – kṣhayāt (a state of reduction, emaciation, wasting), sandhāraṇād (withholding natural urges of the body), raukṣhyād (dryness, roughness), vyāyāmāt (and physical exercise, work, exertion), kṣhudhitasya cha (while feeling hungry) duṣhyanti (are able to vitiate) prāṇavāhīni srotāṁsyanyaiśhca (the *prāṇavahā srotas*, or air network, as well as other *srotases*) dāruṇaiḥ (deeply).

Udakavahā srotas

Fluid network

औष्ण्यादामाद्भयात्
पानादतिशुष्कान्नसेवनात् | अम्बुवाहीनि
दुष्यन्ति तृष्णायाश्चातिपीडनात् || ११

च. वि. ५|११

Auṣhṇyādāmādbhayāt pānādatiśhuṣhkānnasevanāt | Ambuvāhīni duṣhyanti tṛṣhṇāyāśhchātipīḍanāt || 11

Cha. Vi. 5/11

Auṣhṇyād (Heat), āmād (*āma*), bhayāt (fear), pānād (drinking, especially alcohol), atiśhuṣhkānna sevanāt (regular, excessive consumption of extremely dry food), tṛṣhṇāyāśhchātipīḍanāt (and excessive control of thirst) duṣhyanti (are able to vitiate) ambuvāhīni (the *udakavahā srotas*, or fluid network).

Annavahā srotas

Food network

अतिमात्रस्य चाकाले चाहितस्य च भोजनात् | अन्नवाहीनि दुष्यन्ति वैगुण्यात् पावकस्य च || १२

च. वि. ५।१२

Atimātrasya chākāle chāhitasya cha bhojanāt | Annavāhīni duṣhyanti vaiguṇyāt pāvakasya cha || 12

Cha. Vi. 5/12

Ati-mātrasya (Over-eating [too large of a portion size]), chākāle (and at a time) chāhitasya cha bhojanāt (which is inappropriate to eat meals, or eating food which is unwholesome), vaiguṇyāt pāvakasya cha (or consuming food having contradictory qualities [to normal health] and disruptive to proper digestion) duṣhyanti (are able to vitiate) annavāhīni (the *annavahā srotas*, or food network).

Rasavahā srotas

Rasa dhātu network

गुरुशीतमतिस्निग्धमतिमात्रं समश्नताम्| रसवाहीनि दुष्यन्ति चिन्त्यानां चातिचिन्तनात् || १३

च. वि. ५।१३

Guruśhītamatisnigdhamatimātraṁ samaśhnatām | Rasavāhīni duṣhyanti chintyānāṁ chātichintanāt || 13

Cha. Vi. 5/13

Guru (Heavy), śhītam (cold), ati-snigdham (excessively unctuous, oily), ati-mātraṁ (too large, in excessive quantity [meals or food]), samaśhnatām (constantly eating, alternatively, taking a shower or bath after eating), chintyānāṁ (worry), chātichintanāt (and constantly engaged in stressful situations or work) duṣhyanti (are able to vitiate) rasavāhīni (the *rasavahā srotas*, or *rasa dhātu* network).

Raktavahā srotas

Rakta dhātu network

विदाहीन्यन्नपानानि स्निग्धोष्णानि द्रवाणि च | रक्तवाहीनि दुष्यन्ति भजतां चातपानलौ || १४

च. वि. ५।१४

Vidāhīnyannapānāni snigdhoṣhṇāni dravāṇi cha | Raktavāhīni duṣhyanti bhajatāṁ chātapānalau || 14

Cha. Vi. 5/14

Vidāhīni (That which causes a particular type of burning sensation) anna-pānāni (from food and drink), snigdha (or that [food and drink] which is unctuous), uṣhṇāni (hot), dravāṇi cha (or liquidy) bhajatāṁ (which is utilized [consumed] regularly) chātapānalau (along with exposure to the sun) duṣhyanti (is able to vitiate) raktavāhīni (*raktavahā srotas*, or *rakta dhātu* network).

Māṁsavahā srotas

Māṁsa dhātu network

अभिष्यन्दीनि भोज्यानि स्थूलानि च गुरूणि च | मांसवाहीनि दुष्यन्ति भुक्त्वा च स्वपतां दिवा || १५

च. वि. ५।१५

Abhiṣhyandīni bhojyāni sthūlāni cha gurūṇi cha | Māṁsavāhīni duṣhyanti bhuktvā cha svapatāṁ divā || 15

Cha. Vi. 5/15

Abhiṣhyandīni bhojyāni (Food which causes blockage of the exudative channels), sthūlāni (is bulky), cha gurūṇi (and heavy) bhuktvā cha (and is eaten) svapatāṁ divā cha (followed by sleeping during the day) duṣhyanti (is able to vitiate) māṁsavāhīni (*māṁsavahā srotas*, or the *māṁsa dhātu* network).

Medovahā srotas

Medo dhātu network

अव्यायामाद्दिवास्वप्नान्मेद्यानां चातिभक्षणात् | मेदोवाहीनि दुष्यन्ति वारुण्याश्चातिसेवनात् || १६

च. वि. ५।१६

Avyāyāmāddivāsvapnānmedyānāṁ chātibhakṣhaṇāt | Medovāhīni duṣhyanti vāruṇyāśhchātisevanāt || 16

Cha. Vi. 5/16

Avyāyāmād (Avoidance or lack of physical exercise, activity or work), divā-svapnān (sleeping during the day), medyānāṁ chātibhakṣhaṇāt (and consuming too much fatty food), vāruṇyāśhchātisevanāt (and excessive, regular consumption of *vāruṇa*, a specific type of alcoholic preparation) duṣhyanti (are able to vitiate) medovāhīni (*medovahā srotas*, or the *medo dhātu* network).

Asthivahā srotas

Asthi dhātu network

व्यायामादतिसङ्क्षोभादस्थ्नामतिविघट्टनात् | अस्थिवाहीनि दुष्यन्ति वातलानां च सेवनात् || १७

च. वि. ५।१७

Vyāyāmādatisaṅkṣhobhādasthnāmativighaṭṭanāt | Asthivāhīni duṣhyanti vātalānāṁ cha sevanāt || 17

Cha. Vi. 5/17

Vyāyāmād ([Too much] physical exercise, activity, or work), ati-saṅkṣhobhād (excessive agitation, shaking, violent jerks) asthnām (that goes deep into the bones), ati-vighaṭṭanāt (excessive striking, rubbing or breaking apart) vātalānāṁ cha sevanāt (or regular use of foods and activities that provoke *vāta*) duṣhyanti (are able to vitiate) asthivāhīni (*asthivahā srotas*, or the *asthi dhātu* network).

Majjavahā srotas

Majja dhātu network

उत्पेषादत्यभिष्यन्दादभिघातात् प्रपीडनात् | मज्जवाहीनि दुष्यन्ति विरुद्धानां च सेवनात् || १८

च. वि. ५।१८

Utpeṣhādatyabhiṣhyandādabhighātāt prapīḍanāt | Majjavāhīni duṣhyanti viruddhānāṁ cha sevanāt || 18

Cha. Vi. 5/18

Utpeṣhād (Excessive pressure), atyabhiṣhyandād (too much blockage of the exudative channels), abhighātāt (trauma, external attack, damage), prapīḍanāt (compression), viruddhānāṁ cha sevanāt (and regular consumption of food having contradictory properties) duṣhyanti (are able to vitiate) majjavāhīni (*majjavahā srotas*, or the *majja dhātu* network).

Śhukravahā srotas

Śhukra dhātu network

अकालयोनिगमनान्निग्रहादतिमैथुनात् | शुक्रवाहीनि दुष्यन्ति शस्त्रक्षाराग्निभिस्तथा || १९

च. वि. ५।१९

Akālayonigamanānnigrahādatimaithunāt | Śhukravāhīni duṣhyanti śhastrakṣhārāgnibhistathā || 19

Cha. Vi. 5/19

Akāla-yoni-gamanān (Improper timing for

sexual intercourse), nigrahād (improper methods of sexual intercourse), ati-maithunāt (excessive sexual intercourse), śhastra-kṣhāra-agnibhis-tathā (and improper surgical treatments, chemical application of bases, or cauterization) duṣhyanti (are able to vitiate) śhukravāhīni (*śhukravahā srotas*, or the *śhukra dhātu* network).

Mūtravahā srotas

Urinary excretion network

मूत्रितोदकभक्ष्यस्त्रीसेवनान्मूत्रनिग्रहात् | मूत्रवाहीनि दुष्यन्ति क्षीणस्याभिक्षतस्य च || २०

च. वि. ५।१०-२२

Mūtritodakabhakṣhyastrīsevanānmūtran igrahāt | Mūtravāhīni duṣhyanti kṣhīṇasyābhikṣhatasya cha || 20

Cha. Vi. 5/20

Mūtrita (When having the urge to pass urine [and instead]), udaka (drinking water), bhakṣhya (eating food), strī-sevanān (or indulging in sexual intercourse regularly), mūtra-nigrahāt (or restraining the urge to pass urine) kṣhīṇasya (in a debilitated or emaciated person) ābhikṣhatasya cha (or one suffering from chronic disease) duṣhyanti (are able to vitiate) mūtravāhīni (*mūtravahā srotas*, or the urinary excretion network).

Purīṣhavahā srotas

Fecal excretion network

सन्धारणादत्यशनादजीर्णाध्यशनात्तथा | वर्चोवाहीनि दुष्यन्ति दुर्बलाग्नेः कृशस्य च || २१

च. वि. ५।१०-२२

Sandhāraṇādatyaśhanādajīrṇādhyaśhan āttathā | Varchovāhīni duṣhyanti durbalāgneḥ kṛśhasya cha || 21

Cha. Vi. 5/21

Sandhāraṇād (Withholding the urge to pass the bowels), atyaśhanāda (excessive eating in quantity and frequency), jīrṇa-adhyaśhanāt (eating while the previous meal is still digesting), tathā (especially) durbalāgneḥ (in one with a compromised state of *agni*) kṛśhasya cha (or in a weakened, emaciated individual) duṣhyanti (are able to vitiate) varchovāhīni (*purīṣhavahā srotas*, or the fecal excretion network).

Svedavahā srotas

Sweat excretion network

व्यायामादतिसन्तापाच्छीतोष्णाक्रमसेवनात् | स्वेदवाहीनि दुष्यन्ति क्रोधशोकभयैस्तथा || २२

च. वि. ५।१०-२२

Vyāyāmādatisantāpāchchhītoṣhṇākram asevanāt svedavāhīni duṣhyanti krodhaśhokabhayaistathā || 22

Cha. Vi. 5/22

Vyāyāmād (Excessive physical exercise, activity or work), ati-santāpāch (too much exposure to heat), chhīta-uṣhṇā krama sevanāt (regularly going between cold and hot environments), krodha (anger), śhoka (grief), bhayaistathā (and fear) duṣhyanti (are able to vitiate) svedavāhīni (*svedavahā srotas*, or the sweat excretion network).

Sroto duṣhṭi viśheṣha nidāna

Srotas Exudative network of channels	*Viśheṣha nidāna* Specific causative factors	Specific causative factors
Prāṇavahā srotas Air network	• Kṣhaya • Sandhāraṇa •Raukṣhya • Vyāyāmāt kṣhudhitasya cha	• A state of reduction, emaciation, wasting • Withholding natural urges of the body • Dryness, roughness • Physical exercise, work, exertion while feeling hungry
Udakavahā srotas Fluid network	• Auṣhṇya • Āma • Bhaya • Pāna • Ati-śhuṣhkānna sevanāt • Tṛṣhṇāyāśhca atipīḍanāt	• Heat • Āma • Fear • Drinking, especially alcohol • Regular, excessive consumption of extremely dry food • Excessive control of thirst
Annavahā srotas Food network	• Ati-mātrasya • Chākāle • Chāhitasya cha bhojanāt • Vaiguṇyāt pāvakasya cha	• Over-eating [too large of a portion size] • Eating at inappropriate times • Eating food which is unwholesome • Consuming food having contradictory qualities [to normal health] and disruptive to proper digestion
Rasavahā srotas Rasa dhātu network	• Guru • Śhīta • Ati-snigdha • Ati-mātra • Samaśhnatā • Chintyānā • Chātichintanāt	• Heavy • Cold • Excessively unctuous, oily • Too large, in excessive quantity • Constantly eating (alternatively, taking a shower or bath after eating) • Worry • Constantly engaged in stressful situations or work
Raktavahā srotas Rakta dhātu network	• Vidāhīni anna-pānāni • Snigdha • Uṣhṇāni dravāṇi cha • Bhajatāṁ chātapānalau	• That which causes a particular type of burning sensation from food and drink • Food that is too unctuous, oily • Food that is too hot or liquidy • Utilized regularly along with exposure to the sun

Māṁsavahā srotas Māṁsa dhātu network	• Abhiṣhyandīni bhojyāni • Sthūlāni cha gurūṇi • Bhuktvā cha svapatāṁ divā cha	• Food which causes blockage of the exudative channels • Food which is bulky and heavy • Eating followed by sleeping during the day
Medovahā srotas Medo dhātu network	• Avyāyāma • Divā-svapna • Medyānāṁ chātibhakṣhaṇāt • Vāruṇyāśhcha ati-sevanāt	• Avoidance or lack of physical exercise • Sleeping during the day • Consuming too much fatty food • Excessive, regular consumption of vāruṇa, a specific type of alcoholic preparation
Asthivahā srotas Asthi dhātu network	• Vyāyāma • Ati-saṅkṣhobha asthnām • Ati-vighaṭṭanāt • Vātalānāṁ cha sevanāt	• Too much physical exercise • Excessive agitation, shaking, violent jerks that goes deep into the bones • Excessive striking, rubbing or breaking apart • Regular use of foods and activities that provoke vāta
Majjavahā srotas Majja dhātu network	• Utpeṣha • Atyabhiṣhyanda • Abhighāta • Prapīḍana • Viruddhānāṁ cha sevanāt	• Excessive pressure • Too much blockage of the exudative channels • Trauma, external attack, damage • Compression • And regular consumption of food having contradictory properties
Śhukravahā srotas Śhukra dhātu network	• Akāla-yoni-gamana • Nigraha • Ati-maithuna • Śhastra-kṣhāra-agnibhis-tathā	• Improper timing for sexual intercourse • Improper methods of sexual intercourse • Excessive sexual intercourse • Improper surgical treatments, chemical application of bases, or cauterization
Mūtravahā srotas Urinary excretion network	• Mūtrita udaka, bhakṣhya, strī-sevanān • Mūtra-nigrahāt • Kṣhīṇasya ābhikṣhatasya cha	• When having the urge to pass urine and instead drinking water, eating food or indulging in sexual intercourse regularly • Restraining the urge to pass urine • In a debilitated or emaciated person or one suffering from chronic disease

Purīṣhavahā srotas Fecal excretion network	• Sandhāraṇād • Atyaśhanāda • Jīrṇa-adhyaśhanāt • Tathā durbalāgneḥ kṛśhasya cha	• Withholding the urge to pass the bowels • Excessive eating in quantity and frequency • Eating while the previous meal is still digesting • Especially in one with a compromised state of *agni* or in a weakened, emaciated individual
Svedovahā srotas Sweat excretion network	• Vyāyāma • Ati-santāpa • Śhīta-uṣhṇā krama sevanāt • Krodha • Śhoka • Bhaya	• Excessive physical exercise • Too much exposure to heat • Regularly going between cold and hot environments • Anger • Grief • Fear

TEST YOURSELF

Learn, review and memorize key terms from this section.

sroto duṣhṭi nidāna

samānya nidāna

abhiṣhyandi

anabhiṣhyandi

viśheṣha nidāna

Chapter 11: Review

ADDITIONAL READING

Read and review the references listed below to expand your understanding of the concepts in this chapter. Write down the date that you complete your reading for each. Remember that consistent repetition is the best way to learn. Plan to read each reference at least once now and expect to read it again as you continue your studies.

References marked with (skim) can be read quickly and do not require commentary review.

CLASSICS		1st read	2nd read
Charaka	Cha. Sū. 30/12 Cha. Vi. 5/		
Suśhruta	Su. Sā. 9/ Su. Śhā. 4/33		
Aṣhṭāṅga Hṛdaya	AH Su. 13/23-35 AH Sā. 3/41-48		
Bhāva Prakāśha	BP Pū. 6(I)/235		

JOURNALS & CURRENT RESOURCES

QUESTIONS & ANSWERS

Record your questions for this chapter here for further research and discussion.

Question:

Answer:

Question:

Answer:

Question:

Answer:

SELF-ASSESSMENT

1. Which of the following definitions describe the *srotases*?
   a. Flows by oozing or exuding
   b. Innumerable outcomes of vitiation caused by the *doṣhas* and *dhātus*
   c. Rooted from the heart spreading out to the major channels
   d. Supplies nutrition to the *dhātus* during *dhātu pariṇāma*
   e. All of the above

2. Charaka describes physical characteristics of the *srotases* as
   a. Flowing and constantly moving
   b. Pulsating and constantly moving
   c. Similar color, size, shape and length of its own *dhātu*
   d. A and C
   e. B and C

3. Why does Charaka state there are an infinite number of *srotases*?
   a. Aggregation of the *srotases* is believed to produce a human being
   b. Individuals are a product of their own unique factors
   c. Ability to effuse nutrition to the *doṣhas*, resulting in *prakopa* and *praśhamana*
   d. A and B
   e. A and C

4. What does *Punarvasu Ātreya* say about the classification of 13 *srotases*?
   a. They become known through measurable features of aggravation
   b. For those who understand the science more *srotases* will be inferred
   c. It is sufficient to understand only the 13 *srotases*
   d. Each *srotas* has its own root
   e. All of the above

5. According to Charaka what moves throughout the entire body in all the *srotases* and acts as their channels of passage?
   a. All components of the mind
   b. Expressions of the *indriyas*
   c. *Vāta, pitta, kapha*
   d. *Chetanā*
   e. All of the above

6. Which *srotas* is responsible for taste and appetite?
   a. *Annavahā srotas*
   b. *Medovahā srotas*
   c. *Raktavahā srotas*
   d. *Rasavahā srotas*
   e. *Svedovahā srotas*

7. Which *srotas* is responsible for smooth or rough skin?
   a. *Annavahā srotas*
   b. *Medovahā srotas*
   c. *Asthiavahā srotas*
   d. *Rasavahā srotas*
   e. *Svedovahā srotas*

8. Which of the *sroto duṣhṭi lakṣhaṇas* is directly responsible for accumulation?
   a. *Atipravṛtti*
   b. *Saṅga*
   c. *Sirā granthi*
   d. *Vimārga gamana*
   e. All of the above

9. Which *sroto duṣhṭi nidāna* is created by cloudy, heavy *dravya*?
   a. *Abhiṣhyandi*
   b. *Samānya*
   c. *Viśheṣha*
   d. *Anabhiṣhyandi*
   e. All of the above

10. Which *srotas* is most affected by heavy, cold *dravya*?
    a. *Annavahā srotas*
    b. *Mūtravahā srotas*
    c. *Purīṣhavahā srotas*
    d. *Rasavahā srotas*
    e. *Svedovahā srotas*

CRITICAL THINKING

1. Explain how the *rasavahā srotas* fulfill the functions of *prakṛa rasa dhātu* through two examples.

2. How are the *dhātuvagnis* involved with the *srotases* of each *dhātu*?

3. Compare and contrast the *mūtra vṛddhi lakṣhaṇas* with the *mūtra sroto duṣhṭi lakṣhaṇas.*

4. Which *āhāraja* type of *sroto duṣhṭi viśheṣha nidāna* is most likely to affect multiple *srotases*? Why?

5. How does *asthivahā srotas* demonstrate the *āśhraya-āśhrayi bhāva*?

Chapter 12 : Doṣha-dūṣhya sammūrchhana

KEY TERMS

doṣha	dūṣhya	sammūrchhana	ṣhaṭ kriya kāla
doṣha svabhāva	nidāna	saptadūṣhya	

The concept of *doṣha-dūṣhya sammūrchhana* ties together all of the components covered in this Unit and puts them into action. This can be considered the starting point for pathological manifestations and when it occurs, it may result in an infinite number of possible outcomes based on severity, complexity, sequence, manifestation, and more. Earlier stages of *doṣha-dūṣhya sammūrchhana* easily demonstrate the uniqueness of individuals in clinical presentation. At the same time, a well developed *doṣha-dūṣhya sammūrchhana* can produce a very common, well-known outcome in the form of a named manifestation of a pathology which can present very similarly across a wide population.

PARIBHĀṢHĀ

Each component term in the phrase *doṣha-dūṣhya sammūrchhana* provides insight into the processes that happen within this concept. Review each term below.

Doṣha

Recall that *doṣha* is defined as:

Doṣha   दूष्यन्ति इति दोसाः

Dūṣhyanti iti dosāḥ

Doṣha is that which has the potential to vitiate, pollute, or make impure.

Charaka provides a very clear and concise example of this:

तेषां सर्वेषामेव वातपित्तश्लेष्माणो दुष्टा दूषयितारो भवन्ति, दोष स्वभावात् ।

च. शा. ६।१८

Teṣhāṁ sarveṣhāmeva vātapittaśhleṣhmāṇo duṣhṭā dūṣhayitāro bhavanti, doṣha svabhāvāt ||

Cha. Śhā. 6/18

And out of all of the (formed components of the body), *vāta, pitta* and *śhleṣhma* are the ones which are responsible for *dūṣhayat* (vitiating, corrupting, destroying) when they themselves are in a state of *duṣhṭa* (being vitiated, impure, not right, abnormal). That is *doṣha svabhāva* (the nature of the *doṣhas*).

Dūṣhya

Dūṣhya refers to that which can be corrupted, soiled, defiled, disgraced or ruined. In the context of Āyurveda, this can refer to any *dhātu*, especially the *sapta-dhātus*. Vāgbhaṭa uses the concept of *dūṣhya* to define the *sapta-dhātus* in the beginning of *Aṣhṭāṅga Hṛdaya*:

रसासृङ्मांसमेदोस्थिमज्जशुक्राणि धातवः ।
सप्त दूष्याः ... ॥

अ. हृ. सू. १।१३

Rasāsṛṅmāṁsamedosthimajjaśhukrāṇi dhātavaḥ |
Sapta dūṣhyāḥ ... ||

AH Sū. 1/13

The *sapta dūṣhyas* (seven which can be vitiated) are *rasa, rakta, māṁsa, medas, asthi, majja* and *śhukra*.

Sammūrchana

The term *sammūrchhana* refers to the act of congealing or thickening, increasing, spreading or accumulating. Within Āyurveda, *sammūrchhana* refers to the process of the *doṣhas* and *dūṣhyas* conglomerating and building up at a specific location within the body. This happens only when *doṣhas* are in a *vaikṛta* state.

In *Aṣhṭāṅga Saṅgraha*, Vāgbhaṭa describes how the *doṣha*s come into a *vaikṛta* state. He says that:

वैकृतास्तु गर्भादभिनिस्सृरस्याहाररसस्य मलाः सम्भवन्ति । प्राकृतेष्ववरोहन्ति ।

अ. सं. शा. ८।५

Vaikṛtāstu garbhādabhinissṛrasyāhārarasasya malāḥ sambhavanti |
Prākṛteṣhvavarohanti |

AS. Śhā. 8/12

Garbhādabhi (From the moment of birth), *vaikṛtāstu* (the *doṣhas* are formed) *āhārarasa* (from the conversion of *āhārarasa*) to *malāḥ* (the waste products). *Arohanti* (They, the vitiated *doṣhas*, grow from, contininuously increase) *prākṛti* (from the normal, baseline state, or healthy ones).

In order for *sammūrchhana* to occur, the *doṣhas* and *dūṣhyas* must have a place to gather and grow. In *Aṣhṭāṅga Hṛdaya*, Vāgbhaṭa identifies the normal locations of the *doṣhas* in this specific context.

तत्रास्थनि स्थितो वायुः, पित्तं तु स्वेदरक्तयोः ।
श्लेष्मा शेषेषु, तेनैषामाश्रयाश्रयिणां मिथः ॥

अ. हृ. सू. ११।२६

Tatrāsthani sthito vāyuḥ, pittaṁ tu svedaraktayoḥ |
Śhleṣhmā śheṣheṣhu, tenāiṣhāmāśhrayāśhrayeṇāṁ mithaḥ ||

AH Sū. 11/26

Tatrāsthani sthito vāyuḥ (And so, *vāta* is located in the *asthi*), *pittaṁ tu svedaraktayoḥ* (*pitta* is located in the *sveda* and *rakta*), and *śhleṣhmā śheṣheṣhu* (kapha is located in the rest of them, ie, the *āśhraya*, or containers). This is the relationship according to *āśhraya-āśhrayi* (container and resident).

The commentator Hemādri elaborates on this by explaining that:

दूष्याणां वृद्धि क्षयहेत्वादिविज्ञानार्थ दोषदूष्ययोः आश्रयाश्रयिभावम् आह तत्र इति ।

हेमद्रि

Dūṣhyāṇāṁ vṛddhi kṣhayahetvādivijñānārtha doṣhadūṣhyayoḥ āśhrayāśhrayibhāvam āha tatra iti |

Hemādri

Thus, it is explained that the *āśhraya-āśhrayi bhāva* (relationship between the container and the contained) is that of *doṣha* and *dūṣhya* (the vitiator and that which is being vitiated). The *dūṣhya* (that which is vitiated) experiences *vṛddhi* and *kṣhaya* (increase and decrease) according to the *hetu-ādi vijñānārtha* (known causative factors, etc).

The process of *sammūrchhana* increases and decreases according to the supply of inputs as causative factors for vitiation, known as *nidāna*. When more causative factors are provided to the body, they result in an increase in the *doṣhas* with the capacity to vitiate or pollute. Because of the inherent *āśhraya-āśhrayi* relationship between the *doṣhas* and the *dūṣhyas* (as listed above), these locations have a more likely chance of becoming early *dūṣhyas*. They are more likely to be vitiated first because of close proximity.

Finally, Vāgbhaṭa provides a clear summary of the process of *doṣha-dūṣhya sammūrchhana*:

दोषा दुष्टा रसैर्धातून् दूषयन्स्युभये मलान् ॥ ३५
अधो द्वे, सप्त शिरसि, खानि स्वेदवहानि च ।
मल मलायनानि स्युर्यथास्वं तेष्वतो गदाः ॥

अ. हृ. सू. ११।३६

Doṣhā duṣhṭā rasairdhātūn dūṣhayasyubhaye malān || 35
Adho dve, sapta śhirasi, khani svedavahāni ca |
Mala malāyanāni syuryathāsvaṁ teṣhvato gadāḥ ||

AH Sū. 11/36

The *doṣhas* [cause the] *duṣhṭā* (vitiation of) *rasairdhātūn* rasa, etc *dhātus*. *Dūṣhayasyubhaye* (The two together, then go on to vitiate) *malān* (the malas). Altogether, they then go on to vitiate *adho dve* (the two lower channels of waste elimination, for *mūtra* and *purīṣha*), *sapta śhirasi* (the seven channels of waste elimination in the head), *khani svedavahāni ca* (and the channels of *sveda*). *Teṣhvato gadāḥ* (Related disorders) *syuryathāsvaṁ* (develop in the very same place) *mala malāyanāni* (as the channels of waste).

Essentially, the conglomeration of *doṣha-dūṣhya sammūrchhana* creates an accumulation of waste materials that the body naturally attempts to excrete. If these wastes cannot be completely removed, they linger and act as the precursors to disease.

Vāgbhaṭa also provides a very succinct analogy to paint a picture of the process of *doṣha-dūṣhya sammūrchhana*. Its terse depth and breadth can be best understood when the entire process has been well-studied and experienced in practice.

क्षिप्यमाणः खवैगुन्याद्रसः सज्जति यत्र सः ।
यस्मिन्विकारं कुरुते खे वर्षमिव तोयदः ॥
दोषाणामपि चैवं स्यादेकदेशप्रकोपणम्

अ. हृ. सू. ११।६९

Kṣhipyamāṇaḥ khavaigunyādrasaḥ sajjati yatra saḥ |
Yasminvikāram kurute khe varṣhamiva toyadaḥ ||
Doṣhāṇāmapi caivaṁ syādekadeśhaprakopaṇam |

AH Śhā. 3/69-70

Just as rain clouds pour down when stopped in the sky, *rasa dhātu* promotes the growth of disease in any location where its normal flow has become stagnant. Likewise, the *doṣhas* also undergo excessive aggravation when they are stopped or restricted in one place.

The concept of *doṣha-dūṣhya sammūrchhana* is elaborated in its complete state by Suśhruta in Su. Sū. 21/ as *ṣhaṭ kriya kāla* (the six stages of pathology). Suśhruta's explanations move deeper into pathology and will be covered in the context of therapeutic management. This chapter is meant to serve as a basic introduction to the topic from the perspective of healthy physiology.

TEST YOURSELF

Learn, review and memorize key terms from this section.

doṣha

dūṣhya

sammūrchhana

saptadūṣhya

nidāna

ṣhaṭ kriya kāla

Chapter 12: Review

ADDITIONAL READING

Read and review the references listed below to expand your understanding of the concepts in this chapter. Write down the date that you complete your reading for each. Remember that consistent repetition is the best way to learn. Plan to read each reference at least once now and expect to read it again as you continue your studies.

References marked with (skim) can be read quickly and do not require commentary review.

CLASSICS		1st read	2nd read
Charaka	Cha. Śhā. 6/18		
Suśhruta	Su. Sū. 21/		
Aṣhṭāṅga Hṛdaya	AH Sū. 1/13 AH Sū. 11/26 AH Sū. 11/35-36 AH Śhā. 3/69-70		
Bhāva Prakāśha			

JOURNALS & CURRENT RESOURCES

QUESTIONS & ANSWERS

Record your questions for this chapter here for further research and discussion.

Question:

Answer:

Question:

Answer:

Question:

Answer:

SELF-ASSESSMENT

1. Which of the following describes *doṣha-dūṣhya sammūrchhana*?
   a. Early stages demonstrate the uniqueness of individuals
   b. Infinite number of outcomes based on many manifestations
   c. Starting point for pathological manifestations
   d. Well developed stages produce a well-known outcome of the pathology
   e. All of the above

2. What is the definition of *doṣha svabhāva*?
   a. *Doṣha-dūṣhya sammūrchhana*
   b. Nature of the *doṣhas*
   c. State of *duṣhṭa*
   d. *Vāta*, *pitta* and *kapha*
   e. All of the above

3. Which of the following is responsible for vitiating, corrupting or destroying?
   a. *Doṣha-dūṣhya sammūrchhana*
   b. *Doṣha* as a *duṣhya*
   c. *Duṣhṭa* in a state of *doṣha*
   d. *Vāta*, *pitta* and *kapha*
   e. All of the above

4. Which of the following describes *dūṣhya*?
   a. Corruption of the *saptadhātus*
   b. *Doṣha svabhāva*
   c. What is corrupted by *vāta, pitta* and *śhleṣhma*
   d. Both A and C
   e. Both B and C

5. From an Āyurvedic perspective, the term *sammūrchhana* refers to?
   a. Accumulating
   b. Congealing or thickening
   c. Conglomerating at a specific location
   d. Increasing
   e. All of the above

6. According to Vāgbhaṭa, *doṣha vikṛti* occurs
   a. During the conversion of *āhārarasa* to *malā*
   b. Because of vitiated *doṣha*
   c. From the moment of birth as *prākṛti* deviates from its normal state
   d. Both B and C
   e. All of the above

7. In the relationship of *āśhraya-āśhrayi*, Vāgbhaṭa states which of the following?
   a. *Vāta* is located in *asthi*
   b. *Pitta* resides in *sveda* and *rakta*
   c. *Kapha* resides in the remaining *dhātus* and *malas*
   d. B and C only
   e. All of the above

8. The *āśhraya-āśhrayi bhāva* of *doṣha* and *dūṣhya* is?
   a. *Doṣha-dūṣhya sammūrchhana*
   b. *Doṣha* is the vitiator and *dūṣhya* is that which is vitiated
   c. *Doṣha svabhāva*
   d. *Duṣhṭa* in a state of *doṣha*
   e. *Vāta*, *pitta* and *kapha*

9. The process of *sammūrchhana* increases and decreases according to the supply of causative factors for vitiation. This is known as
   a. *Āśhraya-āśhrayi bhāva*
   b. *Doṣhas and dūṣhyas*
   c. *Kṣhaya* and *vṛddhi*
   d. *Nidāna*
   e. All of the above

10. The conglomeration of *doṣha-dūṣhya sammūrchhana* is created
    a. When accumulated waste materials are not excreted from the body
    b. *Doṣhas* undergo excessive aggravation and are stopped or restricted in one place
    c. Throughout *ṣhaṭ kriya kāla*
    d. When *doṣhas* are continuously supplied with factors that promote their unhealthy growth
    e. All of the above

CRITICAL THINKING

1. Considering all of the information in the previous chapters, define and explain the terms *doṣha, dūṣhya* and *sammūrchhana* in your own words.

2. How many *dūṣhyas* could exist? List as many as possible using their correctly transliterated Sanskrit terms accompanied by their meanings.

3. Is *doṣha-dūṣhya sammūrchhana* more likely to occur in a state of *doṣha vṛddhi* or *kṣhaya*? Explain your reasoning with citations (if necessary) and examples.

4. Draw a picture of the analogy of *doṣha-dūṣhya sammūrchhana* provided by Vāgbhaṭa. Label the events using correctly transliterated Sanskrit terms and their meanings.

5. Draw a picture of *doṣha-dūṣhya sammūrchhana* and how its process occurs in the body. Include labels for all events, including all of those which occur before the actual process of *sammūrchhana*.

UNIT II

शारीर

Śārīra

(Study of the human body)

Chapter 13 : Classical perspectives and definitions

KEY TERMS

adhiṣhṭhāna	chikitsā puruṣha	śharīra	śharīra vichaya
aṅga	karma puruṣha	śhārīra	Śhārīra-sthāna
chetanā	pañcha mahābhūta		

The study of the human body was always considered an important and mandatory component of education and training according to classical educational standards. In both the *Charaka sampradāya* and *Suśhruta sampradāya*, students are required to become competent in all of the anatomical knowledge appropriate for the *sampradāya*. A good portion of this information is found in the *Śhārīra-sthāna* of each *saṁhitā*. As each *sampradāya* has a specific focus, the content of *Śhārīra-sthāna* differs somewhat in presentation, organization and content. There are obvious, varying opinions on perspectives, such as the number of bones in the body. These differences are easily acceptable once the full classification system is understood and the perspective is clear.

ŚHĀRĪRA AND ŚHARĪRA

One of the first key distinctions that must be understood is the difference between the two terms *śhārīra* and *śharīra*. Notice that the only difference between the two terms is the presence of a long first a. This seemingly small change has very large implications. The term *śhārīra* refers to the study of the body from an anatomical perspective (and physiological, to some extent), while the term *śharīra* refers to the actual body itself. Notice that the name of the section of each text is *Śhārīra-sthāna* (having the first long a), meaning the section on the study of the body. Contextually, this single difference can have very significant implications.

The scope of *śhārīra* in the classics did not draw a hard line between what is considered today as the study of human anatomy and the study of human physiology. The *śharīra* was always considered to be one entity and its structure and function are interdependent and inseparable. This concept has already been demonstrated throughout Unit I of this volume, especially in the review of *doṣha, dhātu* and *mala*.

TEST YOURSELF

Learn, review and memorize key terms from this section.

śhārīra

____

śharīra

____

Śhārīrasthāna

____

PARIBHĀṢHĀ

Charaka defines *śharīra* as:

तत्र शरीरं नाम चेतनाधिष्ठानभूतं
पञ्चमहाभूतविकारसमुदायात्मकं
समयोगवाहि ।

च. शा. ६।४

Tatra śharīraṁ nāma chetanādhiṣhṭhānabhūtaṁ pañchamahābhūtavikārasamudāyātmakaṁ samayogavāhi |

Cha. Śhā. 6/4

And so, *śharīra* is named as the *adhiṣhṭhāna* (place, location of) *chetanā* (consciousness) and *pañcha mahābhūta*. It is *samudāyātmaka* (by its own nature, the collecting place where) *vikāra* (disease) *samyogavāhi* (congregates, combines or occurs).

Suśhruta provides a more specific definition:

एवं विवर्धितः स यदा हस्तपादजिह्वाघ्राणकर्णनितम्बादिभिरङ्गैरुपेतस्तदा "शरीरं" इति संज्ञां लभते ।

सु. शा. ५।३

Evaṁ vivardhitaḥ sa yadā hastapādajihvāghrāṇakarṇanitambādibhiraṅgairupetastadā "śharīraṁ" iti saṁjṇāṁ labhate |

Sū. Śhā. 5/3

And so, as the embryo grows (as described in the previous *śhloka*), the *aṅga* (limbs) *upeta* (unite, come together), with the *hasta* (hands), *pāda* (feet), *jihva* (tongue), *ghrāṇa* (nose), *karṇa* (ears), *nitamba* (buttocks), *ādi* (etc. becoming visible). At this stage, (the fetus) *saṁjñā labhate* (is said to be known as) "*śharīra*."

From these two definitions, it is clear that the *śharīra*, or physical body is considered to be formed during fetal development and persist throughout an entire lifetime. While *chetanā* is present, *śharīra* is deemed to be alive and functioning, and the object of Āyurveda as *karma puruṣha*, or *chikitsā puruṣha* (Chapters two and four).

The study of the human body is also considered as the concept of *śharīra vichaya*, described by Charaka in Cha. Śhā. 6/3. In this line and its commentary, the importance of the study is stressed and the reasons as well.

शरीरविचयः शरीरोपकारार्थमिष्यते ।

च. शा. ६।३

Śharīravichayaḥ śharīrapakārārthamiṣhyate |

Cha. Śhā. 6/3

Śharīra vichaya (the enumeration, arrangement of the body) *iṣhyate* (is what is wanted) *upakāra* (to help bring forth) *ārtha* (the result, goal, desired achievement) regarding efforts to maintain *śharīra*.

Clearly, an in-depth, comprehensive and thorough study of the body is required in order to effect proper therapeutic actions for it. The level of depth of knowledge must be commensurate with the expectations for any professional healthcare level.

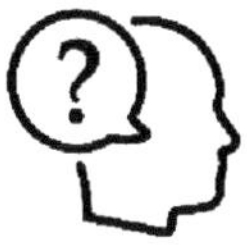

TEST YOURSELF

Learn, review and memorize key terms from this section.

adhiṣhṭhāna ________

chetanā ________

pañcha mahābhūta ________

aṅga ________

karma puruṣha ________

chikitsā puruṣha ________

śharīra vichaya ________

Chapter 13: Review

ADDITIONAL READING

Read and review the references listed below to expand your understanding of the concepts in this chapter. Write down the date that you complete your reading for each. Remember that consistent repetition is the best way to learn. Plan to read each reference at least once now and expect to read it again as you continue your studies.

References marked with (skim) can be read quickly and do not require commentary review.

CLASSICS		1st read	2nd read
Charaka	Cha. Śhā. 6/3-4 Cha. Śhā. (skim)		
Suśhruta	Su. Śhā. 5/3 Su. Śhā. (skim)		
Aṣhṭāṅga Hṛdaya	AH Śhā. (skim)		
Bhāva Prakāśha			

JOURNALS & CURRENT RESOURCES

Journal article: *Concepts of Human Physiology in Ayurveda*, Kishor Patwardhan

QUESTIONS & ANSWERS

Record your questions for this chapter here for further research and discussion.

Question:

Answer:

Question:

Answer:

Question:

Answer:

SELF-ASSESSMENT

1. In *Charaka Saṁhitā* (translated by RK Sharma and Bhagwan Dash), *Śhārīra-sthāna* is found in which printed volume?
   a. Volume I
   b. Volume II
   c. Volume III
   d. Volume IV
   e. Volume V

2. In *Suśhruta Saṁhitā* (translated by GD Singhal et al), *Śhārīra-sthāna* is found after which *sthāna*?
   a. *Sūtra-sthāna*
   b. *Nidāna-sthāna*
   c. *Chikitsā-sthāna*
   d. *Kalpa-sthāna*
   e. *Uttara-tantra*

3. In *Suśhruta Saṁhitā* (translated by KR Srikantha Murthy), *Śhārīra-sthāna* is found before which *sthāna*?
   a. *Sūtra-sthāna*
   b. *Nidāna-sthāna*
   c. *Chikitsā-sthāna*
   d. *Kalpa-sthāna*
   e. *Uttara-tantra*

4. The main goal of *śharīra vichaya* is
   a. To maintain *chetanā*
   b. To maintain *śharīra*
   c. To maintain the *doṣhas*
   d. To maintain the *dhātus*
   e. To maintain the *malas*

5. In the context of *śharīra*, *karma puruṣha* is
   a. bound by its own karma and unchangeable.
   b. a human body in developing stages.
   c. the study of anatomy.
   d. the study of physiology.
   e. the scope of practice for Āyurveda.

6. Students of the *Charaka sampradāya* could apply knowledge of *śharīra vichaya* for
   a. Understanding normal form or function
   b. Assessing abnormal form or function
   c. Determining appropriate management
   d. All of the above
   e. None of the above

7. Based on *prākṛta doṣha lakṣhaṇas*, which *doṣha* is most likely to produce a stable, physical form of the *śharīra*?
   a. *vāta*
   b. *pitta*
   c. *kapha*
   d. *rajas*
   e. *tamas*

8. In a normal, healthy *śharīra*, *pitta doṣha* is primarily located
   a. In the heart
   b. In the bladder
   c. In the eyes
   d. In the umbilical area
   e. In the stomach

9. Which *doṣha* is responsible for transporting other *doṣhas* throughout the *śharīra*?
   a. *vāta*
   b. *pitta*
   c. *kapha*
   d. *rajas*
   e. *tamas*

10. Which of the following regularly need to be eliminated from the *śharīra*?
   a. *doṣhas*
   b. *dhātus*
   c. *malas*
   d. Both A and C
   e. None of the above

CRITICAL THINKING

1. From the individual perspectives of the *Charaka sampradāya* and the *Suśhruta sampradāya*, name at least three reasons why the study of *śharīra* would be so important. If using classical sources to answer this question, cite them.

2. Compare and contrast the organization, structure and high-level (brief) content found in Charaka's, Suśhruta's and the *Aṣhṭāṅga Hṛdaya*'s *Śhārīrasthāna*.

3. Compare and contrast Charaka's definition of *śharīra* with his definition of *āyu*.

4. Describe at least three interesting, notable or important *śhlokas* from each of *Śhārīrasthāna* in the additional reading.

5. Define the terms "*Śhārīra*" and "*śharīra*" from the Monier-Williams dictionary. Explain the difference in your own words.

Chapter 14 : Āyu (Life span)

KEY TERMS

annāda
bāla
jīrṇa
kṣhīrānāda
kṣhīrapa
madhya
parihāṇi
paripakva
sampūrṇatā
vārdhaka
vayas
vivardhamāna
yauvana
yuga

Āyu is the term used to indicate vitality, life and lifespan. The scientific framework of Āyurveda allows for an approximate prediction of life in quantity and quality. These possible outcomes take into account known factors about the individual based on their physical and mental presentation, along with other significant history and living conditions.

Each classical author included a framework for categorizing life span in terms of quantity or duration. Some authors additionally provided specific instructions on how to measure an individual's lifespan using the framework of Āyurveda. This chapter covers the possible outcomes of such assessments in terms of their categorical results. The process of assessment and factors required to be analyzed will be covered in later volumes of this series.

VAYAS

The term *vayas* refers to a period of life or age of an individual. In the context of Āyurveda it is used to categorize all periods of life as normally seen in practice. Compare the categorization methods of significant authors on the following page.

Charaka notes in Cha. Vi. 8/122 that the general or average lifespan of the current era should be considered approximately 100 years. Some may live longer or shorter than this depending on their individual factors and circumstances.

Charaka recommends that the basis for calculating *vaya*s as its stages of life be according to each individual assessment because of these variations. For example, if an individual is assessed to have a shorter lifespan (less than the standard 100 years), each of the periods of life should be adjusted accordingly.

Review the following chart to compare various authors' perspectives on *vayas* and its divisions for a 100-year lifespan.

Cha. Vi. 8/122	*Bāla*			*Madhya*				*Jīrṇa*
	Paripakva	*Vivardhamāna*		30-60 years				60-100 years
	0-16	16-30						
Su. Sū. 35/29	*Bālya*			*Madhya*				*Vṛddha*
	Kṣhīrapa	*Kṣhīrānnāda*	*Annāda*	*Vṛddhi*	*Yauvana*	*Sampūrṇatā*	*Parihāṇi*	
	0-1	1-2	2-16	16-20	20-30	30-40	40-70	70+
AH Śhā. 3/105	*Bāla*			*Madhya*				*Vṛddhi*
	0-16			16-70				70+
BP Pū. 4/42	*Bālya*			*Madhyama*				*Vārdhaka*
	Dugdhāśhī	*Dugdhānnāśhī*	*Annāśhī*	*Vṛddhi*	*Yuvā*	*Pūrṇa*	*Kṣhaya*	
	0-1	1-2	2-16	16-20	20-30	30-40	40-70	70+

TEST YOURSELF

Learn, review and memorize key terms from this section.

annāda

bāla

jīrṇa

kṣhīrānāda

kṣhīrapa

madhya

parihāṇi

paripakva

sampūrṇatā

vārdhaka

vayas

vivardhamāna

yauvana

yuga

Chapter 14: Review

ADDITIONAL READING

Read and review the references listed below to expand your understanding of the concepts in this chapter. Write down the date that you complete your reading for each. Remember that consistent repetition is the best way to learn. Plan to read each reference at least once now and expect to read it again as you continue your studies.

References marked with (skim) can be read quickly and do not require commentary review.

CLASSICS		1st read	2nd read
Charaka	Cha. Vi. 8/122		
Suśhruta	Su. Sū. 35/29		
Aṣhṭāṅga Hṛdaya	AH Śhā. 3/105		
Bhāva Prakāśha	BP Pū. 4/42		

JOURNALS & CURRENT RESOURCES

QUESTIONS & ANSWERS

Record your questions for this chapter here for further research and discussion.

Question:

Answer:

Question:

Answer:

Question:

Answer:

SELF-ASSESSMENT

1. The *vayas* most closely related to *vāta doṣha* is
   a. *bāla*
   b. *madhya*
   c. *jīrṇa*
   d. All of the above
   e. None of the above

2. Which author(s) recognize age brackets for early childhood nutrition and weaning?
   a. Charaka
   b. Suśhruta
   c. Vāgbhaṭa
   d. Bhāvamiśhra
   e. Both B and D

3. According to Vāgbhaṭa, the name of the third and final *vayas* may also be a synonym for
   a. normal *doṣhas*
   b. increased *doṣhas*
   c. decreased *doṣhas*
   d. All of the above
   e. None of the above

4. Which component of *āyu* tends to decay especially in the *vṛddha* stage of life?
   a. *śharīra*
   b. *lakṣhaṇas*
   c. *sattva*
   d. *ātma*
   e. All of the above

5. Each author's *vayas* classification begins *madhya* at the age of 16, except
   a. Charaka
   b. Suśhruta
   c. Vāgbhaṭa
   d. Bhāvamiśhra
   e. None of the above

6. The generally accepted lifespan for the current *yuga* is
   a. 75 years
   b. 80 years
   c. 90 years
   d. 100 years
   e. 125 years

7. Individuals under the age of 30 would be managed in the specialized department of
   a. *Kāyachikitsā*
   b. *Viṣha Gara*
   c. *Kumāra Bhṛtya*
   d. *Bhūta Vidya*
   e. *Śhālākya Tantra*

8. *Vājīkaraṇa* would be most appropriate for an individual in which *vayas*?
   a. *Bāla*
   b. *Madhya*
   c. *Jīrṇa*
   d. *Vārdhaka*
   e. All of the above

9. According to Charaka, an individual with a lifespan of 75 would begin *madhya* at the age of
   a. 18 years
   b. 20.25 years
   c. 22.5 years
   d. 24 years
   e. 25 years

10. According to Suśhruta, an individual with a lifespan of 75 would begin *madhya* at the age of
   a. 11 years
   b. 12 years
   c. 13 years
   d. 14 years
   e. 15 years

CRITICAL THINKING

1. Compare the descriptions of each stage of life provided by the four classical authors. Using any two references (any two authors), note the similarities and differences in their classification method and description of life stages.

2. Consider that a client has been assessed as having a shorter than normal (average) life span of 100 years. Instead, their lifespan may be approximately 80 years. Using Charaka's and Suśhruta's classifications for *vayas*, calculate the age range of the individual throughout each stage of life.

3. Identify and explain the influence of each *doṣha* in each of the classifications of *vayas* in this chapter.

4. If an individual has a very short life span (about 30 years or less) how should their stages of life and age ranges be calculated? Can you cite a classical reference to support your answer?

Chapter 15 : Garbha vijñāna (Embryology)

KEY TERMS

ārtava	garbha vijñāna	rajodarśhana	śhuddha śhukra lakṣhaṇas
duṣhṭa ārtava lakṣhaṇas	garbhadāna	ṛtukāla	śhukra
duṣhṭa śhukra lakṣhaṇas	garbhiṇi	ṛtumati	yamala
garbha	garbhotpatti	śhuddha ārtava lakṣhaṇas	yoni
	puṁsavana		

The study of *garbha vijñāna*, or embryology begins well before the actual conception takes places according to classical literature. The stage of planning and preparing for conception is just as important as the pregnancy itself. Charaka emphasizes this in Cha. Śhā. 8/4 and 8/17 with specific instructions on preparing the female and male bodies through *śhodhana*, or the expulsion of *doṣhas* from the body. He specifically recommends:

स्त्रीपुंसौ स्नेहस्वेदाभ्यामुपपद्य,
वमनविरेचनाभ्यां संशोध्य, क्रमेण
प्रकृतिमापादयेत् ।

च. शा. ८।४

Strīpuṁsau snehasvedābhyāmupapadya, vamanavirecanābhyāṁ saṁśhodhya, krameṇa prakṛtimāpādayet |

Cha. Śhā. 8/4

Both the woman and the man should undergo *sneha* and *sveda* (therapies to induce lubrication and sudation), followed by *saṁśhodhana* (proper therapies to expel *doṣhas* from the body) of *vamana* and/or *virecana*, as required. The *prakṛti* should be restored to normal following these procedures.

This should be followed by additional therapies including the two types of *basti* along with specific (and appropriate) types of foods. When the preparation for conception is done well, the couple is able to conceive easily just like a clean, strong cloth can take up dye with even a small application.

The purpose of *saṁśhodhana* in the preparation for conception is to eliminate any *doṣhas* which may not only interfere with the process of conception, but also in the development of the fetus. This is especially important in the woman's body as the majority of factors over the course of fetal development are attributed to her state of health. By eliminating *doṣhas* before conception, the body is in its best state to promote a healthy fetus. This process of *saṁśhodhana* is only one part of the complete preparation. Additionally, the menstrual cycle must be assessed and brought to its normal, healthy state.

ṚTU KĀLA (FERTILE PERIOD)

Menarche was generally considered to begin at the age of 12 with regular menstrual cycles continuing to around 50 years according to classical literature (AH Śhā. 1/7). Reproduction was considered ideal for a male at age 25 and female at age 16 (AH Śhā. 1/8). Each month was initiated by the appearance of *rajodarśhana* (menstruation) in women with specific characteristics to indicate the normal, healthy state of the reproductive organs, or otherwise.

Rajodarśhana, or active menstruation, was stated to last for three days according to Su. Śhā. 3/6 (commentary).

Counting from the onset of menses, the fourth day up to the fifteenth day was considered to be the appropriate time for fertilization. This period of fertility is called *ṛtu kāla*. On the sixteenth day, *yoni saṅkocha* occurs, which involves the mouth of the uterus, or the cervix, constricting and closing. From this point until the start of the next cycle, *ṛtu kāla* is over and the woman is not normally fertile (Su. Śhā. 3/6, commentary).

Use the table of references below to identify the key concepts related to *ṛtu kāla* and read directly from the classical texts to understand each author's opinions, recommendations and perspectives.

Concept with nearest English equivalent	Ref. from Cha.	Ref. from Su.	Ref. from AH	Ref. from BP
Rajodarśhana, rajasrāva Menstruation			AH Śhā. 1/7, 1/22	BP Pū. 3/1
Ṛtumati lakṣhaṇas Characteristics of a menstruating woman		Su. Śhā. 3/7-8	AH Śhā. 1/20	
Ṛtumati charya Regimen during menses	Cha. Śhā. 8/5		AH Śhā. 1/23-26	BP Pū. 3/3-11
Ṛtu kāla Fertile period		Su. Śhā. 2/33, 3/6	AH Śhā. 1/21, 1/27	BP Pū. 3/2, 3/38

TEST YOURSELF

Learn, review and memorize key terms from this section.

garbha vijñāna

____

ṛtukāla

____

rajodarśhana

____

yoni

____

ṛtumati

____

ASSESSMENT OF ŚHUKRA AND ĀRTAVA

In order for a healthy conception to take place, the reproductive components of both the male and female were to be assessed and corrected to normalcy, if necessary. The male's *śhukra*, or semen, and the female's *ārtava*, or menstrual fluids, were analyzed and compared to specific characteristics known as the *śhuddha śhukra* and *śhuddha ārtava lakṣhaṇas*.

Concept with nearest English equivalent	Ref. from Cha.	Ref. from Su.	Ref. from AH	Ref. from BP
Śhuddha ārtava lakṣhaṇas Pure menstrual blood	Cha. Chi. 30/226	Su. Śhā. 2/17, 3/10	AH Śhā. 1/18	
Śhuddha śhukra lakṣhaṇas Pure semen	Cha. Śhā. 2/4 (bhūta, rasa)	Su. Śhā. 2/11	AH Śhā. 1/17-18	
Duṣhṭa/vikṛta ārtava lakṣhaṇas Unhealthy menstrual blood	Cha. Chi. 30/		AH Śhā. 1/10-12	
Duṣhṭa/vikṛta śhukra lakṣhaṇas Unhealthy semen			AH Śhā. 1/10-12	

TEST YOURSELF

Learn, review and memorize key terms from this section.

śhukra

ārtava

śhuddha śhukra lakṣhaṇas

śhuddha ārtava lakṣhaṇas

duṣhṭa śhukra lakṣhaṇas

duṣhṭa ārtava lakṣhaṇas

GARBHOTPATTI (PROCREATION)

The term *garbhotpatti* includes two terms which refer to:

Garbha	The embryo and developing fetus
Utpatti	The process, procedure, formation of

Together, garbhotpatti includes conception and development of the fetus. A thorough review of classical opinions about this stage reveals that there were many considerations both before and after the actual moment of conception. Use the following table of references to read directly from the classical texts about each of these stages and understand each author's opinions and perspectives on the topics.

Concept with nearest English equivalent	Ref. from Cha.	Ref. from Su.	Ref. from AH	Ref. from BP
Garbhadāna Conception ceremony	Cha. Śhā. 8/5-14		AH Śhā. 1/27-33	
Varṣha Proper age			AH Śhā. 1/8-9	
Maithuna Intercourse	Cha. Śhā. 4/7, 8/6-8		AH Śhā. 1/34	BP Pū. 3/12-26, 28-30
Garbha sambhāva sāmagri Factors for *garbha*		Su. Śhā. 2/33		
Garbhotpatti Conception	Cha. Śhā. 8/5		AH Śhā. 1/1-2	BP Pū. 3/12
Sadyo gṛhita garbhiṇi Signs of conception	Cha. Śhā. 2/23	Su. Śhā. 3/13	AH Śhā. 1/35-36	BP Pū. 3/42
Garbha Conception, definition	Cha. Śhā. 4/5	Su. Śhā. 5/3		
Garbha pañcha mahābhūtas *Bhautika* composition	Cha. Śhā. 2/26-27			
Garbha saṁbhāva Factors responsible for *garbha*	Cha. Śhā. 3/			BP Pū. 3/316-319
Role of *ojas*	Cha. Sū. 30/9-11			
Garbha liṅgotpatti kāraṇa Fetal sex determination	Cha. Śhā. 2/12-15, 2/24-27	Su. Śhā. 3/5, 3/12	AH Śhā. 1/5, 1/69-72	
Abnormal development of fetus	Cha. Śhā. 2/17-21, 2/29-30			

Influencing specific characteristics of the child				
Concept with nearest English equivalent	Ref. from Cha.	Ref. from Su.	Ref. from AH	Ref. from BP
Strī-purușha Parental characteristics	Cha. Śhā. 8/18, 2/12			
General methods	Cha. Śhā. 8/9-14		AH Śhā. 1/32	
Puṁsavana Producing a male child	Cha. Śhā. 8/19		AH Śhā. 1/37	
Varṇa Complexion	Cha. Śhā. 8/15			
Sattva Mental disposition	Cha. Śhā. 8/16			

Special variations of the embryo during early stages of development				
Concept with nearest English equivalent	Ref. from Cha.	Ref. from Su.	Ref. from AH	Ref. from BP
Yamala garbha Twins	Cha. Śhā. 2/16		AH Śhā. 1/6	BP Pū. 3/39
Napuṁsaka Eunuch				

TEST YOURSELF

Learn, review and memorize key terms from this section.

garbha

garbhotpatti

garbhadāna

garbhiṇi

puṁsavana

yamala

Chapter 15: Review

ADDITIONAL READING

Read and review the references listed below to expand your understanding of the concepts in this chapter. Write down the date that you complete your reading for each. Remember that consistent repetition is the best way to learn. Plan to read each reference at least once now and expect to read it again as you continue your studies.

Use the additional references throughout this chapter and record what you've completed.

CLASSICS	1st read	2nd read
Charaka		
Suśhruta		
Aṣhṭāṅga Hṛdaya		
Bhāva Prakāśha		

JOURNALS & CURRENT RESOURCES

Journal article: *Contribution of Ayurveda to the Modern Embryology*, Dr.Deepa MD et al

QUESTIONS & ANSWERS

Record your questions for this chapter here for further research and discussion.

Question:

Answer:

Question:

Answer:

Question:

Answer:

SELF-ASSESSMENT

1. *Ṛtu kāla* is classically considered to begin and last for
   a. 12-16 days from the onset of menses
   b. The onset of menses thru 16 days
   c. The 4th day after the onset of menses to the 15th day
   d. The ovulation period
   e. None of the above

2. The first 3 days of *ṛtumati charya* include all of the following except
   a. Observing celibacy
   b. Sleeping on the ground
   c. Avoiding bathing
   d. Ābhyaṅga
   e. Eating from an unbroken vessel

3. *Śhuddha ārtava lakṣhaṇas* state that *ārtava*
   a. Does not stain clothes
   b. Resembles rabbit's blood
   c. Resembles liquid shellack
   d. Is profuse in quantity
   e. A, B, and C

4. *Śhuddha śhukra lakṣhaṇas* state that *śhukra*
   a. Resembles the color of a crystal
   b. Is fluid
   c. Has the odor of honey
   d. Is sweet
   c. All of the above

5. What are the *garbha sambhāva sāmagri*?
   a. Ovulation period
   b. Body of uterus
   c. Nutrition of embryo
   d. Fertilised ovum
   e. All of the above

6. What does *garbhotpatti* include?
   a. Creation of the universe
   b. Conception and development of the fetus
   c. Conception only
   d. Fertilization of the egg only
   e. None of the above

7. What are the classical signs of conception?
   a. Elimination of the ejaculated semen from the uterus
   b. Salivation
   c. Heaviness
   d. Drowsiness
   e. B, C, and D

8. What is the meaning of *puṁsavana*?
   a. The therapeutic process of conceiving a female baby
   b. The procedure to conceive a male baby
   c. The process of conception
   d. The process of purifying reproductive tissue
   e. None of the above

9. What is the role of *ojas* in conception and fetal development?
   a. It is the essence of the slimy material formed at the onset of fertilization that initially nourishes the embryo
   b. Upon fertilization the *ātma* lodges in the *ojas* created by the union of sperm and ovum
   c. Entrance of ojas into the heart of the embryo manifests the cardiac activities
   d. All of the above
   e. None of the above

10. Where do the four sources of the four *mahābhūtas* in a fetus come from?
    a. *Ap, pṛthvi, tejas, vāyu*
    b. *Ap, pṛthvi, tejas, ākāṣha*
    c. The mother's ovum, the father's sperm, the mother's *āhāra,* the fetus' *ātma*
    d. Diet, lifestyle, ojas, the soul
    e. None of the above

CRITICAL THINKING

1. Compare and contrast the definitions of *garbha* from Charaka and Suśhruta.

2. Review the *ṛtumati lakṣhaṇas* from various classical sources. Explain how these *lakṣhaṇas* describe a presentation of a "normal" menses and why specific *ṛtumati charya* recommendations are appropriate.

3. Consider the recommended age for reproduction given in the classics. Describe an analogy using *loka-puruṣha sāmya* which explains and supports the reasoning for the classical age recommendations.

4. Are you aware of any current scientific evidence that may support or disprove the classical practice of *puṁsavana*? Could this practice be explained today?

5. Compare and contrast the *sadyo gṛhita garbhiṇi lakṣhaṇas*. Explain how these *lakṣhaṇas* describe a presentation of "normal" early pregnancy. Which *lakṣhaṇas* could indicate a problem, or unhealthy state of pregnancy?

6. Classically, the first trimester was considered a time that could greatly influence the developing embryo. How could this perspective affect recommendations for early pregnancy management today?

Chapter 16 : Prasūti vijñāna (Pregnancy)

KEY TERMS

aparā	garbha	garbhiṇi lakṣhaṇas	prasava māsa
āsanna prasava	garbha poṣhaṇa	māsa-anumāsika	sūtikā
āvi	garbha vṛddhi-kara bhāva	mātṛjādi bhāvas	sūtikā gāra
bhāva	garbhiṇi	prasava kāla	sūtikopachara
dauhṛdaya	garbhiṇi chārya		

Pregnancy is a complex process even in its healthiest, normal state. Classical study and practice of pregnancy management is considered a very specialized area which requires a comprehensive, deep study paired with thorough experience. Here, an introductory overview of the process along with important literature is covered. Use the following table of references to read directly from the classics about each of the significant topics and understand each author's opinions and perspectives.

GARBHIṆI (MOTHER)

Garbhiṇi, the mother, provides the most important support to the developing fetus. She is responsible for contributing three out of the six factors described by Charaka in Cha. Śhā. 3/. The six *bhāvas*, often refered to as the *mātṛjādi bhāvas*, and their contributing factors include:

Bhāva	Explanation
Mātṛja	Factors derived from the mother include most of the soft organs of the body: *tvak* (skin), *lohita* (blood), *māṁsa* (muscle), *medas* (fat), *nābhi* (umbilicus), *hṛdaya* (heart), *kloma* (?), *yakṛt* (liver), *plīhā* (spleen), *vṛkka* (two kidneys), *basti* (urinary bladder), *purīṣhādhāna* (rectum), *āmāśhaya* (stomach), *pakvāśhaya* (intestines), *uttara guda* (upper part of the anal canal), *adha guda* (lower part of the anal canal), *kṣhudrāntra* (small intestines), *sthūlāntra* (large intestines), *vapā* (mesentery), *vapāvahana* (omentum).
Pitṛja	Factors derived from the father include many of the harder structures of the body: *keśha* (hair on the head), *śhmaśhru* (facial hair), *nakha* (nails), *loma* (bodily hair), *danta* (teeth), *asthi* (bones), *sirā* (veins), *snāyu* (ligaments), *dhamani* (arteries), *śhukra* (semen).
Ātma	Factors derived from the soul include characteristic features and behaviors of the individual, most notably *sukha* (happiness), *duḥkha* (unhappiness), *ichchhā* (desires), *dveṣha* (aversions), *chetana* (consciousness), *dhṛti* (courage), *buddhi* (intellect), *smṛti* (memory), *ahaṅkāra* (ego), *prayatna* (effort).
Sātmya	Factors derived from regular, wholesome habits followed by the mother include *ārogya* (consistent health, absence of disease), *anālasya* (consistent absence of laziness), *alolupatva* (consistent absence of desires or greed), *indriya prasāda* (clarity of sense organs), *svara-varṇa-bīja saṁpat* (excellent characteristics of voice, complexion and reproductive seed), *praharṣha* (desire to procreate).
Rasa	Factors derived from *rasa*, the nourishing, expressed juice produced as the first result of the mother's consumed food, include *śharīrasya-ābhinivṛtti-abhivṛddhi* (manifestation and growth of the physical body), *prāṇa-anubandha* (continuous attachment of life), *tṛpti* (satisfaction, contentment), *puṣhṭi* (healthy growth, filling out the body), *utsāha* (enthusiasm).
Sattva	Factors derived from the mental disposition of the individual include *bhakti* (likings, devotion towards), *śhīla* (conduct, behavior), *śhauca* (purity, cleanliness), *dveṣha* (aversions), *smṛti* (memory), *moha* (delusion, detachment from), *yoga* (attachment towards), *mātsarya* (strong desire not to part with), *śhaurya* (bravery), *bhaya* (fear), *krodha* (anger), *tandra* (drowsiness, tiredness, apathy), *utsāha* (enthusiasm), *taikṣhṇya* (sharpness, acuity), *mārdava* (softness), *gāmbhīrya* (seriousness), *mana-āvasthitatva* (instability of the mind).

Garbhiṇi is responsible for the *mātṛja, sātmyaja* and *rasaja* factors prior to conception, at the moment of conception and throughout the duration of the pregnancy.

Use the table of references below to understand the classical opinions on *garbhiṇi* and recommendations in a healthy, normal pregnancy.

Concept with nearest English equivalent	Ref. from Cha.	Ref. from Su.	Ref. from AH	Ref. from BP
Garbhiṇi lakṣhaṇas Characteristics of a pregnant woman	Cha. Śhā. 2/23-25	Su. Śhā. 3/14-15	AH Śhā. 1/50-52	BP Pū. 3/43-44
Garbhiṇi chārya Routine for the healthy pregnant woman	Cha. Śhā. 8/20-21, 8/32	Su. Śhā. 10/3-4	AH Śhā. 1/43-48, 50-68	BP Pū. 3/330-339
Dauhṛdaya Fetal heart beat	Cha. Śhā. 4/15-19	Su. Śhā. 3/18	AH Śhā. 1/52-54	BP Pū. 3/294-304

TEST YOURSELF

Learn, review and memorize key terms from this section.

garbhiṇi

---

bhāva

---

mātṛjādi bhāvas

---

garbhiṇi lakṣhaṇas

---

garbhiṇi chārya

---

dauhṛdaya

GARBHA (FETUS)

The term *garbha* is used to denote the embryo from the moment of conception through complete fetal development and delivery. Classical literature explains the significant developments of a normal, healthy *garbha* during each month of gestation. The recommendations for the mother during each month are intended to support this development and the health of both.

Anatomically, the development of the fetus has also been described in detail. Although the organs and other body parts may not have been directly visible during earlier stages, classical authors recognize they are present and will develop at their appropriate times.

Concept with nearest English equivalent	Ref. from Cha.	Ref. from Su.	Ref. from AH	Ref. from BP
Normal development of *garbha*	Cha. Śhā. 6/22, 25-26	Su. Śhā. 3/31		BP Pū. 3/315, 3/289-293
Garbha vṛddhi-kara bhāva Causative factors for formation of *garbha*	Cha. Śhā. 4/27	Su. Śhā. 4/38, 4/57-61	AH Śhā. 3/4-6	
Garbha poṣhaṇa Nourishment of fetus	Cha. Śhā. 6/23	Su. Śhā. 3/31	AH Śhā. 1/56	BP Pū. 3/321
Māsa-anumāsika, Garbha vṛddhi krama Month-by-month fetal development	Cha. Śhā. 4/9-25	Su. Śhā. 3/18-30	AH Śhā. 1/54-57	BP Pū. 3/289-308

TEST YOURSELF

Learn, review and memorize key terms from this section.

garbha

---

garbha vṛddhi-kara bhāva

---

garbha poṣhaṇa

---

māsa-anumāsika

PRASAVA KĀLA (LABOR AND DELIVERY)

Prasava kāla, the period for labor and delivery, was considered normal in the 9th, 10th, 11th or 12th months most likely based on a 28-day lunar calendar. Chakrapāṇi comments on Cha. Śhā. 4/25 that the ninth and tenth months are ideal, while the eleventh and twelfth months are only slightly abnormal with little risk to the fetus. Prior to delivery, many arrangements were to be made including the construction of the *sūtikā gāra*, or maternity chambers. The mother was advised to enter the *sūtikā gāra* during the 8th month and make herself comfortable there to prepare for delivery. She would generally remain in the chambers for six weeks after delivery and when menses returned, she would no longer be considered *sūtikā* (recently delivered)

Concept with nearest English equivalent	Ref. from Cha.	Ref. from Su.	Ref. from AH	Ref. from BP
Prasava māsa Normal delivery time	Cha. Śhā. 4/25, 6/24	Su. Śhā. 3/30	AH Śhā. 1/66	BP Pū. 3/340
Sūtikā gāra Maternity home	Cha. Śhā. 8/33-35	Su. Śhā. 10/5	AH Śhā. 1/73	BP Pū. 3/341
Prasava kāraṇa Cause for onset of labor		Su. Ni. 8/7-8		
Prajāyinī lakṣhaṇa Early signs of labor		Su. Śhā. 10/6		
Prajanana kāla, *Āsanna prasava lakṣhaṇa* 1st stage of labor	Cha. Śhā. 8/36		AH Śhā. 1/74-76	
Upasthita prasava 2nd stage of labor		Su. Śhā. 10/7		BP Pū. 3/342-343
Parivartita garbha Process of fetal descent	Cha. Śhā. 8/39		AH Śhā. 1/80	
Prasava vidhi Normal delivery process	Cha. Śhā. 6/24, 8/37-40	Su. Śhā. 10/8-9	AH Śhā. 1/77-82	BP Pū. 3/344-350
Āvī Contractions	Cha. Śhā. 8/37	Su. Śhā. 10/9	AH Śhā. 1/80-82	
Aparā pātana Placental delivery	Cha. Śhā. 8/41, 8/44		AH Śhā. 1/89-91	BP Pū. 3/349

TEST YOURSELF

Learn, review and memorize key terms from this section.

prasava kāla

prasava māsa

sūtikā gāra

sūtikā

āsanna prasava

āvi

aparā

SŪTIKOPACHARA (CARE OF THE MOTHER AFTER DELIVERY)

The woman who has just delivered is called *sūtikā* in the classics. Opinions vary on the duration of this name. According to Suśhruta and Vāgbhaṭa, the woman should be considered *sūtikā* for six weeks while adhering to a restricted diet and lifestyle to help restore her *dhātus* to normal. Other texts like *Bhāvaprakāśha*, *Kāśhyapa Saṁhitā* and *Yogaratnākara* are in agreement with this general statement and also state that the period of *sūtikā* may last for one, four or six months depending on the needs of the woman. Some authors state that other references consider the period to be complete when normal menstruation returns.

The six-week period of puerperium in Western Medicine aligns with the typical six-week period of *sūtikā*. Classically, the dietary and lifestyle restrictions, along with external body treatments intend to restore the mother's body to its pre-pregnancy state and help prevent many possible diseases which can easily begin to form during this time. Disorders which do take hold in the body are generally considered to vary between difficult to cure to incurable.

A review of classical references for recommendations of diet, lifestyle and treatments reveals that there are a significant variety of opinions on how to best manage *sūtikā* to reinstate normal strength of *dhātus* and prevent disease. These variations can all be considered potentially valid because their application depends on many factors. *Kāśhyapa* adds that the approach to management be customized according to the *deśha*, or geographical environment of the mother. In drier regions, more oil is appropriate while in damper regions oil should be sparingly used or avoided altogether.

Concept with nearest English equivalent	Ref. from Cha.	Ref. from Su.	Ref. from AH	Ref. from BP
Sūtikaya, Sūtikopachara Management of mother	Cha. Śhā. 8/48	Su. Śhā. 10/16-20	AH Śhā. 1/94-100	BP Pū. 4/2-6

TEST YOURSELF

Learn, review and memorize key terms from this section.

sūtikā

____

sūtikopachara

____

Chapter 16: Review

ADDITIONAL READING

Read and review the references listed below to expand your understanding of the concepts in this chapter. Write down the date that you complete your reading for each. Remember that consistent repetition is the best way to learn. Plan to read each reference at least once now and expect to read it again as you continue your studies.

Use the additional references throughout this chapter and record what you've completed.

CLASSICS	1st read	2nd read
Charaka		
Suśhruta		
Aṣhṭāṅga Hṛdaya		
Bhāva Prakāśha		

JOURNALS & CURRENT RESOURCES

1. Normal labor and delivery (Western): https://www.youtube.com/watch?v=Elh3krhcbTo
2. Labor and delivery video (Western): https://www.youtube.com/watch?v=dYu-0rOnLpA
3. Fetal circulation: https://www.youtube.com/watch?v=-IRkisEtzsk

QUESTIONS & ANSWERS

Record your questions for this chapter here for further research and discussion.

Question:

Answer:

Question:

Answer:

Question:

Answer:

SELF-ASSESSMENT

1. What are the *mātṛjādi bhāvas*?
   a. Six factors contributing to the formation and development of the fetus
   b. Qualities of the mother of the fetus
   c. *Tvak, lohita, māṁsa, medas*
   d. All of the above
   e. None of the above

2. Which factors are derived from *pitṛ* in the developing embryo and fetus?
   a. *Loma*
   b. *Danta*
   c. *Asthi*
   d. All of the above
   e. None of the above

3. Which factors are derived from the *ātma* in the developing embryo and fetus?
   a. *Sukha and duḥkha*
   b. *Ichchhā* (desires) and *dveṣha* (aversions)
   c. *Chetana, dhṛti* (courage), *ahaṅkāra*
   d. *Buddhi, smṛti*
   e. All of the above

4. Which factors are derived from *mātṛ*?
   a. Most of the soft organs of the body
   b. *Māṁsa, medas, tvak, lohita* (blood)
   c. *Hṛdaya, yakṛt, plīhā, vṛkka, basti, purīṣhādhāna, āmāśhaya, pakvāśhaya*
   d. All of the above
   e. None of the above

5. Which three *bhāvas* does the *garbhiṇi* provide to the developing fetus?
   a. *Mātṛja, pitṛja,* and *sātmya bhāva*
   b. *Mātṛja, sattva,* and *sātmya bhāva*
   c. *Mātṛja, rasa,* and *sātmya bhāva*
   d. *Ātma, pitṛja,* and *sātmya bhāva*
   e. None of the above

6. What does *dauhṛdaya* indicate?
   a. The fetus' senses are manifest and its mind associates with feelings and desires from its previous life
   b. The fetal heartbeat is detectable
   c. The heart of the fetus is connected to the heart of the *garbhiṇi*
   d. The *garbhiṇi*'s cravings now indicate fetal cravings and should be satisfied
   e. All of the above

7. According to Charaka, during the first four months of pregnancy what should be consumed regularly by the *garbhiṇi?*
   a. *Śhali* rice
   b. Ghee
   c. Milk
   d. Medicated ghee
   e. All of the above

8. What is classically recommended for the *garbhiṇi* to do during the 9th month of pregnancy?
   a. *Anuvāsana basti* using oil prepared with sweet herbs
   b. Insert cotton swabs soaked in oil into her vagina to oleate the uterus and genital tract
   c. Take yoga classes
   d. A and B
   e. None of the above

9. What are signs of impending delivery and birth?
   a. Pain in the groin, region of the bladder, pelvis, sides of the chest and back
   b. Looseness in the eyes
   c. Feeling in the chest as if a knot is being untied
   d. Feeling as if something is coming down from the pelvis
   e. All of the above

10. What is classically included in *sūtikopachara*?
    a. She should be sprinkled with warm water.
    b. Once she feels hungry, ghee, oil, *vasā* and/or *mājja* should be given along with *paṇcakola* spices.
    c. Her belly should be anointed with ghee and oil and wrapped tightly with a long cloth.
    d. Gruel prepared with *pippali* should be consumed in proper quantity
    e. All of the above

CRITICAL THINKING

1. Explain the importance of the 4th and 8th months of fetal development.
2. Review the recommendations for *garbhiṇi chārya*, the routine for the pregnant woman, provided in the classics. Identify three recommendations which could be relevant today and explain why.
3. Watch video #1 (animation of normal labor and delivery) and describe any similarities that you notice with classical explanations of labor and delivery.

Chapter 17 : Bāla prakaraṇa (Management of birth and childhood)

KEY TERMS

bāla prakaraṇa	jāta	saṁskāra	stanya
dhātri	kumāra gāra		

After the birth of *jāta*, a normal, healthy newborn, the classics specify key procedures to stabilize the child immediately. Many of these procedures are followed today in a similar fashion using modernized tools and facilities such as clearing the airway including nose and throat, bathing the newborn, providing an initial feeding (immunization, or protection), and more.

Throughout childhood, the classics also specify several *samskāras*, which can be considered similarly to milestones in development. Many of these are very closely intertwined with current, cultural Hindu religious customs. For a basic overview of *samskāras*, read the article *Āyurvedic and traditional Hindu childhood samskāra offer methodical life guidance*, by Pravin Masram et al.

TEST YOURSELF

Learn, review and memorize key terms from this section.

bāla prakaraṇa

---

jāta

---

saṁskāra

---

stanya

---

dhātri

---

kumāra gāra

Concept with nearest English equivalent	Ref. from Cha.	Ref. from Su.	Ref. from AH	Ref. from BP
Nābhi nāḍī chedana Cutting the umbilical cord	Cha. Śhā. 8/44	Su. Śhā. 10/12	AH Utt. 1/5	
Jāta Management of newborn	Cha. Śhā. 8/42-43, 46-47	Su. Śhā. 10/13, 10/23	AH Utt. 1/1-5	BP Pū. 4/1
Jāta karma Birth rituals, rites	Cha. Śhā. 8/46-47	Su. Śhā. 10/13	AH Utt. 1/1-4	
Āyu Assessment of life span	Cha. Śhā. 8/51		AH Utt. 1/24	
Prāśhana Initial feeding		Su. Śhā. 10/15	AH Utt. 1/8-14	
Stanya Breastmilk	Cha. Śhā. 8/52-58	Su. Śhā. 10/14	AH Utt. 1/15-20	BP Pū. 4/7-35
Dhātri Wet nurse	Cha. Śhā. 8/52-58	Su. Śhā. 10/25-27	AH Utt. 1/16-17	BP Pū. 4/24-29
Kumāra gāra Nursery	Cha. Śhā. 8/59-63			
Bālopachāra Care of the child	Cha. Śhā. 8/64	Su. Śhā. 10/46-47	AH Utt. 1/25-28, 1/40-45	
Nāmakaraṇa Naming ceremony	Cha. Śhā. 8/50	Su. Śhā. 10/24	AH Utt. 1/22-23	
Annaprāśhana Weaning		Su. Śhā. 10/49	AH Utt. 1/37-39	BP Pū. 4/36
Karṇa vedhana Ear piercing		Su. Sū. 16/3	AH Utt. 1/28-36	

Chapter 17: Review

ADDITIONAL READING

Read and review the references listed below to expand your understanding of the concepts in this chapter. Write down the date that you complete your reading for each. Remember that consistent repetition is the best way to learn. Plan to read each reference at least once now and expect to read it again as you continue your studies.

Use the additional references throughout this chapter and record what you've completed.

CLASSICS	1st read	2nd read
Charaka		
Suśhruta		
Aṣhṭāṅga Hṛdaya		
Bhāva Prakāśha		

JOURNALS & CURRENT RESOURCES

Āyurvedic and traditional Hindu childhood samskāra offer methodical life guidance, by Pravin Masram et al.

QUESTIONS & ANSWERS

Record your questions for this chapter here for further research and discussion.

Question:

Answer:

Question:

Answer:

Question:

Answer:

SELF-ASSESSMENT

1. What is the proper procedure for cutting the umbilical cord according to Suśhruta?
   a. The umbilical cord should be ligated four *aṅgula* from the umbilicus then cut
   b. The umbilical cord should be ligated eight *aṅgula* from the umbilicus, cut and hung loosely from the infant's neck with a string
   c. The umbilical cord should be clamped and cut with sharp scissors
   d. The umbilical cord should be ligated 2 *aṅgula* from the umbilicus using string, then cut
   e. None of the above

2. Management of newborns includes
   a. Cleaning the mouth with ghee and rock salt
   b. Cutting the umbilical cord
   c. Sprinkling cold water on the newborn in summer or warm water in winter
   d. Postnatal rites and feeding *ghṛta* and honey with gold dust
   e. All of the above

3. When does milk production commence after normal labor and birth?
   a. Right after the baby is born
   b. Three to five days after the baby is born
   c. Within one week
   d. Upon commencement of nursing
   e. None of the above

4. What characteristic feature is not utilized in classical assessment of life span for a newborn?
   a. Hair
   b. Tongue
   c. Skin
   d. Genitals
   e. None of the above

5. What dravya does Suśhruta recommend to feed to the newborn twice before the initial breastfeeding?
   a. *Ghṛta* and honey in the quantity that fits in the newborn's palm
   b. *Ghṛta* and gold flakes
   c. Honey and salt
   d. Substances with *madhura rasa* cooked into ghee
   e. None of the above

6. Which *lakṣhaṇas* indicate *vāta* vitiation in breast milk?
   a. Exceedingly white color, excessively sweet *anurasa* with salty after taste
   b. Blackish or reddish color, astringent *anurasa,* clear, not unctuous, frothy
   c. Blackish, blueish, yellowish or coppery in color, bitter *anurasa*, sour or pungent after taste, excessively hot
   d. Yellowish color, salty *anurasa*, sweet after taste, heavy
   e. None of the above

7. Which characteristics are important when choosing a wet nurse for a newborn?
   a. Youthful, free of disease, kind, born in the same locality
   b. Irreverent of children, having birthed only daughters, born into a different caste
   c. Excellent quality and quantity of breastmilk, skillful in service, clean
   d. Both A and C
   e. None of the above

8. Why are newborns given two names during their naming ceremony?
   a. One is based upon the *nākṣhatra* or constellation in which the child was born
   b. One is the name by which he would be called or known by in the family or society, known as the *ābhiprāyika*
   c. One is based upon the family's historical ties to their familial temple
   d. Both A and B
   e. All of the above

SELF-ASSESSMENT

9. According to Suśhruta, which food should first be given for weaning?
   a. Cooked fruit
   b. Fresh fruit
   c. Light and beneficial cereals
   d. Easy to digest rice and dal mixed together
   e. All of the above

10. When should *karṇa vedhana* be done on an infant?
    a. 2-3 months old
    b. 4-5 months old
    c. 6-7 months old
    d. 8-9 months old
    e. 10-12 months old

CRITICAL THINKING

1. Compare the classical recommendations for management of the newborn. Different authors have provided similar instructions but in various orders. Provide possible explanations for these differences.

2. Cite a medical definition for colostrum and explain where it fits in the management of the newborn and mother.

3. In caring for the newborn and child, what general similarities could be found between classical intentions and current practices of any tradition or culture?

4. Review the types of foods and method recommended for weaning. What could be considered relevant for practical application today?

5. Could the classical *samskāras* be compared to a similar process in other religions? Explain.

Chapter 18 : Prakṛti

KEY TERMS

bhautika prakṛti	eka-doṣha	prakṛti	śhleṣhmalā
deha prakṛti	mānasika prakṛti	sama-doṣha	vātalā
doṣhika prakṛti	pittalā	śharīrika prakṛti	vikṛti
dvi-doṣha			

Prakṛti can be considered the unique, base constitution that is set within an individual from the moment of conception. It is influenced by the ratio and proportion of *bhūtas* provided by the mother, father and additional factors at the moment of conception and is influenced during gestation.

NIRUKTI & PARIBHĀṢHĀ

To better understand the term p*rakṛti*, first review its etymology and definitions.

Nirukti

The term *prakṛti* derives from the Sanskrit *dhātu* √ *kṛ*, which indicates:

√ kṛ — to do, make, perform, accomplish, cause, effect, prepare, undertake

to execute, carry out (as an order or command)

to manufacture, prepare, work at, elaborate, build

to form or construct one thing out of another (abl. or instr.)

to employ, use, make use of (instr.)

to compose, describe

to cultivate

The *dhātu* √ *kṛ* is prefixed by *pra-* which indicates:

pra- — before

forward, in front, on, forth (mostly in connection with a verb, esp. with a verb of motion which is often to be supplied)

Finally, the term ends with *-ti* which is shortened by its conjoining *sandhi* from *iti*:

-ti — for iti (after k / ā)

iti — in this manner, thus (in its original signification, iti refers to something that has been said or thought, or lays stress on what precedes)

often equivalent to “as you know”

As a complete term, *prakṛti* indicates that which is made or created first. It is the design or plan for the individual’s construction and character, and is executed as such. This initial plan is set from the beginning of life and does not change throughout the duration of life. It is only towards the end of life that alterations may arise. Any changes that do manifest are meant to signal that the end of life is approaching. Suśhruta states this as:

प्रकोपो वाऽन्यथाभावो क्षयो वा नोपजायते । प्रकृतीनां स्वभावेन जायते तु गतायुषः ॥ ७८

विषजातो यथा कीटो न विषेण विपद्यते ।
तद्वत्प्रकृतयो मर्त्यं शक्नुवन्ति न बाधितुम् ॥

सु. शा. ४।७९

Prakopo vā ' nyathābhāvo kṣhayo vā nopajāyate | Prakṛtīnāṁ svabhāvena jāyate tu gatāyuṣhaḥ ||
Viṣhajāto yathā kīṭo na viṣheṇa vipadyate | Tadvatprakṛtayo martyaṁ śhaknuvanti na bādhitum

Su. Śhā. 4/78-79

Prakopo (Aggravation) vā (or) ' nyathābhāvo (change from normal state) kṣhayo vā (or decrease) na-upajāyate (does not just happen on its own). Prakṛtīnāṁ svabhāvena jāyate (When a natural change does occur to the *prakṛti*) tu (that [indicates]) gata-āyuṣhaḥ (life, lifespan or vitality is going away).

Paribhāṣhā

Suśhruta provides a very clear and concise definition of seven types of *prakṛti*.

सप्त प्रकृतयो भवन्ति - दोषैः पृथक्, द्विशः, समस्तैश्च ॥

सु. शा. ४।६२

Sapta prakṛtayo bhavanti - doṣhaiḥ pṛthak, dviśhaḥ, samastaiśhcha ||

Su. Śhā. 4/62

Sapta (The seven) prakṛtayo ([types of] *prakṛti*) bhavanti (are) - doṣhaiḥ (each *doṣha*) pṛthak (separately), dviśhaḥ (two together), samastaiśhcha (and all three in normal, healthy state).

The seven types of *prakṛti* are:

Eka-doṣha	*Vāta*
	Pitta
	Kapha
Dvi-doṣha	*Vāta-Kapha*
	Vāta-Pitta
	Pitta-Kapha
Sama-doṣha	*Vāta-Pitta-Kapha*

More complex definitions available in the classics convey the understanding of the functions and practical application of *prakṛti*.

समपित्तानिलकफाः केचिद्गर्भादि मानवाः ।
दृश्यन्ते वातलाः केचित्पित्तलाः श्लेष्मलास्तथा || ३९
तेषामनातुराः पूर्वे वातलाद्याः सदातुराः ।
दोषानुशयिता ह्येषां देहप्रकृतिरुच्यते ||

च. सू. ७। ३९-४०

Samapittānilakaphāḥ kechidgarbhādi mānavāḥ |
Dṛśhyante vātalāḥ kechitpittalāḥ śhleṣhmalāstathā || 39
Teṣhāmanāturāḥ pūrve vātalādyāḥ sadāturāḥ |
Doṣhānuśhayitā hyeṣhāṁ dehaprakṛtiruchyate ||

Cha. Sū. 7/39-40

Certain people maintain a state of *sama pitta*, *anila* and *kapha* from the moment the *garbha* is formed (conception). It is also seen that others have a particular predominance of (*doṣhas* causing a state of) *vātalā*, *pittalā* or *śhleṣhmalā*. Those in the first category are unlikely to regularly be afflicted by disorders, while the people of the second category are always afflicted by *vāta* and the other *doṣhas*. The *deha prakṛti* is known by the *doṣhānuśhayitā* (the predominance of unavoidable *doṣha*).

शुक्रशोणितसंयोगे यो भवेद्दोष उत्कटः ।
प्रकृतिर्जायते ... ॥

सु. शा. ४।६३

Śhukraśhoṇitasaṁyoge yo
bhaveddoṣha utkaṭaḥ |
Prakṛtirjāyate ... ||

Su. Śhā. 4/63

Śhukra-śhoṇita-saṁyoge yo (At the time of union of sperm and ovum) bhaved-doṣha (whichever *doṣha*) utkaṭaḥ (is above or exceeding its normal limit) prakṛtir-jāyate (is that which wins out as the *prakṛti*).

Charaka provides a more comprehensive definition and explanation in the context of assessment of an individual's state of health. Understanding and determining *prakṛti* is considered one of the main factors in a thorough assessment.

तत्रप्रकृत्यादीन्भावाननुव्याख्यास्यामः |
तद्यथा- शुक्रशोणितप्रकृतिं,
कालगर्भाशयप्रकृतिं,
आतुराहारविहारप्रकृतिं,
महाभूतविकारप्रकृतिंचगर्भशरीरमपेक्षते |
एतानियेनयेनदोषेणाधिकेनैकेनानेकेनवास
मनुबध्यन्ते, तेनतेनदोषेणगर्भोऽनुबध्यते;
ततःसासादोषप्रकृतिरुच्यतेमनुष्याणांगर्भा
दिप्रवृत्ता | तस्माच्छलेष्मलाःप्रकृत्याकेचित्,
पित्तलाःकेचित्, वातलाःकेचित्,
संसृष्टाःकेचित्, समधातवःकेचिद्भवन्ति | ...

च. वि. ८।९५

Tatra prakṛtyādīn
bhāvānanuvyākhyāsyāmaḥ | Tadyathā -
śhukraśhōṇitaprakṛtiṁ,
kālagarbhāśhayaprakṛtiṁ,
āturāhāravihāraprakṛtiṁ,
mahābhūtavikāraprakṛtiṁ cha
garbhaśharīramapekṣhate | Etāni hi
yena yena doṣheṇādhikenaikenānekena
vā samanubadhyante, tena tena
doṣheṇa garbho ' nubadhyate; tataḥ sā
sā doṣhaprakṛtiruchyate manuṣhyāṇāṁ
garbhādipravṛttā |
Tasmāchchhleṣhmalāḥ prakṛtyā kechit,
pittalāḥ kechit, vātalāḥ kechit,
saṁsṛṣhṭāḥ kechit, samadhātavaḥ
kechidbhavanti | ...

Cha. Vi. 8/95

Tatra (And so,) prakṛtyādīn bhāvānanu (the principles of *prakṛti* and its related factors) vyākhyāsyāmaḥ (are now going to be explained) - tadyathā (as follows) – śhukra (sperm) śhōṇita (and ovum) prakṛtiṁ (result in the *prakṛti*), kāla (time or timing of conception) garbhāśhaya (in the uterus) prakṛtiṁ (result in the *prakṛti*), ātura (the health [of the mother]) āhāra ([her] diet) vihara (and all activities) prakṛtiṁ (result in the *prakṛti*), mahābhūta (the gross elements) vikāra (and any disease or dysfunction) prakṛtiṁ (result in *prakṛti*) cha (and) garbhaśharīram (the body of the fetus) apekṣhate (is produced in this way). Etāni hi yena yena doṣheṇādhikenaikenānekena vā (Thus, the *doṣhas*, either singly or in combination) samanubadhyante (become permanently attached), tena tena doṣheṇa garbho ' nubadhyate (and become the *doṣhas* of the fetus from then on); tataḥ sā sā doṣha-prakṛtir-uchyate (and so, these very *doṣhas* are called the *doṣha-prakṛti*) manuṣhyāṇāṁ (of human beings) garbhādi-pravṛttā (originating from the development of the fetus and its related factors). Tasmāch-chhleṣhmalāḥ prakṛtyā kechit (Some of these *prakṛti* are predominant in *śhleṣhma* and are referred to as *śhleṣhmalā*), pittalāḥ kechit (some are predominant in *pitta* and referred to as *pittalā*), vātalāḥ kechit (some are predominant in *vāta* and are known as *vātalā*), saṁsṛṣhṭāḥ kechit (some are predominant in a mixed combination and are known as *saṁsṛṣhṭā*), samadhātavaḥ kechid-bhavanti (and some maintain a state of normal equilibrium of the supportive systems and are called *samadhātu*).

Vāgbhaṭa explains an important point along with his definition of *prakṛti* by including a classification of low, medium and best types of *prakṛti*.

शुक्रार्तवस्थैर्जन्मादौ विषेणेव विषक्रिमेः ॥
९
तैश्च तिस्रः प्रकृतयो हिनमध्योत्तमाः पृथक् ।
समधातुः समस्तासु श्रेष्ठा, निन्द्या द्विदोषजाः
॥

अ. हृ. सू. १।१०

Śhukrārtavasthairjanmādau viṣheṇeva viṣhakrimeḥ ||
Taiśhcha tisraḥ praṛtayo hinamadhyottamāḥ pṛthak |
Samadhātuḥ samasthāsu śhreṣhṭhā, nindyā dvidoṣhajāḥ ||

AH Sū. 1/10

Śhukrārtava-sthair-janmādau ([The *doṣhas*] Being in both the sperm and the ovum, they both give rise to it [*prakṛti*]) viṣheṇeva viṣhakrimeḥ (just as poisonous worms arise from poison itself). Taiśhcha tisraḥ praṛtayo (From each of these three [*doṣhas*] hinamadhyottamāḥ pṛthak (come the [three] distinct levels of low, medium and best, respectively [ie, *vāta*, *pitta*, *kapha*]). Samadhātuḥ (The state of equilibrium of the supportive systems of the body) samasthāsu (is that which arises from a healthy, normal state) śhreṣhṭhā (and is best), nindyā (the worst is) dvidoṣhajāḥ (the combination born out of two *doṣhas*).

The interpretation of this succinct statement provides insight into the comparison of *doṣhas* and *prakṛti*. The order described is:

Hina (Low)	*Vāta* *Vāta-Kapha*
Madhyama (Medium)	*Pitta* *Vāta-Pitta*
Uttama (Best)	*Kapha* *Pitta-Kapha* *Tridoṣha* (*Samadhātu*)

The low, medium and best levels are to be considered in the context of an individual's resilience, general state of health, ability to tolerate variations in diet and lifestyle, capacity for physical work, mental state and more. Within each of these levels, there is a wide spectrum of possibilities for each presentation of *prakṛti*.

Vāgbhaṭa later adds that because of the strength of *vāta* to produce disequilibrium and disease, it is considered the most dangerous of the *tridoṣha* (AH Śhā. 3/84)

Charaka explains the combinations of *doṣhas* as *saṁsarga* (two *doṣhas*) and *sannipāta* (three *doṣhas*):

(प्रायः) शारीरदोषाणामेकाधिष्ठानीयानां सन्निपातः संसर्गो वा समानगुणत्वात्; दोषा हि दूषणैः समानाः ||

च. वि. ६। १०

(Prāyaḥ) śhārīradoṣhāṇām ekādhiṣhṭhānīyānāṁ sannipātaḥ saṁsargo vā samānaguṇatvāt; doṣhā hi dūṣhaṇaiḥsamānāḥ ||

Cha. Vi. 6/10

(Prāyaḥ) (For the most part), śhārīra-doṣhāṇām (the *doṣhas* of the body) ekādhiṣhṭhānīyānāṁ (which are located in one place) sannipātaḥ saṁsargo vā (all combine together, or combine in two) samānaguṇatvāt (based on the similarities in their characteristics); doṣhā hi (the *doṣhas* themselves) dūṣhaṇaiḥsamānāḥ (are the same as or similar to that which they are vitiating).

Charaka also makes clear the distinction between recognizing *prakṛti* versus *vikṛti*. The technical terms of *vātalā*, *pittalā* and *śhleṣhmalā* refer to the predominance of *doṣha* indicating a state of *vikṛti* rather than *prakṛti*.

न च विकृतेषु दोषेषु प्रकृतिस्थत्वमुपपद्यते,
तस्मान्नैताः प्रकृतयः सन्ति ... ||

च. वि. ६।१३

Na cha vikṛteṣhu
doṣheṣhuprakṛtisthatvamupapadyate,
tasmānnaitāḥ prakṛtayaḥ santi ... ||

Cha. Vi. 6/13

Prakṛti-sthatvam (To be in a state of normal, healthy *prakṛti*) upapadyate (is possible) na cha vikṛteṣhu doṣheṣhu (only when none of the doṣhas are in a state of *vikṛti*), tasmān (therefore), na-itāḥ (these [individuals] cannot) prakṛtayaḥ santi (be in a state of *prakṛti*).

TEST YOURSELF

Learn, review and memorize key terms from this section.

prakṛti

eka-doṣha

dvi-doṣha

sama-doṣha

vikṛti

vātalā

pittalā

śhleṣhmalā

BHEDA

Charaka and Suśhruta provide unique perspectives on the general classifcations of *prakṛti*. Each of these has important practical applications for clinical assessments.

Śharīrika prakṛti

Charaka indirectly explains two top-level classifications of *prakṛti* through the concept of *doṣhas* as *śharīrika* and *mānasika*. Understanding the relationship between the *doṣhas* and *prakṛti* is significant here as it lays the foundation for connecting the two locations of disease in the body and mind.

Śharīrika prakṛti is synonymous with *deha*, or *dehika prakṛti*, and *doṣhika prakṛti*.

तत्र त्रयः शरीरदोषा वातपित्तश्लेष्माणः, ते
शरीरं दूषयन्ति; द्वौ पुनः सत्त्वदोषौ
रजस्तमश्च, तौ सत्त्वं दूषयतः | ताभ्यां च
सत्त्वशरीराभ्यां दुष्टाभ्यां विकृतिरुपजायते,
नोपजायते चाप्रदुष्टाभ्याम् ||

च. शा. ४।३४

Tatra trayaḥ śharīradoṣhā
vātapittaśhlēṣhmāṇaḥ, te śharīraṁ
dūṣhayanti; dvau punaḥ sattvadoṣhau
rajastamaśhcha, tau sattvaṁ
dūṣhayataḥ | tābhyāṁ cha
sattvaśharīrābhyāṁ duṣhṭābhyāṁ
vikṛtirupajāyate, nopajāyate
chāpraduṣhṭābhyām ||

Cha. Śhā. 4/34

Tatra (And so) trayaḥ (the three) śharīradoṣhā (*doṣhas* of the body [are]) vāta-pitta-śhlēṣhmāṇaḥ (*vāta*, *pitta* and *kapha*), te (these three) dūṣhayanti ([have the tendency to] vitiate, pollute or disturb) śharīraṁ (the body); dvau punaḥ (likewise, the two) sattva-doṣhau (*doṣhas* of *sattva*, ie, *manas*, the mind [are]) rajas-tamaśh-cha (*rajas* and *tamas*), tau (they both) dūṣhayataḥ ([have the tendency to] vitiate, pollute or disturb) sattvaṁ (the *sattva*, or normal, healthy discernment). Tābhyāṁ cha sattva-śharīrābhyāṁ (Either or both of these, the mind and/or body) duṣhṭābhyāṁ (become vitiated) vikṛtir-upajāyate (when *vikṛti* arises or exists), na-upajāyate cāpraduṣhṭābhyām ([disease itself] does not exist without either or both of these being vitiated).

In the subclassification of *śharīrika prakṛti*, the types include the three *doṣhas* singly, and in combination. Detailed *lakṣhaṇas* for *vāta*, *pitta* and *śhleṣhma* are described in the classics, while the authors state that combinations should be understood by the various mixtures of their features.

The question naturally arises then regarding the *doṣhas* and their influence on *prakṛti* and *vikṛti*. Should these *doṣhas* be considered the same or distinct causative factors? Chakrapāṇi discusses this in the commentary of Cha. Sū. 17/62.

Mānasika prakṛti

Charaka then explains *mānasika prakṛti* and its classifications as three main types:

त्रिविधं खलु सत्त्वं - शुद्धं, राजसं,
तामसमिति| तत्र शुद्धमदोषमाख्यातं
कल्याणांशत्वात्, राजसं सदोषमाख्यातं
रोषांशत्वात्, तामसमपि सदोषमाख्यातं
मोहांशत्वात् | तेषां तु त्रयाणामपि
सत्त्वानामेकैकस्य भेदाग्रमपरिसङ्ख्येयं
तरतमयोगाच्छरीरयोनिविशेषेभ्यश्चान्योन्यानु
विधानत्वाच्च | शरीरं ह्यपि
सत्त्वमनुविधीयते, सत्त्वं च शरीरम् | ...

च. शा. ४।३६

Trividhaṁ khalu sattvaṁ - śhuddhaṁ,
rājasaṁ, tāmasamiti | Tatra
śhuddhamadoṣhamākhyātaṁ
kalyāṇāṁśhatvāt, rājasaṁ
sadoṣhamākhyātaṁ roṣhāṁśhatvāt,
tāmasamapisadoṣhamākhyātaṁ
mohāṁśhatvāt | ...

Cha. Śhā. 4/36

Trividhaṁ khalu sattvaṁ (The three types of mental state, or mind are) - śhuddhaṁ (clean, pure [*sattva*, or discernment]), rājasaṁ (initiation, action), tāmasam-iti (and inertia). Tatra (And so), śhuddham (the clean, pure type of *sattva*) adoṣhamākhyātaṁ (does not cause or create *doṣhas*, or vitiating factors) kalyāṇāṁśhatvāt (due to its natural component of benevolence, generosity, virtuousness), rājasaṁ (the initiating or action type of mental state) sa-doṣhamākhyātaṁ (is perpetually associated with *doṣhas*) roṣhāṁśhatvāt (due to its natural component of anger, fury, passion, rage, desire) tāmasam-api (and the inertia type of mental state) sa-doṣhamākhyātaṁ (is perpetually associated with *doṣhas*) mohāṁśhatvāt (due to its natural component of confusion, delusion, ignorance, inability to discriminate).

The three main types of *mānasika prakṛti* are

described as *sattva*, *rajas* and *tamas* (or *sattvika*, *rājasika* and *tāmasika*). Additionally, each of these three is demonstrated through several character examples using personality types that were well-known to the authors and readers of the classical texts. Review Cha. Śhā. 4/37-39 for a complete description.

Suśhruta includes an explanation of *mānasika prakṛti* along with descriptions of their profiles and characteristic features in Su. Śhā. 4/81-98. Vāgbhaṭa includes similar descriptions in AH Śhā. 3/7.

Bhautika Prakṛti

Suśhruta states that many scholars also recognize *prakṛti* based on the *pañcha mahābhūtas*:

प्रकृतिमिह नराणां भौतिकीं केचिदाहुः
पवनदहनतोयैः कीर्तितास्तास्तु तिस्रः ।
स्थिरविपुलशरीरः पार्थिवश्च क्षमावान्
शुचिरथ चिरजीवी नाभसः खैर्महद्भिः ॥

सु. शा. ४।८०

Prakṛtimiha narāṇaṁ bhautikīṁ kechidāhuḥ pavanadahanatoyaiḥ kīrtitāstāstu tisraḥ | Sthiravipulaśharīraḥ pārthivaśhcha kṣhamāvāñ śhuchiratha chirajīvī nābhasaḥ khairmahadbhiḥ ||

Su. Śhā. 4/80

Prakṛtimiha (In the context of *prakṛti*), narāṇaṁ (many people) bhautikīṁ (consider the *bhūtas* [as the explanation]) kechidāhuḥ (some of which) pavana-dahana-toyaiḥ (*vāta*, *pitta* and *kapha*) kīrtitāstāstu (have already been mentioned) tisraḥ (as the three [*doṣhas*]). Sthira-vipula-śharīraḥ (Stability, and a strong body) pārthivaśhcha ([are found in those predominant of] *pṛthvi mahābhūta*) kṣhamāvāñ (along with tolerance, patience, forbearance); śhuchir-atha (purity, cleanliness in all things), chira-jīvī ([and] a long life) nābhasaḥ ([are found in those predominant of ākāśha *mahābhūta*)] khairmahadbhiḥ (along with large, hollow spaces in the cavities of the body).

Here, Suśhruta directly connects the *doṣhas* to the *pañcha mahābhūtas* and briefly explains the *lakṣhaṇas* of those which have not yet been explained as part of the *tridoṣhas*.

Charaka provides insight into the logic behind the concept of *bhautika prakṛti* by describing the contributions that each *mahābhūta* makes to the development of *garbha*.

तत्रास्याकाशात्मकं शब्दः श्रोत्रं लाघवं
सौक्ष्म्यं विवेकश्च, वाय्वात्मकं स्पर्शः स्पर्शनं
रौक्ष्यं प्रेरणं धातुव्यूहनं चेष्टाश्च शारीर्यः,
अग्न्यात्मकं रूपं दर्शनं प्रकाशः
पक्तिरौष्ण्यं च, अबात्मकं रसो रसनं शैत्यं
मार्दवं स्नेहःक्लेदश्च, पृथिव्यात्मकं गन्धो
घ्राणं गौरवं स्थैर्यं मूर्तिश्चेति ॥

च. शा. ४।१२

Tatrāsyākāśhātmakaṁ śhabdaḥ śhrotraṁ lāghavaṁ saukṣhmyaṁ vivekaśhcha, vāyvātmakaṁ sparśhaḥ sparśhanaṁ raukṣhyaṁ preraṇaṁ dhātuvyūhanaṁ cheṣhṭāśhcha śhārīryaḥ, agnyātmakaṁ rūpaṁ darśhanaṁ prakāśhaḥ paktirauṣhṇyaṁ cha, abātmakaṁ raso rasanaṁ śhaityaṁ mārdavaṁ snehaḥ kledaśhcha, pṛthvyātmakaṁ gandho ghrāṇaṁgauravaṁ sthairyaṁ mūrtiśhcheti ||

Cha. Śhā. 4/12

Tatrāsyākāśhātmakaṁ (And so [in the garbha] that which derives from *ākāśha* includes) śhabdaḥ (sound), śhrotraṁ (sense of hearing, ears), lāghavaṁ (lightness), saukṣhmyaṁ (minuteness), vivekaśhcha (and discrimination, distinction, the power of separation), vāyvātmakaṁ (that which derives from *vāyu* includes) sparśhaḥ (sensation, tangibility), sparśhanaṁ (the sense of touch), raukṣhyaṁ (dryness), preraṇaṁ (initiation, impulse), dhātuvyūhanaṁ (separation, distinction and development of the supportive systems of the body), cheṣhṭāśhcha śhārīryaḥ (and all actions of the body), agnyātmakaṁ (that which derives from *agni* includes) rūpaṁ (visible form), darśhanaṁ (the sense of sight), prakāśhaḥ (shine, luster, brightness), paktirauṣhṇyaṁ cha (the capacity to digest, and heat), abātmakaṁ (that which derives from *ap* includes) raso (flavor, taste), rasanaṁ (the sense of taste), śhaityaṁ (coolness), mārdavaṁ (softness), snehaḥ (unctuousness, oiliness) kledaśhcha (and moisture), pṛthvyātmakaṁ (that which derives from *pṛthvi* includes) gandho (smells, odors), ghrāṇaṁ (the sense of smell), gauravaṁ (heaviness), sthairyaṁ (stability) mūrtiśhcheti (and anything which takes on physical form).

Use the following tables to review the *bhautika prakṛti lakṣhaṇas* in detail.

Nābhasa prakṛti lakṣhaṇas with nearest English equivalent	Cha. Śhā. 4/12	Su. Śhā. 4/80
Śhuchir-atha Purity, cleanliness in all things		✓
Chira-jīvī A long life		✓
Khairmahadbhiḥ Large, hollow spaces in the cavities of the body		✓
Śhabdaḥ Sound	✓	
Śhrotraṁ Sense of hearing, ears	✓	
Lāghavaṁ Lightness	✓	
Saukṣhmyaṁ Minuteness	✓	
Viveka Discrimination, distinction, the power of separation	✓	

Vāyavya prakṛti lakṣhaṇas with nearest English equivalent	Cha. Śhā. 4/12	Su. Śhā. 4/80
Sparśhaḥ Sensation, tangibility	✓	
Sparśhanaṁ The sense of touch	✓	
Raukṣhyaṁ Dryness	✓	
Preraṇaṁ Initiation, impulse	✓	
Dhātuvyūhanaṁ Separation, distinction and development of the supportive systems of the body	✓	
Cheṣhṭāśhcha śhārīryaḥ And all actions of the body	✓	

Āgneya prakṛti lakṣhaṇas with nearest English equivalent	Cha. Śhā. 4/12	Su. Śhā. 4/80
Rūpaṁ Visible form	✓	
Darśhanaṁ The sense of sight	✓	
Prakāśhaḥ Shine, luster, brightness	✓	
Pakti The capacity to digest	✓	
Uṣhṇyaṁ Heat	✓	

Āpya prakṛti lakṣhaṇas with nearest English equivalent	Cha. Śhā. 4/12	Su. Śhā. 4/80
Raso Flavor, taste	√	
Rasanaṁ The sense of taste	√	
Śhaityaṁ Coolness	√	
Mārdavaṁ Softness	√	
Snehaḥ Unctuousness, oiliness	√	
Kledaśhcha And moisture	√	

Pārthiva prakṛti lakṣhaṇas with nearest English equivalent	Cha. Śhā. 4/12	Su. Śhā. 4/80
Sthira Stability		√
Vipula-śharīraḥ A strong body		√
Kṣhamāvāñ Tolerance, patience, forbearance		√
Gandho Smells, odors	√	
Ghrāṇaṁ The sense of smell	√	
Gauravam Heaviness	√	
Sthairyaṁ Stability	√	
Mūrtiśhcheti And anything which takes on physical form	√	

TEST YOURSELF

Learn, review and memorize key terms from this section.

śharīrika prakṛti

---

deha prakṛti

---

doṣhika prakṛti

---

mānasika prakṛti

---

bhautika prakṛti

ŚHARĪRIKA PRAKṚTI LAKṢHAṆAS

Charaka and Suśhruta each discuss the *śharīrika prakṛti lakṣhaṇas* in a unique way. Each author's opinion is discussed separately to convey their original perspective.

Read additional descriptions from AH Śhā. 3/83-104 and BP Pū. 4/51+.

Charaka's perspective

Charaka connects the *guṇas* to the production of specific characteristics and features for each of the three *doṣhas* (as *vātalā*, *pittalā* or *śhleṣhmalā*). He states that the presence of these *guṇas* not only causes the manifestation of specific features, but also affects the individual's overall strength, quantity and quality of life. Review these statements for each of the three *doṣhas*:

For *vātalā*:

तएवङ्गुणयोगाद्वातलाःप्रायेणाल्पबलाश्चा
ल्पायुषश्चाल्पापत्याश्चाल्पसाधनाश्चाल्पधनाश्च
भवन्ति ||

च. वि. ८।९८

Ta evaṅguṇayogādvātalāḥ
prāyeṇālpabalāśhchālpāyuṣhaśhchālpā
patyāśhchālpasādhanāśhchālpadhanāś
hcha ||

Cha. Vi. 8/98

Ta evaṅguṇa-yogād (Due to the natural associations with these *guṇas*), vātalāḥ (in those who tend to have increased *vāta*) prāyeṇa (they generally [experience]) alpa-balā-śhcha (low physical strength, resilience) alpa-āyuṣha-śhcha (and a low lifespan, quality of life, vitality) alpa-apatyā-śhcha (and low, few or no children) alpa-sādhanā-śhcha (and low, little or no means [to further their goals]) alpa-dhanā-śhcha (and litte wealth).

For *pittalā*:

तएवङ्गुणयोगात्पित्तलामध्यबलामध्यायुषो
मध्यज्ञानविज्ञानवित्तोपकरणवन्तश्चभवन्ति
||

च. वि. ८।९७

Ta evaṅguṇayogāt pittalā madhyabalā
madhyāyuṣho
madhyajñānavijñānavittopakaraṇavanta
śhcha bhavanti ||

Cha. Vi. 8/97

Ta evaṅguṇa-yogāt (Due to the natural associations with these *guṇas*), pittalā (in those who tend to have increased *pitta* [they generally experience]) madhya-balā (moderate physical strength, resilience), madhya-āyuṣho (moderate lifespan, quality of life, vitality), madhya jñāna, vijñāna, vitta upakaraṇa vanta-śhcha bhavanti (and moderate amounts of intellectual knowledge, scientific knowledge, wealth (possessions), tools and means (to further their goals).

<u>For *śhleṣhmalā*</u>:

तएवङ्‌गुणयोगाच्छलेष्मलाबलवन्तोवसुम
न्तोविद्यावन्तओजस्विनःशान्ताआयुष्मन्तश्च
भवन्ति ||

च. वि. ८।९६

Ta evaṅguṇayogāchchhleṣhmalā
balavanto vasumanto vidyāvanta
ojasvinaḥ śhāntā āyuṣhmantaśhcha
bhavanti ||

Cha. Vi. 8/96

Ta evaṅguṇayogāt (Due to the natural associations with these *guṇas*), śhleṣhmalā (in those who tend to have increased *kapha* [they generally experience]) bala-vanto (well-proportioned physical strength, resiliance), vasumanto (wealth), vidyā-vanta (well-proportioned aquired knowledge), ojasvinaḥ (lively, energetic character), śhāntā (serenity, peacefulness), āyuṣhmantaśhcha bhavanti (and a long, healthy, fulfilling life).

These explanations also support the grading of *doṣhas* from lowest to highest (or best).

In terms of combinations of *doṣhas*, Charaka states that these characteristics should be assessed based on their myriad combinations. An individual in a state of normal health is considered *samadhātu*. Here, characteristics of all three *doṣhas* are found operating in their normal, *prākṛta* state (Cha. Vi. 8/99-100).

Review the following tables to understand how the *guṇas* contribute to the character, behaviors and actions of each type of individual.

Vātalā lakṣhaṇas (Cha. Vi. 8/98)

Guṇas of *vātalā*	Produces	Nearest English equivalent
Rūkṣha Dry	• Rūkṣha, apachita, alpa śharīrā • Pratata rūkṣha, kṣhāma, sanna-sakta jarjarasvarā • Jāgarūkā	• Dry, thin, weak body • Constantly dry, weak (debilitated), low (sunk in), stuck, broken (hollow) voice • Awake (alert, occupied)
Laghu Light	• Laghu, chapala gati, cheṣhṭa, āhāra, vyāhārā	• Light, unstable (constantly moving, fidgeting) gait, physical actions, food (in any manner), speech
Chala Moving	• Anavasthita sandhi, akṣhi, bhrū, hanu, oṣhṭha, jihvā, śhiraḥ, skandha, pāṇi, pādāḥ	• Instability in the joints, eyes, eyebrows, jaw, lips, head, shoulder and clavicular region, hands and feet
Bahu Abundant	• Bahu pralāpa, kaṇḍarā, sirā, pratānāḥ	• Abundance of talk, tendons, branches (networks) of veins
Śhighra Quick	• Śhrīghra samārambha, kṣhobha, vikārāḥ • Śhīghra trāsa, rāga, virāgāḥ • Śhruta grāhiṇo alpa smṛtaya	• Quick initiation of actions, emotions (irritation, agitation), and disease • Quick to become afraid (anxious), like and dislike • Hears and grasps quickly but remembers little
Śhīta Cold	• Śhītā sahiṣhṇavaḥ • Pratata śhītaka, udvepaka, stambha	• Low tolerance for cold • Constantly feels cold, shivering (trembling), and stiffness
Paruṣha Rough	• Paruṣha kēśha, śhmaśhru, roma, nakha, daśhana, vadana, pāṇi, pādāḥ	• Rough (stiff, hard) hair on the head, beard, body hair, nails, teeth, mouth (or face), hands and feet
Viśhada Clear	• Sphuṭita aṅga, āvayavāḥ • Satata sandhi-śhabda-gāmina	• Cracking of bodily limbs and parts • Constantly producing sounds from the joints when walking (moving around)

Pittalā lakṣhaṇas (Cha. Vi. 8/97)

Guṇas of *pittalā*	Produces	Nearest English equivalent
Uṣhṇa Hot	• Uṣhṇā sahā • Uṣhṇa mukhāḥ • Sukumāra avadāta gātrāḥ • Prabhūta viplu, vyaṅga, tila, piḍakāḥ • Kṣhut, pipāsā vantaḥ • Kṣhipra valī, palita, khālitya doṣhāḥ • Prāyo mṛdu, alpa kapila śhmaśhru, loma, keśhāśhcha	• Always feeling hot • Heat around the face and mouth • Delicate, beautiful body (easily prone to disorders by heat) • Many moles, freckles, marks pimples • Constantly hungry and thirsty • Early wrinkles, greying, balding • Generally soft, thin, tawny (red, light brown) beard, body and head hair
Tīkṣhṇa Sharp	• Tīkṣhṇa parā kramāḥ • Tīkṣhṇa agnayaḥ • Prabhūta āśhana, pānāḥ • Klēśha āsahiṣhṇavō • Dandaśhūkāḥ	• Sharp (fiery, piercing) courage, strength, bravery • Sharp (quick) *agni* • Excessive intake of food and drink • Low tolerance for stress • Acrid, incisive
Drava Liquid	• Śhithila, mṛdu sandhi, māṁsāḥ • Prabhūta sṛṣhṭa sveda, mūtra, purīṣhāśhcha	• Loose (lax) and soft joints and muscles • Excessive (constant) output of sweat, urine and feces
Visra Bad smelling	• Prabhūta pūti kakṣha, āsya, śhiraḥ, śharīra gandhāḥ	• Excessive foul smell from the armpits, mouth, head and body
Amla Sour	• Tvād alpa śhukra, vyavāya, āpatyāḥ	• Less reproductive capacity, sex drive and children
Kaṭuka Pungent	• Same as *amla*	• Same as *amla*

Śhleṣhmalā lakṣhaṇas (Cha. Vi. 8/96)

Guṇas of *śhleṣhmalā*	Produces	Nearest English equivalent
Snigdha Oily	• Snigdha aṅgāḥ	• Unctuous (well-lubricated) bodily limbs
Śhlakṣhṇa Smooth	• Śhlakṣhṇa aṅgāḥ	• Smooth bodily limbs
Mṛdu Soft	• Dṛṣhṭi sukha • Sukumāra, avadāta gātrāḥ	• Pleasant appearance • Delicate, beautiful body
Madhura Sweet	• Prabhūta śhukra, vyavāya, āpatyāḥ	• High reproductive capacity, strong sex drive and many children
Sāra Flowing	• Sāra • Saṁhata • Sthira śharīrāḥ	• High quality *sāra* • Proper compact form of the body • Stable body
Sāndra Dense	• Upachita, paripūrṇa, sarva aṅgāḥ	• Robust (thick, big, thriving), fully developed (perfect) limbs and parts of the entire body
Manda Slow	• Manda cheṣhṭa, āhāra, vyāhārāḥ	• Slow in all physical actions, food (in any manner), speech
Stimita Stable	• Aśhīghra ārambha, kṣhobha, vikārāḥ	• Not quick to initiate any action, to become angry (or emotional), or disease
Guru Heavy	• Sāra ādhiṣhṭhitāva • Sthita gatayaḥ	• Energetic output is directed (purposeful, steadfast) • Stability in movement
Śhīta Cold	• Alpa kṣhut, tṛṣhṇā, santāpa, sveda doṣhāḥ	• Less (infrequent) trouble (discomfort, disorders) due to hunger, thirst, heat, sweat
Vijjala Slimy	• Suśhliṣhṭa sāra sandhi bandhanāḥ	• Well-bound and developed joints and all of their bindings (connective structures)
Achchha Clear	• Prasanna darśhana, ānanāḥ • Prasanna, snigdha varṇa, svarāśhcha	• Pleasant look and face • Pleasant, unctuous (supple, not dry) outward appearance (complexion), and voice

Suśhruta's perspective

Suśhruta describes *prakṛti lakṣhaṇas* using characteristics, physical behaviors, mental state, emotions, dreams and similes. Review the original statements and then use the following tables which list the *lakṣhaṇas* grouped into categories.

Notice Suśhruta's use of the phrases *vāta prakṛti*, *pitta prakṛti* and *kapha prakṛti*. While Charaka clearly mentioned that these phrases do not correctly convey the intention of *prakṛti* and its involvement of the *doṣhas* into a state of *vikṛti*, Suśhruta and other authors have used them. Always keep in mind the distinction between states of *prakṛti* and *vikṛti* as they have significant impacts in every aspect of therapeutic application.

For *vāta prakṛti*:

तत्र वातप्रकृति; प्रजागरूकः शीतद्वेषी दुर्भगः स्तेनो मत्सर्यनार्यो गन्धर्वचित्तः स्फुटितकरचरनोऽल्परूक्षश्मश्रुनखकेशः क्राथी दन्तखादी च भवति ॥ ६४

अधृतिरदृढसौहृदः कृतघ्नः कृशपरुषो धमनीततः प्रलापी ।
द्रुतगतिरटनोऽनवस्थितात्मा वियति च गच्छति सम्भ्रमेण सुप्तः ॥ ६५

अव्यवस्थितमतिश्चलदृष्टिर्मन्दरत्नधनसञ्चय मित्रः । किञ्चिदेव विलपत्यनिबद्धं मारुतप्रकृतिरेष मनुष्यः ॥ ६६

(वातिकाश्चाजगोमायुशशाखूष्ट्रशुनां तथा ।
गृध्रकाकखरादीनामनूकैः कीर्तिता नराः ॥ ६७)

सु. शा. ४।६४-६७

Tatra vātaprakṛti prajāgarūkaḥ śhītadveṣhī durbhagaḥ steno matsaryanāryo gandharvichittaḥ sphuṭitakaracharano ' lparūkṣhaśhmaśhrunakhakeśhaḥ krāthī dantakhādī cha bhavati || 64

Adhṛtiradṛḍhasauhṛdaḥ kṛtaghnaḥ kṛśhaparuṣho dhamanītataḥ pralāpī |
Drutagatiraṭano ' navasthitātmā viyati cha gachchhati sambhrameṇa suptaḥ || 65

Avyavasthitamatiśhchaladṛṣhṭirmandara tnadhanasañchaya mitraḥ | Kiñchideva vilapatyanibaddhaṁ mārutaprakṛtireṣha manuṣhyaḥ || 66

(Vātikāśhchājagomāyuśhaśhākhuṣhṭraśh unāṁ tathā |
Gṛdhrakākakharādīnāmanūkaiḥ kīrtitā narāḥ || 67)

Su. Śhā. 4/64-67

Tatra vātaprakṛti (And so, *vātaprakṛti* [is one who]) prajāgarūkaḥ (always seems wide awake), śhītadveṣhī (hates cold), durbhagaḥ (is unlucky, ugly), steno (is a thief) matsaryanāryo (jealous of others, never satisfied by others) gandharvichittaḥ (loves music), sphuṭita-kara-charano (prone to cracks in the hands and feet), ' lpa-rūkṣha-śhmaśhru-nakha-keśhaḥ (has scanty and dry beard, nails and hair on the head), krāthī (is malicious), danta-khādī cha bhavati (and grinds their teeth). || 64

Adhṛtir ([One who is] unsteady) adṛḍha (and unreliable) sauhṛdaḥ (as a friend), kṛtaghnaḥ (ungrateful), kṛśha (weak) paruṣho (and harsh), dhamanītataḥ (with abundant veins visible through the skin) pralāpī (and talks a lot unnecessarily). Drutagatiraṭano ([He] walks quickly) ' navasthitātmā viyati cha (and yet wanders without direction) gachchhati sambhrameṇa suptaḥ (even in dreams he walks around agitated or anxious). || 65

Avyavasthitam ([He is]) uncertain, disorganized, unsettled), atiśh-chala-dṛṣhṭir (the eyes and gaze move too much), manda ratna dhana (slow [if at all to build up] precious jewels and wealth), sañchaya mitraḥ (and has very few friendships). Kiñchid-eva (Thus, these things and) vilapati (constant chatter), anibaddhaṁ (that is incoherent) māruta-prakṛtireṣha (represents vātaprakṛti) manuṣhyaḥ (in humans). || 66

Vātikāśhcha (Due to vāta), āja (goat), gomāyu (jackal), śhaśha (rabbit), ākhu (mouse, rat) uṣhṭra (camel), śhunāṁ (dog) tathā (and even) gṛdhra (vulture), kāka (crow), kharā (donkey, mule), dīnāmanūkaiḥ kīrtitā narāḥ (are the personalities and natural characteristics found in humans).

<u>For *pitta prakṛti*:</u>

पित्तप्रकृतिस्तु स्वेदनो दुर्गन्धः
पीतशिथिलाङ्गास्ताम्रनखनयनतालुजिह्वौष्ठ
पाणिपादतलो दुर्भगो
वलीपलितखालित्यजुष्टो बहुभुगुष्णद्वेषी
क्षिप्रकोपप्रसादो मध्यबलो मध्यायुश्च भवति
॥ ६८

मेधावी निपुणमतिर्विगृह्य वक्ता तेजस्वी
समितिषु दुर्निवारवीर्यः । सुप्तः सन्
कनकपलाशकर्णिकारान् सम्पश्येदपि च
हुताशविद्युदुल्काः ॥ ६९

न भयात् प्रणमेदनतेष्वमृदुः प्रणतेष्वपि
सान्त्वनदानरुचिः । भवतीह सदा
व्यथितास्यगतिः स भवेदिह
पित्तकृतप्रकृतिः ॥ ७०

(भुजङ्गोलूकगन्धर्वयक्षमार्जारवानरैः ।
व्याघ्रर्क्षनकुलानूकैः पैत्तिकास्तु नराः स्मृताः
॥ ७१)

सु. शा. ४।६८-७१

Pittaprakṛtistu svedano durgandhaḥ
pītaśhithilāṅgāstāmranakhanayanatāluji
hvoṣhṭhapāṇipādatalo durbhago
valīpalitakhālityajuṣhṭo
bahubhuguṣhṇadveṣhī
kṣhiprakopaprasādo madhyabalo
madhyāyuśhcha bhavati || 68

Medhāvī nipuṇamatirvigṛhya vaktā
tejasvī samitiṣhu durnivāravīryaḥ |
Suptaḥ san kanakapalāśhakarṇikārān
sampaśhyedapi cha
hutāśhavidyudulkāḥ || 69

Na bhayā praṇamedanateṣhvamṛduḥ
praṇateṣhvapi sāntvanadānaruchiḥ |
Bhavatīha sadā vyathitāsyagatiḥ sa
bhavediha pittakṛtaprakṛtiḥ || 70

(
Bhujaṅgolūkagandharvayakṣhamārjārav
ānaraiḥ | Vyāghrarkṣhanakulānūkaiḥ
paittikāstu narāḥ smṛtāḥ || 71)

Su. Śhā. 4/68-71

Pittaprakṛtistu (And so, *pittaprakṛti* [is one who]) svedano (constantly sweats), durgandhaḥ (body produces a bad smell), pīta-śhithila-aṅgās (bodily limbs are yellowish and loose or lax), tāmra nakha, nayana, tālu, jihva, oṣhṭha, pāṇi, pāda, talo (has a coppery color of nails, eyes, palate, tongue, lips, palms of the hands and soles of the feet) durbhago (is ugly), valī palita khālitya (prone to premature wrinkles, greying and balding), juṣhṭo (frequent) bahu (excessive) bhug (meals, eating), uṣhṇa-dveṣhī (hates heat), kṣhipra (quickly) kopa (increases agitation) prasādo (and calms down), madhya-balo (medium physical strength), madhya-āyuśhcha bhavati (and moderate lifespan, vitality). || 68

Medhāvī (Intelligent), nipuṇam (clever, astute), atirvigṛhya (too aggressive, independent), vaktā-tejasvī (spirited, winning orator) samitiṣhu (who is brave and aggressive), dur-nivāra vīryaḥ (and has the power to defeat in any way necessary). Suptaḥ (While dreaming), san (he sees) kanaka (gold, treasures), palāśha (green, red like leaves and flowers), karṇikārān (earrings of gold, jewelry), sampaśhyedapi (abundance of riches, wealth) cha hutāśhavidyudulkāḥ (and fire and lightening). || 69

Na bhayā (Does not give into fear), praṇamedanateṣhv-amṛduḥ (harsh on those who are disobedient), praṇateṣhvapi sāntvanadānaruciḥ (yet peaceful with those who are obedient). Bhavatīha sadā vyathita-āsya-gatiḥ (Always troubled by diseases of the mouth), sa bhavediha pittakṛtaprakṛtiḥ (this is how *pittaprakṛti* is). || 70

Bhujaṅga (Snake), ulūka (owl), gandharva (a type of demigod), yakṣha (a type of demigod), mārjāra (cat), vānaraiḥ (monkey), vyāghra (tiger), rkṣha (bear), nakula (mongoose) ānūkaiḥ paittikāstu narāḥ smṛtāḥ (are the types of characters that a *paittika* man naturally represents).

For *kapha prakṛti*:

श्लेष्मप्रकृतिस्तु दूर्वेन्दीवरनिस्त्रिंशार्द्रारिष्टकशरकाण्डानाम न्यतमवर्णः सुभगः प्रियदर्शनो मधुरप्रियः कृतज्ञो धृतिमान् सहिष्णुरलोलुपो बलवांश्चरग्राही दृढवैरश्च भवति ॥ ७२

शुक्लाक्षः स्थिरकुटिलालिनीलकेशो लक्ष्मीवान् जलदमृदङ्गसिंहघोषः । सुप्तः सन् सकमलहंसचक्रवाकान् सम्पश्येदपि च जलाशयान् मनोज्ञान् ॥ ७३

रक्तान्तनेत्रः सुविभक्तगात्रः स्निग्धच्छविः सत्त्वगुणोपपन्नः । क्लेशक्षमो मानोयिता गुरूणां ज्ञेयो बलासप्रकृतिर्मनुष्यः ॥ ७४

(दृढशास्त्रमितिः स्थिरमित्रधनः परिगण्य चिरात् प्रददाति बहु । परिनिश्चितवाक्यपदः सततं गुरुमानकरश्च भवेत् स सदा ॥ ७५

ब्रह्मरुद्रेन्द्रवरुणैः सिंहाश्वगजगोवृषैः । तार्क्ष्यहंससमानूकाः श्लेष्मप्रकृतयो नराः ॥ ७६)

सु. शा. ४।७२-७६

Śhleṣhmaprakṛtistu dūrvandīvaranistriṁśhārdrāriṣhṭakaśharakāṇḍānāmanyatamavarṇaḥ subhagaḥ priyadarśhano madhurapriyaḥ kṛtajño dhṛtimān sahiṣhṇuralolupo balavāṅśhcharagrāhī dṛḍhavairaśhcha bhavati || 72

Śhuklākṣhaḥ sthirakuṭilālinīlakeśho lakṣhmīvān jaladamṛdaṅgasiṁhaghoṣhaḥ | Suptaḥ san sakamalahaṁsachakravākān sampaśhyedapi cha jalāśhayān manojñān || 73

Raktāntanetraḥ suvibhaktagātraḥ snighdhachchhaviḥ sattvaguṇopapannaḥ | Kleśhakṣhamo mānoyitā gurūṇaṁ jñeyo balāsaprakṛtimanuṣhyaḥ || 74

(Dṛḍhaśhāstramitiḥ sthiramitradhanaḥ parigaṇya chirāt pradadāti bahu | Pariniśhchitavākyapadaḥ satataṁ gurumānakaraśhcha bhavet sa sadā || Brahmarudrendravaruṇaiḥ siṁhāśhvagajagovṛṣhaiḥ | Tārkṣhyahaṁsasamānūkāḥ śhleṣhmaprakṛtayo narāḥ || 76)

Su. Śhā. 4/72-76

Śhleṣhmaprakṛtistu (And so, *kaphaprakṛti* [is one who]) dūrvan dīvaranistriṁśhārdrāriṣhṭaka (like dūrva grass, sky-blue lotus, a sword) śharakāṇḍā (the stem of the śharakāṇḍā plant), nāmanyatamavarṇaḥ (has a color or complexion of these), subhagaḥ (is well-built), priyadarśhano (good-looking), madhurapriyaḥ (enjoys sweets), kṛtajño (is grateful), dhṛtimān (patient), sahiṣhṇuralolupo (tolerant and not greedy), balavāṅśhcharagrāhī (has good physical strength and takes time to grasp), dṛḍhavairaśhcha bhavati (and remembers for a long time). || 72

Śhuklākṣhaḥ (Sclera of the eyes is clean and white), sthira-kuṭilāli-nīla-keśho (hair on the head is strong and stable, curly, deep bluish-black) lakṣhmīvān (is wealthy), jalada-mṛdaṅga-siṁha-ghoṣhaḥ (voice, speech and sounds are like [the roaring of] the ocean, a drum, or a lion), suptaḥ san (when dreaming he beholds [scenes]) sakamala-haṁsa-chakravākān (with lotus, swans, and birds) sampaśhyedapi cha jalāśhayān manojñān (in ponds in his mind). || 73

Raktāntanetraḥ ([He has] red in the inner canthus of the eyes), suvibhakta-gātraḥ (well-proportioned body) snighdhachchhaviḥ (which is supple and good-looking) sattva-guṇopapannaḥ (abundant in *sattva guṇa*), kleśhakṣhamo (handles all types of stress easily), mānoyitā gurūṇaṁ (and is respectful to teachers and elders), jñeyo balāsa-prakṛtimanuṣhyaḥ (is known as *kaphaprakṛti*). || 74

Dṛḍhaśhāstramitiḥ ([He] is steadfast in the *śhāstras*) sthira-mitra-dhanaḥ (stable friendships and wealth), pariganṇya chirāt pradadāti bahu (gives great presents, donations, gifts after long consideration), pariniśhchitavākyapadaḥ (speaks deliberately), satataṁ guru-mānakaraśhcha (always respectful to teachers and elders) bhavet sa sadā. Brahma (*Brahma*), Rudra (Rudra), Indra (Indra), Varuṇaiḥ (Varuṇa), siṁha (lion), aśhva (horse), gaja (elephant) govṛṣhaiḥ (bull) tārkṣhya (eagle), haṁsa (swan), samānūkāḥ śhleṣhmaprakṛtayo narāḥ (are the types of characters that a *kaphaja* man naturally represents).

Vāta prakṛti lakṣhaṇas (Su. Śhā. 4/64-67)

Category	Lakṣhaṇas	Nearest English equivalent
Physical characteristics	• Prajāgarūkaḥ • Śhīta-dveṣhī • Durbhagaḥ • Sphuṭita-kara-charano • Alpa-rūkṣha-śhmaśhru-nakha-keśhaḥ • Adhṛtir, adṛḍha sauhṛdaḥ • Kṛśha • Dhamanītataḥ • Pralāpī • Atiśh-chala-dṛṣhṭir	• Always seems wide awake • Hates cold • Is unlucky, ugly • Prone to cracks in the hands and feet • Has scanty and dry beard, nails and hair on the head • Unsteady, unreliable as a friend • Weak • With abundant veins visible through the skin • Talks a lot unnecessarily • Eyes and gaze move too much
Physical behaviors	• Danta-khādī • Drutagatiraṭano anavasthitātmā viyati cha	• Grinds their teeth • Walks quickly yet wanders without direction
Mental state	• Steno • Krāthī • Kṛtaghnaḥ • Avyavasthitam • Manda ratna dhana • Vilapati anibaddhaṁ	• Is a thief • Is malicious • Ungrateful • Uncertain, disorganized, unsettled • Slow [if at all to build up] precious jewels and wealth • Constantly moaning
Emotions	• Matsaryanāryo • Gandharvichittaḥ • Paruṣho • Sañchaya mitraḥ	• Jealous of others, never satisfied by others • Loves music • Harsh • Has very few friendships
Dreams	• Gachchhati sambhrameṇa suptaḥ	• Even in dreams he walks around agitated or anxious
Similes	• Āja • Gomāyu • Śhaśha • Ākhu • Uṣhṭra • Śhunāṁ • Gṛdhra • Kāka • Kharā	• Goat • Jackal • Rabbit • Mouse, rat • Camel • Dog • Vulture • Crow • Donkey, mule

Pitta prakṛti lakṣhaṇas (Su. Śhā. 4/64-67)

Category	Lakṣhaṇas	Nearest English equivalent
Physical characteristics	• Durgandhaḥ • Pīta-śhithila-aṅgā • Tāmra nakha, nayana, tālu, jihva, oṣhṭha, pāṇi, pāda, talo • Durbhago • Valī, palita, khālitya • Uṣhṇa-dveṣhī • Madhya-āyu • Bhavatīha sadā vyathita-āsya-gatiḥ	• Body produces a bad smell • Bodily limbs are yellowish and loose or lax • Has a coppery color of nails, eyes, palate, tongue, lips, palms of the hands and soles of the feet • Is ugly • Prone to premature wrinkles, greying, balding • Hates heat • Moderate lifespan, vitality • Always troubled by diseases of the mouth
Physical behaviors	• Svedano • Juṣhṭo, bahu bhuk • Madhya-balo	• Constantly sweats • Frequent, excessive meals or eating • Medium physical strength
Mental state	• Medhāvī • Nipuṇam • Atirvigṛhya • Vaktā-tejasvī samitiṣhu dur-nivāra vīryaḥ	• Intelligent • Clever, astute • Too aggressive, independent • Spirited, winning orator who is brave and aggressive and has the power to defeat in any way necessary
Emotions	• Kṣhipra kopa prasādo • Na bhayā • Praṇamedanateṣhv-amṛdu • Praṇateṣhvapi sāntvanadānaruciḥ	• Quickly increases agitation and calms down • Does not give into fear • Harsh on those who are disobedient • Peaceful with those who are obedient
Dreams	• Suptaḥ san kanaka, palāśha, karṇikārān, sampaśhyedapi cha hutāśhavidyudulkāḥ	• While dreaming he sees gold or treasures, green or red-like leaves and flowers, earrings of gold or jewelry, abundance of riches or wealth, fire and lightening
Similes	• Bhujaṅga • Ulūka • Gandharva • Yakṣha • Mārjāra • Vānaraiḥ • Vyāghra • Rkṣha • Nakula	• Snake • Owl • A type of demigod • A type of demigod • Cat • Monkey • Tiger • Bear • Mongoose

Kapha prakṛti lakṣhaṇas (Su. Śhā. 4/64-67)

Category	Lakṣhaṇas	Nearest English equivalent
Physical character-istics	• Dūrvan dīvarani-striṁśhārdrāriṣhṭaka, śharakāṇḍā nāmanyatamavarṇaḥ • Subhagaḥ • Priyadarśhano • Balavān • Śhuklākṣhaḥ • Sthira-kuṭilāli-nīla-keśho • Lakṣhmīvān • Raktāntanetraḥ • Suvibhakta-gātraḥ snighdhachchhaviḥ • Sthira-mitra-dhanaḥ • Parigaṇya chirāt pradadāti bahu	• Has a color or complexion like dūrva grass, sky-blue lotus, a sword, the stem of the śharakāṇḍā plant • Well-built • Good-looking • Good physical strength • Sclera of the eyes is clean and white • Hair on the head is strong and stable, curly, deep bluish-black • Wealthy • Red in the inner canthus of the eyes • Well-proportioned body which is supple and good-looking • Stable friendships and wealth • Gives great presents, donations, gifts after long consideration
Physical behaviors	• Madhura-priyaḥ • Jalada-mṛdaṅga-siṁha-ghoṣhaḥ	• Enjoys sweets • Voice, speech and sounds are like [the roaring of] the ocean, a drum, or a lion
Mental state	• Charagrāhī dṛḍhavairaśhcha • Sattva-guṇopapannaḥ • Kleśhakṣhamo • Dṛḍhaśhāstramitiḥ • Pariniśhchitavākyapadaḥ • Satataṁ guru-mānakaraśhcha	• Takes time to grasp and remembers for a long time • Abundant in *sattva guṇa* • Handles all types of stress easily • Steadfast in the *śhāstras* • Speaks deliberately • Always respectful to teachers and elders
Emotions	• Kṛtajño • Dhṛtimān • Sahiṣhṇuralolupo • Mānoyitā gurūṇaṁ	• Grateful • Patient • Tolerant and not greedy • Respectful to teachers and elders
Dreams	• Suptaḥ san sakamala-haṁsa-chakravākān jalāśhayān manojñān sampaśhyedapi cha	• When dreaming he beholds [scenes] with lotus, swans, and birds in ponds in his mind
Similes	• Brahma, Rudra, Indra, Varuṇa • Siṁha • Aśhva • Gaja • Govṛṣhaiḥ • Tārkṣhya • Haṁsa	• *Brahma*, *Rudra*, *Indra*, Varuṇa • Lion • Horse • Elephant • Bull • Eagle • Swan

Chapter 18: Review

ADDITIONAL READING

Read and review the references listed below to expand your understanding of the concepts in this chapter. Write down the date that you complete your reading for each. Remember that consistent repetition is the best way to learn. Plan to read each reference at least once now and expect to read it again as you continue your studies.

References marked with (skim) can be read quickly and do not require commentary review.

CLASSICS		1st read	2nd read
Charaka	Cha. Sū. 7/39-40 Cha. Vi. 6/10-13 Cha. Vi. 8/95-100 Cha. Śhā. 4/12 Cha. Śhā. 4/34-36		
Suśhruta	Su. Śhā. 4/62-80		
Aṣhṭāṅga Hṛdaya	AH Sū. 1/10 AH Śhā. 3/83-104		
Bhāva Prakāśha	BP Pū. 4/51+		

JOURNALS & CURRENT RESOURCES

1. A History of Indian Philosophy, Volume I, Volume 2, Surendranath Dasgupta, pages 334-337 (https://books.google.com/books?id=NjI9AAAAIAAJ&pg=PA334&lpg=PA334&dq=vatala+pittala&source=bl&ots=5NNO81ASyk&sig=6aGP9YxTay-8OB4jS-AZ3JF_q7M&hl=en&sa=X&ved=0ahUKEwjJ2rjf3v_WAhWJh1QKHd_MDcYQ6AEIKDAA#v=onepage&q&f=false)
2. Journal article (optional): *Prakrti-vada or inherent constitution of an individual*, MM Pandya
3. Journal article: Concept of deha prakriti vis-à-vis human constitution in Ayurveda, J.S. Tripathi and R.H.Singh

QUESTIONS & ANSWERS

Record your questions for this chapter here for further research and discussion.

Question:

Answer:

Question:

Answer:

Question:

Answer:

SELF-ASSESSMENT

1. Which of the following describes *prakṛti*?
   a. Created by a ratio of *bhūtas* from both mother and father
   b. Determined at conception
   c. *Sama-doṣha*
   d. Set at the beginning of life and does not change throughout life
   e. All of the above

2. Which of the following describes *prakṛti* when it has changed?
   a. *Doṣhika prakṛti*
   b. End of life is near
   c. *Vātalā, pittalā, śhleṣhmalā*
   d. *Vikṛti*
   e. All of the above

3. Which of the following is not considered *vātalā*, *pittalā*, or *śhleṣhmalā*?
   a. Always afflicted by one of the *doṣhas*
   b. *Deha prakṛti*
   c. Predominance of *eka-doṣha* that easily vitiates
   d. *Sama-doṣha*
   e. All of the above

4. Which *eka-doṣha* is considered *hina*?
   a. *Kapha*
   b. *Pitta*
   c. *Saṁsṛṣhṭā*
   d. *Tridoṣha*
   e. *Vāta*

5. Which of the following can be considered *doṣhas* or vitiating factors?
   a. *Rajas* and *tamas*
   b. *Vāta, pitta, kapha*
   c. *Vātalā, pittalā, śhleṣhmalā*
   d. All of the above
   e. None of the above

6. Which of the following are responsible for *vāyavya bhautika prakṛti*?
   a. Coolness, moisture, sense of taste
   b. Discrimination, long life, sense of hearing
   c. Heat, luster, sense of sight
   d. Initiation and actions of the body, sense of touch
   e. Stable and strong sense of smell

7. Which of the following are responsible for *āpya bhautika prakṛti*?
   a. Coolness, moisture, sense of taste
   b. Discrimination, long life, hearing
   c. Heat, luster, sense of sight
   d. Initiation and actions of the body, sense of touch
   e. Stable and strong sense of smell

8. Charaka and Suśhruta each discuss the *śharīrika prakṛti lakṣhaṇas* in a unique way. Which of the following best describes Charaka's uniqueness?
   a. *Guṇas* are the cause for manifestation of specific features, strength and lifespan
   b. Uses terms *vāta prakṛti, pitta prakṛti* and *kapha prakṛti*
   c. Uses terms *vātalā, pittalā, śhleṣhmalā*
   d. Both A and B
   e. Both A and C

9. How does Charaka describe the *guṇas* of *vātalā*?
   a. Delicate and beautiful body, premature wrinkles and grey hair, bad smell, sharp, acrid
   b. Ugly, premature wrinkles and grey hair, bad smell and aggressive
   c. Ugly, scanty hair, abundant veins, hates cold, few friends
   d. Unreliable, jealous, malicious, few friends
   e. Weak, cold intolerant, talkative, quick emotions and poor memory

10. How does Suśhruta describe *pitta prakṛti lakṣhaṇas*?
    a. Delicate beautiful body, premature wrinkles and grey hair, bad smell, sharp, acrid
    b. Ugly, premature wrinkles and grey hair, bad smell, aggressive, brave
    c. Ugly, scanty hair, abundant veins, hates cold, few friends
    d. Unreliable, jealous, malicious, few friends
    e. Weak, cold intolerant, talkative, quick emotions and poor memory

CRITICAL THINKING

1. Explain the difference between *prākṛta doṣha lakṣhaṇas* and *prakṛti lakṣhaṇas*.

2. Identify two *deha prakṛti lakṣhaṇas* from any author(s) (with references) and describe how each would be assessed practically.

3. Think of an example of a close friend who is *vātala*, *pittala* or *śhleṣhmalā*. What do you know about them that matches classical descriptions? Include references from various authors.

Chapter 19 : Śharīra saṅkhya avayava

KEY TERMS

aṅguli pramāṇa
añjali pramāṇa
pramāṇa
śharīra aṅga
śharīra aṅga vibhāga
śharīra saṅkhya avayava
śharīra vichaya

Śharīra saṅkhya avayava is the enumeration of all parts and components of the physical body. Classically, this study was included as a major component of *śharīra vichaya* (see Chapter 13). From the perspective of the *Charaka sampradāya*, the goal is to fully understand all of the components of the physical system in their normal state. Only then can therapeutic interventions be properly applied to arrest the progress of abnormalities and reinstate normalcy.

Suśhruta utilizes this knowledge for much of the same purpose, but the application of surgical methodologies requires that the understanding of the physical body be even more advanced. In addition to the organization and enumeration of bodily parts, Suśhruta includes detailed descriptions of procedures for cadaver dissection and specific application of anatomical knowledge in various types of surgeries.

Much of this information is found in the classical texts in clear and direct statements. Therefore, this chapter will require the student to utilize classical resources for further explanation of the topics covered. Reference tables with topics and concepts include specific line numbers from multiple authors wherever possible.

First, a brief overview of the organization of the human body is covered. The major methods of measurement are also described.

ORGANIZATION AND MEASUREMENT

The human body is divided into major and minor parts. The correct division, distinction and measurement of these parts is one of several key components to health and referred to as *pramāṇa* (Cha. Sū. 30/26). The assessment of an individual's *pramāṇa* provides significant clinical insight into their state of health and can be a major indicator of future health.

From the top-most level, the human body is subdivided into six main areas. These are the *śharīra aṅga*, or the body limbs. This initial subdivision is called *śharīra aṅga vibhāga*, or the division of the limbs of the body.

The *six śharīra aṅga* include:

2 *bāhū* - 2 arms

2 *sakthinī* - 2 legs

1 *śhiro-grīva* - 1 head and neck

1 *antarādhi* - 1 trunk

See also AH Śhā. 3/1.

The two primary measuring systems used in *śharīra vichaya* include measurement by length and volume.

Aṅguli pramāṇa measures length on an individualized scale. Classical references do not provide an exact scale, however, in general practice it is set by equating one unit to the width of the individual's thumb at its widest point. Or, with the four fingers of the hand flat, the straight distance across all four proximal interphalangeal joints is measured as four *aṅgula*. One *aṅgula* usually approximates to three-quarters of an inch, or 19.05 millimeters, in a typical South Indian demographic. *Aṅguli* measures length, width, breadth or distance, such as the height of the body.

Añjali pramāṇa measures volume of liquids within the body on an individualized scale. The common practice of creating one *añjali* is to cup the two hands to hold the maximum amount of water possible.

The classics provide extensive lists of ideal measurements for the entire body. However, it must be remembered that these specifications are likely the outcome of long-term study over male-dominant populations of the Indian subcontinent. In order to determine whether these ideal specifications are valid outside of the Indian demographic, large scale studies will need to be performed in a scientific manner.

ŚHARĪRA SAṄKHYA AVAYAVA

The following tables compile classical references related to *śharīra saṅkhya avayava* from popular authors. Note that each author has their own individual variations in their listings and descriptions. This combined view includes the most common bodily components in language that is consistent across authors for easier comparison.

All references are listed in Roman alphabetical order.

Śharīra saṅkhya avayava Enumeration of the body's components	Ref. from Cha.	Ref. from Su.	Ref. from AH	Ref. from BP
Āmāśhaya Upper stomach; organ which holds undigested food	Cha. Vi. 2/15-18			
Aṅga viniśhchaya Cadaver dissection		Su. Śhā. 5/47-49		
Aṅguli pramāṇa Length measurement	Cha. Vi. 8/117			
Añjali pramāṇa Volumetric measurement	Cha. Śhā. 7/15		AH Śhā. 3/80-82	
Āśhaya (*sapta-āśhaya*) Seven viscera		Su. Śhā. 5/8	AH Śhā. 3/9-11	BP Pu. 3/213-218
Asthna, *danta*, *ulukhala*, *nakha* The group of bones, teeth, teeth sockets, nails	Cha. Śhā. 7/6	Su. Śhā. 5/18-23	AH Śhā. 3/16	
Asthi-saṅghāta Conjunctions of bones		Su. Śhā. 5/16	AH Śhā. 3/15	BP Pu. 3/277
Bhautika śharīra Composition of *bhūtas* in the body	Cha. Śhā. 7/16, 4/12		AH Śhā. 3/3	
Dhamani Arterial networks, arteries	Cha. Sū. 30/12 Cha. Śhā. 7/14	Su. Śhā. 9/	AH Śhā. 3/39	BP Pu. 3/264-266
Hṛdaya The heart	Cha. Sū. 30/3-7			
Indriya (adhiṣhṭhāna, *buddhi*, etc) Senses (their locations, processing centers, etc)	Cha. Śhā. 7/7			
Jāla Network structures		Su. Śhā. 5/12	AH Śhā. 3/14-15	BP Pu. 3/273
Jaṭharāgni Main digestive capacity			AH Śhā. 3/49	

Śharīra saṅkhya avayava Enumeration of the body's components	Ref. from Cha.	Ref. from Su.	Ref. from AH	Ref. from BP
Kalā (*sapta kalā*) Seven membranes		Su. Śhā. 4/5-21	AH Śhā. 3/9	BP Pū. 3/219-222
Kaṇḍarā Large *snāyus*		Su. Śhā. 5/11	AH Śhā. 3/14-15	BP Pu. 3/267-268
Keśha Hair on the head	Cha. Śhā. 7/14			
Koṣhṭha Gastro-intestinal tract (mouth to anus)	Cha. Sū. 11/48			
Koṣhṭhāṅga Limbs (organs) of the GIT	Cha. Śhā. 7/10		AH Śhā. 3/12	
Kūrchā Networks of brush-like structures		Su. Śhā. 5/13	AH Śhā. 3/14-15	BP Pu. 3/274
Loma Hair on the body	Cha. Śhā. 7/14			BP Pu. 3/285
Loma kūpa Follicles of the hair on the body				BP Pu. 3/285
Mahā mūla (*Daśha mahā mūla*) Ten major vessels attached to the heart	Cha. Sū. 30/8			
Mahānti chhidrāṇi Major orifices of the body	Cha. Śhā. 7/12	Su. Śhā. 5/10		BP Pu. 3/269-270
Malāyanā Excretory orifices	Cha. Sū. 7/42-43			
Māṁsa rajju Rope-like structures attached to the muscles, fascia		Su. Śhā. 5/14	AH Śhā. 3/14-15	BP Pu. 3/275

Śharīra saṅkhya avayava Enumeration of the body's components	Ref. from Cha.	Ref. from Su.	Ref. from AH	Ref. from BP
Marga (*tri-marga*) Pathways, of three types	Cha. Sū. 11/34, 11/48 Cha. Sū. 17/112-114		AH Sū. 12/44-48	
Marma (107) Sensitive points, congregation points of *prāṇa*	Cha. Śhā. 7/14	Su. Śhā. 6/	AH Śhā. 4/	BP Pu. 3/223-238
Marma (*tri-marma*) Three primary sensitive points	Cha. Chi. 26/			
Paramāṇu Smallest level of division within the body, possibly cells	Cha. Śhā. 7/17			
Peśhi Muscles	Cha. Śhā. 7/14	Su. Śhā. 5/37-41	AH Śhā. 3/17	
Prāṇāyatanāni, *jīvītadhāma*, *daśha āyatanāni* Main locations or seats of life within the body, ten repositories of life	Cha. Śhā. 7/9 Cha. Sū. 29/3-4	Su. Śhā. 4/1	AH Śhā. 3/13	
Pratyāṅga Structures and organs that are ancillary to the *aṅga*	Cha. Śhā. 7/11			
Sandhi Joints	Cha. Śhā. 7/14	Su. Śhā. 5/24-28	AH Śhā. 3/17	BP Pu. 3/239-243
Sevani, or *sīvani* Suture-like structures		Su. Śhā. 5/15	AH Śhā. 3/14-15	BP Pu. 3/276
Sīmantā Sutures of asthi-saṅghāta		Su. Śhā. 5/17	AH Śhā. 3/14-15	BP Pu. 3/278
Sirā Venous networks, veins	Cha. Śhā. 7/14	Su. Śhā. 7/	AH Śhā. 3/18-38	BP Pu. 3/244-257

Śharīra saṅkhya avayava Enumeration of the body's components	Ref. from Cha.	Ref. from Su.	Ref. from AH	Ref. from BP
Śhiras The head	Cha. Sū. 17/12			
Śhmaśhru Beard and mustache hair	Cha. Śhā. 7/14			
Snāyu Ligaments	Cha. Śhā. 7/14	Su. Śhā. 5/29-36	AH Śhā. 3/17	BP Pu. 3/258-263
Srotas (*abhyantara*) Internal, exudative channels	Cha. Vi. 5/	Su. Śhā. 9/	AH Śhā. 3/41-48	BP Pu. 3/271-272
Srotas (*bāhya*) Channels with external openings	Cha. Sū. 30/12		AH Śhā. 3/40	
Tvak (ṣhat tvak) Skin, the six-layered model	Cha. Śhā. 7/4			
Tvak (sapta tvak) Skin, the seven-layered model		Su. Śhā. 4/4	AH Śhā. 3/8	BP Pu. 3/279-284

TEST YOURSELF

Learn, review and memorize key terms from this section.

śharīra saṅkhya avayava

śharīra vichaya

pramāṇa

śharīra aṅga

śharīra aṅga vibhāga

aṅguli pramāṇa

añjali pramāṇa

Chapter 19: Review

ADDITIONAL READING

Read and review the references listed below to expand your understanding of the concepts in this chapter. Write down the date that you complete your reading for each. Remember that consistent repetition is the best way to learn. Plan to read each reference at least once now and expect to read it again as you continue your studies.

References marked with (skim) can be read quickly and do not require commentary review.

CLASSICS		1st read	2nd read
Charaka	Cha. Vi. 5/ Cha. Śhā. 7/		
Suśhruta	Su. Śhā. 4/4-32 Su. Śhā. 5/ Su. Śhā. 6/ Su. Śhā. 7/ Su. Śhā. 9/		
Aṣhṭāṅga Hṛdaya	AH Śhā. 3/ AH Śhā. 4/		
Bhāva Prakāśha	BP Pū. 3/65-97 BP Pū. 3/213-288		

JOURNALS & CURRENT RESOURCES

Journal article: *Scientific study of Charakokta Anguli Pramana in reference to human height*, Shashikant, K, et al

QUESTIONS & ANSWERS

Record your questions for this chapter here for further research and discussion.

Question:

Answer:

Question:

Answer:

Question:

Answer:

SELF-ASSESSMENT

1. Which of the following describes the purpose of *śharīra saṅkhya avayava*?
   a. Anatomical knowledge for surgical application
   b. Organization and enumeration of bodily parts
   c. Understand bodily parts in their normal state for proper therapeutic actions
   d. A and B
   e. All of the above

2. The subdivision of the body into 2 arms, 2 legs, 1 head and 1 trunk, is known as
   a. *Aṅguli pramāṇa*
   b. *Añjali pramāṇa*
   c. *Pramāṇa*
   d. *Śharīra aṅga*
   e. *Śharīra vichaya*

3. The measuring systems used in *śharīra vichaya* include
   a. Length
   b. Volume
   c. Weight
   d. A and B
   e. All of the above

4. *Aṅguli pramāṇa* measures
   a. Height
   b. Individual length
   c. Three-quarters of an inch
   d. A and B
   e. All of the above

5. *Añjali pramāṇa* measures
   a. Individual bodily liquid quantities
   b. Two hands cupped together
   c. Volume
   d. A and B
   e. All of the above

6. What are the potential limitations of classically-defined measurements?
   a. Based on demographics of the Indian subcontinent
   b. Male-dominant
   c. Not based on the current era
   d. Classical authors utilized different measurements
   e. All of the above

7. Which of the following are described by all authors?
   a. *Dhamani, sirā, srotas*
   b. *Marma, sandhi, snāyu*
   c. *Tvak, loma, keśha*
   d. A and B
   e. All of the above

8. The *āmāśhaya* is grouped under which category?
   a. *Asthi*
   b. *Marma*
   c. *Āśhaya*
   d. *Srotas*
   e. *Marga*

9. Which topic did Suśhruta describe that is particularly significant for surgical practice?
   a. Bones, teeth, teeth sockets, nails
   b. Cadaver dissection
   c. Fascia
   d. Muscles
   e. Three pathways

10. What does Charaka include in his classification of *tri-marma*?
    a. Eyes, brain, ears
    b. Head, digestive system, bladder
    c. Heart, head, bladder
    d. A and B
    e. All of the above

CRITICAL THINKING

1. What differences can be seen in the explanation of *śharīra saṅkhya avayava* between the *Charaka sampradāya* and the *Suśhruta sampradāya*? Which school of practice does Vāgbhaṭa seem to follow? Which does Bhāvamiśhra appear to follow?

2. How many bones and bony structures are listed by each author? How can this discrepancy be explained?

3. What is the main difference between *bāhya* and *abhyantara srotas*?

4. Briefly explain Charaka's use of the *tri-marma*. What are they and why have they been selected?

5. Measure your own *aṅgula* using the approaches described in this chapter. What is your height in *aṅgula*?

Chapter 20 : Aṣhṭa vidha sāra

KEY TERMS

aṣhṭa vidha sāra
asthi sāra
avara
bala
daśhavidha parīkṣha
dhātu
dhātu sārata
madhyama
majja sāra
māṁsa sāra
medo sāra
parīkṣha
pramāṇa
rakta sāra
sāra
sattva sāra
śhukra sāra
tvak sāra
uttama

The concept of *aṣhṭa vidha sāra* is explained primarily by Charaka and Suśhruta. Vāgbhaṭa includes a short, concise reference to the topic but does not elaborate it in specific detail.

Charaka includes the explanation within the context of individual clinical assessment using the *daśhavidha parīkṣha* (ten component assessment model). Understanding an individual's *sāra* aids in determining specific approaches in clinical management.

The phrase *aṣhṭa vidha sāra* refers to the eight types of *sāra*. Each of these types intends to assess the state of an individual's *dhātus* in terms of their overall health and condition. In this context, the entire topic is more often referred to as *dhātu sārata*.

ASSESSING SĀRA

The Monier-Williams Dictionary defines the term *sāra* as:

sāra — the core or pith or solid interior of anything

firmness, strength, power, energy

the substance or essence or marrow or cream or heart or essential part of anything, best part, quintessence

a chief ingredient or constituent part of the body (causing the peculiarities of temperament; reckoned to be seven)

Chakrapāṇi defines *sāra* as:

विशुद्धतरो धातुः सारोच्यते ।

चक्र. (च. वि. ८।१०२)

Viṣhuddhataro dhātuḥ sārochyate |

Cakr. (Cha. Vi. 8/102)

Viṣhuddha (The specific, particular or distinct purity, health or quality) taro (in an even better state [than normal]) dhātuḥ (of the *dhātus*) sāra uchyate (is known as *sāra*).

Charaka explains that there are eight types of *sāra*, one for each *dhātu* plus one for *sattva*. Additionally, a given individual may be assessed as having all *sāras* present, as *sarva sāra*, but this is not a separate type.

The assessment of *sāra* provided important clinical information to help determine which one (or more) of an individual's *dhātus* were in healthy, strong states. *Sāra* was intended to be assessed for each *dhātu* to help plan management protocols. Each assessment is graded on a scale of *avara*, *madhyama*, *uttama* (deficient, moderate, excellent) to identify which *dhātus* need improvement.

सारतश्चेति साराण्यष्टौ पुरुषाणां बलमानविशेषज्ञानार्थमुपदिश्यन्ते; तद्यथा - त्वग्रक्तमांसमेदोऽस्थिमज्जशुक्रसत्त्वानीति ||

च. वि. ८।१०२

Sārataśhcheti sārāṇyaṣhṭau puruṣhāṇāṁ balamānaviśheṣhajñānārthamupadiśhyante tadyathā - tvagraktamāṁsamedo ' sthimajjaśhukrasattvānīti ||

Cha. Vi. 8/102

Sārataśhcheti (And the *sārata*) sārāṇy-aṣhṭau (is of eight types) puruṣhāṇāṁ (in individuals) bala (based on strength) māna (measured) viśheṣha (specifically) jñānārtham (through the knowledge of these things [*lakṣhaṇas*]) upadiśhyante (as described [here]); tadyathā (and so they [the eight] are) – tvag (*tvak* [*sāra*]), rakta (*rakta* [*sāra*]), māṁsa (*māṁsa* [*sāra*]), medo (*medo* [*sāra*]), asthi (*asthi* [*sāra*]), majja (*majja* [*sāra*]), śhukra (*śhukra* [*sāra*]), sattvānīti (and finally *sattva* [*sāra*]).

Grading of each of the *sāra* as *avara*, *madhyama*, *uttama* is briefly described by Charaka only through *asāra* and *madhya*:

अतोविपरीतास्त्वसाराः || ११२

च. वि. ८।११२

Atoviparītāstvasārāḥ || 112

Cha. Vi. 8/112

Ato (And so), viparīta-astu (the opposite [of the *lakṣhaṇas* provided]) asārāḥ (should be considered *asāra*, or the absence of healthy *sāra*).

मध्यानांमध्यैःसारविशेषैर्गुणविशेषाव्याख्याताभवन्ति || ११३

च. वि. ८।११३

Madhyānāṁmadhyaiḥsāraviśheṣhairguṇaviśheṣhāvyākhyātābhavanti || 113

Cha. Vi. 8/113

Madhyānāṁ (A moderate amount) madhyaiḥ sāra (or medium level of *sāra*) bhavanti (is assessed by) viśheṣhair-guṇa (presence of specific *guṇas*) viśheṣhā-vyākhyātā (and its specific manifestation).

Charaka states that the purpose of *sāra* assessment is to provide a correct understanding of the individual's *bala* from general and specific perspectives.

इतिसाराण्यष्टौपुरुषाणांबलप्रमाणविशेषज्ञानार्थमुपदिष्टानिभवन्ति || ११४

च. वि. ८।११४

Itisārāṇyaṣhṭaupuruṣhāṇāṁbalapramāṇaviśheṣhajñānārthamupadiṣhṭānibhavanti || 114

Cha. Vi. 8/114

Iti (And so), sārāṇyaṣhṭau (the eight *sāras*) upadiṣhṭāni bhavanti (have been specified, described, instructed) jñānārtham (for knowing these things) viśheṣha (specifically about, or to measure) bala (the strength) pramāṇa (in quantity, or level) puruṣhāṇāṁ (of individuals).

Sāra assessment is considered particularly important within the context of a complete and thorough assessment using the *daśhavidha parīkṣha* because it aids the clinician in proper assessment of other components as well.

कथंनुशरीरमात्रदर्शनादेवभिषङ्मुह्येदयमु पचितत्वाद्बलवान्, अयमल्पबलःकृशत्वात्, महाबलोऽयंमहाशरीरत्वात्, अयमल्पशरीरत्वादल्पबलइति; दृश्यन्तेह्यल्पशरीराःकृशाश्चैकेबलवन्तः; तत्रपिपीलिकाभारहरणवत्सिद्धिः| अतश्चसारतःपरीक्षेतेत्युक्तम् || ११५

च. वि. ८|११५

Kathaṁ nu śharīramātradarśhanādeva bhiṣhaṅmuhyedayamupachitatvādbalav ān, ayamalpabalaḥ kṛśhatvāt, mahābalo ' yaṁ mahāśharīratvāt, ayamalpaśharīratvādalpabala iti; dṛśhyante hyalpaśharīrāḥ kṛśhāśhchaike balavantaḥ; tatra pipīlikābhāraharaṇavat siddhiḥ | Ataśhcha sārataḥ parīkṣhetetyuktam || 115

Cha. Vi. 8/115

Kathaṁ (How, why [is it that]) nu (just) śharīra mātra darśhanād (by looking at the size of the physical body) eva bhiṣhaṅ (even a physician) muhyed (maybe be uncertain as to) ayam (this one [the patient]) upachitatvād balavān ([having] great strength because he is big), ayam ([or] that one [another patient]) alpa balaḥ kṛśhatvāt ([having] less strength because he is thin)? Mahābalo ([Is] great strength) ayaṁ (in one) mahā-śharīratvāt (due to a large body), ayam (and in another) alpaśharīratvād (an emaciated body) alpabala (causes less strength;) iti (is it so?); dṛśhyante (It is seen that) hi (in one with) alpaśharīrāḥ (a weak, thin body) kṛśhāśhchaike (and even emaciation), balavantaḥ (there is great strength) tatra (just like) pipīlikā (a black ant) bhāraharaṇavat siddhiḥ (that can carry immensely heavy loads that seems beyond its ability). Ataśhcha (And likewise), sārataḥ (*sārata*) parīkṣhetet (must be assessed) yuktam (through analysis of all specific factors).

Although Charaka does not explicitly grade the *sāra* themselves, Suśhruta does provide an explanation. He specifies that a general grading of the individual can be done based on the *sāra* assessment where *sattva sāra* is the highest of all, followed by *śhukra sāra* to *tvak sāra* from highest to lowest among the *dhātus*. The benefits of the higher levels result in a longer, healthier lifespan and prosperity. Notice that Charaka lists the *sāras* in order from *tvak* to *sattva* (ie, lowest to highest), while Suśhruta lists them from *sattva* to *tvak* (ie, highest to lowest). He states:

... एषां पूर्वं पूर्वं प्रधानमायुःसौभाग्ययोरिति ||

सु. सू. ३५|१६

... Eṣhāṁ pūrvaṁ pūrvaṁ pradhānamāyuḥsaubhāgyayaoriti ||

Su. Sū. 35/16

Eṣhāṁ (Each of these) pūrvaṁ pūrvaṁ (one after the other [from *sattva sāra* to *tvak sāra*]) pradhānam (is better than the preceeding) āyuḥ (in lifespan, life, vitality), saubhāgyayaoriti (and success, good fortune, beauty).

Suśhruta additionally states the importance of a thorough assessment of *sāra* to provide a complete picture of the individual.

विशेषतोऽङ्गप्रत्यङ्गप्रमाणादथ सारतः । परीक्ष्यायुः सुनिपुणो भिषक् सिध्यति कर्मसु ||

सु. सू. ३५|१७

Viśheṣhto ‘ ṅgapratyaṅgapramāṇādatha sārataḥ | Parīkṣhyāyuḥ sunipuṇo bhiṣhak sidhyati karmasu ||

Su. Sū. 35/17

Viśheṣhto (The specific) aṅga (limbs, parts of the body) pratyaṅga (and their divisions or sub-parts) pramāṇād (must be measured properly) atha sārataḥ (through *sārata* as described). Parīkṣhya (The assessment of) āyuḥ (lifespan, vitality), sunipuṇo (by a truly expert, professional) bhiṣhak (physician) sidhyati (awards him great success) karmasu (in his actions of treatment).

Vāgbhaṭa introduces the concept of *sāra* briefly while describing the ideal characteristics and features for a healthy, successful individual in AH Śhā. 3/107-116. He then states:

त्वग्रक्तादीनि सत्त्वान्तान्यग्र्याण्यष्टौ
यथोत्तरम् । बलप्रमाणज्ञानार्थं
साराण्युक्तानि देहिनाम् ॥ ११७
सारैरुपेतः सर्वः स्यात्परं गौरवसंयुतः ।
सर्वारम्भेषु चाशावान्सहिष्णुः सन्मतिः स्थिरः
॥ ११८

अ. हृ. शा. ३।११७-११८

Tvagraktādīni sattvāntānyagryāṇyaṣhṭau yathottaram | Balapramāṇajñānārthaṁ sārāṇyuktāni dehinām || 117
Sārairupetaḥ sarvaḥ syātparaṁ gauravasaṁyutaḥ | Sarvārambheṣhu chāśhāvānshiṣhṇuḥ sanmatiḥ sthiraḥ || 118

AH Śhā. 3/117-120

Tvag (*Tvak*), raktādīni (and *rakta*, etc) sattvāntāni (through *sattva*) agryāṇi (are the group of the best) aṣhṭau (eight) yatha uttaram (with each one better than the previous). Bala pramāṇa (The measurement of strength) jñānārthaṁ (is known through these things [*lakṣhaṇas*]) sārāṇ (as *sāra*) yuktāni (by a thorough analysis of all specific factors) dehinām (in the body).

Although Vāgbhaṭa does not explicitly list the *sāra lakṣhaṇas* as clearly as Charaka and Suśhruta do, he does provide a description of ideal features of the body in AH Śhā. 3/107-116. Careful analysis of these *lakṣhaṇas* demonstrates many similarities with the *dhātu sāra lakṣhaṇas*.

TEST YOURSELF

Learn, review and memorize key terms from this section.

aṣhṭa vidha sāra ____

dhātu sārata ____

sāra ____

dhātu ____

avara ____

madhyama ____

uttama ____

tvak sāra ____

rakta sāra ____

māṁsa sāra ____

medo sāra ____

asthi sāra ____

majja sāra ____

śhukra sāra ____

sattva sāra ____

bala ____

pramāṇa
daśhavidha parīkṣha
parīkṣha

SĀRA LAKṢHAṆAS

Review the *dhātu sāra lakṣhaṇas* from Charaka and Suśhruta in the following tables. Consider each component and its possible methods of clinical assessment.

Tvak sāra lakṣhaṇas	Cha. Vi. 8/103	Su. Sū. 35/16
Snigdha, śhlakṣhṇa, mṛdu, prasanna (tvak) Skin is supple, smooth, soft and pleasing to look at	✓	✓
Sūkṣhma, alpa, gambhīra, sukumāra loma Bodily hair is very fine, less (sparse), deeply-rooted and delicate (pleasant to look at)	✓	✓
Saprabha eva cha tvak And the skin is full of luster, glowing, brilliant	✓	
Produces:		
Sukha Happiness, contentment	✓	
Saubhāgya Good fortune, success, beauty	✓	
Aiśhvarya Prosperity, wealth, power	✓	
Upabhōga Pleasure, enjoyment, contentment through eating	✓	
Buddhi Intelligence	✓	
Vidya Learned knowledge, wisdom	✓	
Ārogya Absence of disease	✓	
Praharṣhaṇa Pleasure, excitement, sensual pleasure	✓	
Ānya-āyuṣhyatvaṁ cha And above all else, longevity, full lifespan, quality of life	✓	

Rakta sāra lakṣhaṇas	Cha. Vi. 8/104	Su. Sū. 35/16
Karṇa, akṣhi, mukha, jihvā, nāsa, oṣhṭha, pāṇi-pāda tala, nakha, lalāṭa, mehana - snigdha, rakta varṇa, śhrīmad-bhrājiṣhṇu The ears, eye area, face, tongue, nose, lips, soles of the hands feet, nails, forehead and genital organs are unctuous (thick, moist), reddish color, and sexy	√	√
Produces:		
Sukham Happiness, contentment	√	
Uddhatāṁ medhāṁ Arrogant, sharp mental state and intelligence	√	
Manasvitvaṁ Magnanimous, wise	√	
Saukumāryam Delicate, tender body	√	
Anati-balam Not too strong	√	
Akleśha-sahiṣhṇutvam Intolerant to stress, difficult situations, work	√	
Uṣhṇāsahiṣhṇutvaṁ cha And intolerant to heat	√	

Māṁsa sāra lakṣhaṇas	Cha. Vi. 8/105	Su. Sū. 35/16
Śhaṅkha, lalāṭa, kṛkāṭikā, akṣhi, gaṇḍa, hanu, grīvā, skandha, udara, kakṣha, vakṣha, pāṇi-pāda sandhaya - sthira, guru, śhubha, māṁsa-upacitā The temples, forehead, nape of the neck, eye area, cheeks, jaw, neck, shoulders, abdomen, axillae, chest, joints of the arms and legs are stable, heavy, beautiful, and covered with well-developed muscles	✓	
Achchhidra gātraṁ Absence of hollow, empty, defective, faulty, undeveloped areas of the body		✓
Gūḍha asthi, sandhi māṁsa upachita Well-covered bones and joints by well-developed muscles		✓
Produces:		
Kṣhamāṁ Tolerance, forbearance, patience	✓	
Dhṛtimalaulyaṁ Steady, firm courage (self-control)	✓	
Vittaṁ Acquisitions, property, wealth, money	✓	
Vidyāṁ Acquired knowledge, wisdom	✓	
Sukham Happiness, contentment	✓	
Ārjavam Honesty, sincerity, straight-forwardness	✓	
Ārogyaṁ Absence of disease	✓	
Balamāyuśhcha dīrghamācha Strength throughout one's long lifespan	✓	

Medo sāra lakṣhaṇas	Cha. Vi. 8/106	Su. Sū. 35/16
Varṇa, svara, netra, keśha, loma, nakha, danta, oṣhṭha, mūtra, purīṣheṣhu viśheṣhataḥ sneho The complexion, voice, eyeballs, hair on the head, body hair, nails, teeth, lips, urine and stools are unctuous (greasy, oily)	√	
Snigdha mūtra, sveda, svara Unctuous or oily urine and sweat, and a smooth voice		√
Bṛhat śharīra Big, bulky body		√
Āyāsa asahiṣhṇuta Incapable of tolerating stress, work, difficulties		√
Produces:		
Vitta Acquisitions, property, wealth, money	√	
Aiśhvarya Prosperity, wealth, power	√	
Sukha Happiness, contentment	√	
Upabhoga Pleasure, enjoyment, contentment through eating	√	
Pradānāni Generosity	√	
Ārjavam Honesty, sincerity, straight-forwardness	√	
Sukumāra upachāratāṁ cha And delicate, tender in their approach and interactions	√	

Asthi sāra lakṣhaṇas	Cha. Vi. 8/106	Su. Sū. 35/16
Pārṣhṇi, gulpha, jānu, aratni, jatru, cibuka, śhiraḥ, parva-sthūlāḥ, sthūla-asthi, nakha, dantāśhchā The heels, ankles, knees, elbows, collar bones, chin, head, small joints (of the hands and feet), nails and teeth are thick-boned (strong, heavy)	✓	
Mahā śhiraḥ, skandha Large (big) head and shoulder area		✓
Dṛḍha danta, hanu, asthi, nakha Strong teeth, jaw, bones and nails		✓
Produces:		
Temaha utsāhāḥ Extremely excitable, enthusiastic	✓	
Kriyāvantaḥ Always very active	✓	
Kleśhasahāḥ High tolerance for stress	✓	
Sāra, sthira śharīrā Solid, stable body	✓	
Bhavanti āyuṣhmantaśhcha And endowed with longevity, full lifespan, quality of life	✓	

Majjā sāra lakṣhaṇas	Cha. Vi. 8/106	Su. Sū. 35/16
Mṛdvaṅgā balavantaḥ The limbs are soft (supple) yet strong	√	
Snigdha varṇa svarāḥ The complexion and voice are unctuous (smooth)	√	
Sthūla dīrgha vṛtta sandhayaśhcha The joints are thick (heavy, well-set), long and round	√	
Mahā śhiraḥ, skandha Large (big) head and shoulder area		√
Dṛḍha danta, hanu, asthi, nakha Strong teeth, jaw, bones and nails		√
Akṛśha, uttama bala Not (too) thin or lean, with high levels of strength		√
Snigdha, gambhīra svara Smooth, deep voice		√
Saubhāgya upapanna Good fortune		√
Mahā netra Large eyes		√
Produces:		
Dīrghāyuṣho Long lifespan	√	
Balavantaḥ Excellent strength	√	
Śhruta Astute listener (and comprehends well through listening)	√	
Vitta Acquisitions, property, wealth, money	√	
Vijñāna Acquired scientific knowledge	√	
Āpatya Children	√	
Sammāna bhājaśhcha And recognized for his portion of honor	√	

Śhukra sāra lakṣhaṇas	Cha. Vi. 8/109	Su. Sū. 35/16
Saumyāḥ A saumya appearance (soft, gentle, pleasing, with good looks)	✓	
Saumya prekṣhiṇaḥ Soft, gentle look (of the eyes)	✓	
Kṣhīra-pūrṇa-lochana Eyes that look as though they are full of milk	✓	
Iva praharṣha bahulāḥ Abundant interest, excitement	✓	
Snigdha, vṛtta, sāra, sama-saṁhata, śhikharadaśhanāḥ, prasanna, snigdha, varṇa svara Unctuous, round, strong, even (symmetrical), attractive, pleasant and smooth complexion and voice	✓	
Ābhrājiṣhṇavo Alluring, charming, magnetic appearance (personality)	✓	
Mahā-sphicaśhcha Large buttocks	✓	
Snigdha, saṁhata, śhveta asthi, danta, nakha Supple, proportionate (compact, well-formed) and white bones, teeth and nails		✓
Bahula kāma, prajaṁ Abundant sexual desire and children		✓
Produces:		
Strīpriya Enjoy sexual pleasures (and women enjoy them)	✓	
Upabhogā Pleasure, enjoyment, contentment through eating	✓	
Balavantaḥ Excellent strength	✓	
Sukha Happiness, contentment	✓	
Aiśhvarya Prosperity, wealth, power	✓	
Ārogya Absence of disease	✓	

Vitta Acquisitions, property, wealth, money	√	
Sammāna āpatya bhājaśhcha Recognized for honor and many children	√	

Sattva sāra lakṣhaṇas	Cha. Vi. 8/110	Su. Sū. 35/16
Smṛti-manto Good memory	✓	✓
Bhakti-mantaḥ Good dedication	✓	✓
Kṛtajñāḥ Appreciation, gratefulness	✓	
Prājñāḥ Wisdom	✓	✓
Śhuchayo Cleanliness, purity	✓	✓
Maha-utsāhā Abundant enthusiasm	✓	
Dakṣhā Skill	✓	
Dhīrāḥ Courage, concentration of mind	✓	
Samara-vikrāntayō Bravery, steadfast attitude in conflict	✓	
Dhinastyakta-viṣhādāḥ Absence of sorrow	✓	
Suvyavasthita gati Confident gait	✓	
Gambhīra buddhi Depth of intellect	✓	
Cheṣhṭāḥ kalyāṇābhi niveśhinaśhcha Engages in correct (benevolent) actions sincerely	✓	✓
Śhauryopetaṁ Endowed with heroism		✓
Produces:		
Teṣhāṁ sva-lakṣhaṇair-evaguṇā vyākhyātāḥ Their *lakṣhaṇas* (as explained above) indicate the characteristics produced	✓	

Sarva sāra lakṣhaṇas	Cha. Vi. 8/110	Su. Sū. 35/16
Sarvaiḥ sārair upētāḥ puruṣhā bhavanti Characteristics of all of the *sāras*, including *sattva sāra*	√	
Atibalāḥ Too much strength	√	
Parama sukha The best (ultimate) level of happiness, contentment	√	
Yuktāḥ kleśha sahāḥ Sensible tolerance for stress; knows limits and acts accordingly	√	
Sarvārambha iṣhvātmani jāta pratyayāḥ Commences all desires with calculated ideas, plans thoroughly	√	
Kalyāṇa abhiniveśhinaḥ Benevolent intentions		
Sthira samāhita śharīrāḥ Stable, well-bound and built body	√	
Susamāhita gatayaḥ Well-coordinated movements	√	
Sānunāda snigdha gambhīra mahāsvarāḥ His sound is smooth and deep with a great (bellowing) voice	√	
Produces:		
Sukha Happiness, contentment	√	
Aiśhvarya Prosperity, wealth, power	√	
Vitta Acquisitions, property, wealth, money	√	
Upabhoga Pleasure, enjoyment, contentment through eating	√	
Sammāna bhājomandajaraso Recognized for honorable work	√	
Manda vikārāḥ Slow to develop disease	√	
Prāyastulya guṇa vistīrṇāpatyāśh chirajīvinaśhcha Same characteristics in their children who live long lives	√	

Chapter 20: Review

ADDITIONAL READING

Read and review the references listed below to expand your understanding of the concepts in this chapter. Write down the date that you complete your reading for each. Remember that consistent repetition is the best way to learn. Plan to read each reference at least once now and expect to read it again as you continue your studies.

References marked with (skim) can be read quickly and do not require commentary review.

CLASSICS		1st read	2nd read
Charaka	Cha. Vi. 8/102-115		
Suśhruta	Su. Sū. 35/16-17		
Aṣhṭāṅga Hṛdaya	AH Śhā. 3/107-120		
Bhāva Prakāśha			

JOURNALS & CURRENT RESOURCES

QUESTIONS & ANSWERS

Record your questions for this chapter here for further research and discussion.

Question:

Answer:

Question:

Answer:

Question:

Answer:

SELF-ASSESSMENT

1. Which of the following best describes *aṣhṭa vidha sāra*?
   a. Determines specific approaches in clinical management
   b. Health assessment of individual *dhātus*
   c. Measured on a scale of *avara*, *madhyama*, *uttama*
   d. Refers to eight types of *sāra*
   e. All of the above

2. The term *sāra* is defined as
   a. Distinct purity or quality of health
   b. Firmness, strength, power, energy
   c. The *dhātus*
   d. A and B
   e. B and C

3. Which of the following best describes the term *sarva sāra*?
   a. All the *dhātus*
   b. All the best *sāras* are present
   c. Seven types of *sāra*
   d. A and B
   e. B and C

4. Which of the following best describes *asāra*?
   a. *Avara*
   b. *Madhyama*
   c. *Uttama*
   d. A and B
   e. B and C

5. Suśhruta specifies a general grading of an individual's *sāra* can be based on
   a. *Sattva sāra* is the highest of all
   b. *Uttama sāra* from *sattva* to *tvak sāra*
   c. *Uttama sāra from tvak to sattva sāra*
   d. A and B
   e. A and C

6. Vāgbhaṭa (AH Śhā. 3/107-116) describes the ideal qualities for health and claims an endowed individual will attain
   a. Comfortable life
   b. Desires achieved
   c. One hundred years of life
   d. Wealth
   e. All of the above

7. *Tvak sāra* which has glowing soft skin with fine body hair, produces
   a. *Ārogya*
   b. *Buddhi*
   c. *Sukha*
   d. *Vidya*
   e. All of the above

8. *Māṁsa sāra* which is stable and well developed produces
   a. Active with high tolerance for stress
   b. Intolerant to heat and stress
   c. Long lifespan and children
   d. Pleasure, enjoyment, contentment through eating
   e. Strength, happiness and absence of disease

9. *Majjā sāra* which has large eyes and smooth deep voice produces
   a. Active with high tolerance for stress
   b. Intolerant to heat and stress
   c. Long lifespan and children
   d. Pleasure, enjoyment, contentment through eating
   e. Strength, happiness and absence of disease

10. *Sattva sāra lakṣhaṇas* produce
    a. Courage and bravery
    b. Prosperity, wealth, power
    c. Similar characteristics found in their children
    d. Slow to develop disease
    e. Wisdom, skill and good memory

CRITICAL THINKING

1. The *aṣhṭa vidha sāra* include many *lakṣhaṇas* which then produce an outcome for an individual who has that type of *sāra*. Explain how this may be possible.

2. What could be some of the benefits of assessing the *aṣhṭa vidha sāra* for an individual in a clinical setting?

3. Which of the *aṣhṭa vidha sāra* may produce an individual more likely to have a long lifespan? What is a possible connection between a long lifespan and each of these *dhātus?*

4. If an individual has a single *dhātu sāra*, what possibly happens to the subsequent *dhātus*, after that *sāra*? Would they be more likely to be high quality or deficient? Use *dhātu pariṇāma* to explain your answer.

5. Why is *sattva sāra* considered to be the best of all *aṣhṭa vidha sāra*? Consider Chapters 23, 24 and 26 in your answer.

Chapter 21 : Saṁhanana

KEY TERMS			
alpa	daśhavidha parīkṣha	madhya avastha	saṁhanana
bala	deha	pramāṇa	uttama
bālya avastha	madhya	sama	vṛddha avastha

The concept of *saṁhanana* is explained briefly in the classics primarily by Charaka. It refers to the compactness of the physical body as an outcome of well-developed *dhātus* through proper, healthy nourishment and growth. Practical application and clinical assessment of *saṁhanana* requires melding together many parameters that can be assessed individually through *pramāṇa* and *śharīra saṅkhya avayava*.

UNDERSTANDING SAṀHANANA

The Monier-Williams Dictionary states that the term *saṁhanana* is formed by a combination of *saṁ* plus the Sanskrit *dhātu* √ *han* suffixed with *-na* (producing *hanana*). These terms indicate:

saṁ (sam)	with, together with, along with, together, altogether (used as a preposition or prefix to verbs and verbal derivatives
	expressing "conjunction," "union," "thoroughness," "intensity," "completeness"
√ han	to strike, beat, pound, hammer
-na	indicating the production of an action, the doing of such action

Coalescing these components into the term *saṁhanana* produces various meanings. In the context of Āyurveda only certain meanings are applicable.

saṁhanana	compact, solid, firm
	making compact or solid
	striking together
	the act of striking together
	hardening
	solidity, compactness, robustness, strength, muscularity
	firmness, steadfastness
	the body (as having the limbs well compacted)

When considering these definitions and meanings, understanding *saṁhanana* can be likened to forging a sword. Striking one object with another creates a specific shape and presses the form of the struck object into a hardened, compact, stable position. *Saṁhanana* can be considered both the process of making the sword (or body into a specific, compact shape) as well as its measurable outcome.

Saṁhanana can be expressed in Āyurveda as:

Formation	the process of development of the physical body into a compact, stable and well-formed shape
Assessment	measurements of specific

attributes and features of the body that can indicate the level or degree of proper, compact development

Both the formation and assessment of *saṁhanana* are closely related. The correct understanding of one provides relevant information to the other.

Formation of *saṁhanana* occurs and changes throughout an individual's lifespan. The ability of the physical body to achieve a higher level of *saṁhanana* is largely based on the individual's current stage of life. For example, in *bālya avastha* the physical body is expected to grow and develop to attain its maximum capacity in terms of size. However, the level of *saṁhanana* generally remains low. During *madhya avastha*, an individual generally has the capacity to attain their maximum or best state of *saṁhanana*. And in *vṛddha avastha*, *saṁhanana* usually declines.

The means by which the formation of *saṁhanana* can be determined is currently measurable and comparable to classical records only. The specific types of measurements of the body using length, volume and count are recorded in various *saṁhitās*. While this information stands as a valuable record of the time, its practicality and implementation are not confirmed to be accurate today for a general audience.

Many factors must be considered when using specific classical measurements of *pramāṇa*. Most importantly, were these measurements recorded based only on the demographic population of the Indian subcontinent? Did they include both male and female measurements? What was the age or life period considered to best represent the recorded measurements?

The divergence of normal standards in ethnic subpopulations is well-recognized today as are distinctions for sex, age and other factors. Application of classical standards for normal *saṁhanana* need to be reassessed, researched and developed in order to be practically applicable today.

In light of the preceding, a review of the classical references of *saṁhanana* in terms of their assessment and practical application will be provided here as a background to the concept. Measuring the formation of *saṁhanana* in context of *pramāṇa* has been covered in Chapter 19.

Charaka discusses the concept of *saṁhanana* briefly in a few references throughout the entire treatise. He introduces the concept through its synonyms and basic means of assessment in three graded levels.

संहननतश्चेतिसंहननं, संहतिः,
संयोजनमित्येकोऽर्थः ।
तत्रसमसुविभक्तास्थि, सुबद्धसन्धि,
सुनिविष्टमांसशोणितं,
सुसंहतंशरीरमित्युच्यते ।
तत्रसुसंहतशरीराःपुरुषाबलवन्तः,
विपर्ययेणाल्पबलाः,
मध्यत्वात्संहननस्यमध्यबलाभवन्ति || ११६

च. वि. ८।११६

Saṁhananataśhcheti saṁhananaṁ, saṁhatiḥ, saṁyojanamityeko ' rthaḥ | Tatra samasuvibhaktāsthi, subaddhasandhi, sunivișhṭamāṁsaśhōṇitaṁ, susaṁhataṁ śharīramityuchyate | Tatra susaṁhataśharīrāḥ puruṣhā balavantaḥ, viparyayeṇālpabalāḥ, madhyatvāt saṁhananasya madhyabalā bhavanti || 116

Cha. Vi. 8/116

Saṁhananataśhcheti (And so *saṁhanana* is assessed [considering the context of the previous *śhloka*'s descriptions of *sāra*) ityeko ' rthaḥ ([and it] is also known by one of the following synonyms) saṁhananaṁ (*saṁhanana*), saṁhatiḥ (*saṁhati*), saṁyojanam (*saṁyojana*). Tatra (And so) ityuchyate (it is said to be) sama (normal, complete) suvibhaktāsthi (well-divided, symmetrical skeletal structure and bones), subaddha (well-bound) sandhi (joints), suniviṣhṭa (well-developed, properly situated) māṁsa (muscular structures and muscle) śhōṇitaṁ ([and] blood, vascular system, supportive system to *māṁsa*), susaṁhataṁ (properly compacted, well-developed) śharīram (body [overall]). Tatra (And so) susaṁhata (a properly compacted, well-developed) śharīrāḥ (physical body) puruṣhā (in human beings) balavantaḥ ([results in] increased strength), viparyayeṇa (the opposite [results in]) alpa [less, reduced) balāḥ (strength), madhyatvāt ([and] a moderate amount) saṁhananasya (of *saṁhanana* [results in]) madhya (a medium amount) balā (of strength) bhavanti (is how it is explained).

Reviewing this section of *śhlokas* in detail provides a good picture of *saṁhanana* and a concise explanation of its assessment. Note that contextually, this explanation of *saṁhanana* has been provided after the detailed description of *dhātu sārata* (covered in this volume in Chapter 20). This placement implies that the high-quality characteristics found in *dhātu sārata* can also be interpreted within the context of *saṁhanana*.

Saṁhanana is also understood through the synonyms of:

saṁhati	striking together, closure
	compactness, solidity
	keeping together, saving, economy
	a compact mass, bulk, heap, collection, multitude
saṁyojana	the act of joining or uniting with

The assessment of *saṁhanana* is done by analyzing the characteristics, qualities and features of all of the following in their state of *sama* (normal, complete development):

suvibhakta asthi
: well-divided, symmetrical skeletal structure and bones

subaddha sandhi
: well-bound joints

suniviṣhṭa māṁsa śhōṇitaṁ
: well-developed, properly situated muscular structures and muscle and blood, vascular system, supportive system to *māṁsa*

susaṁhataṁ śharīram
: properly compacted, well-developed body, overall

The assessment of *saṁhanana* can be graded on three scales. The methodology for grading should use the individual's normal, healthy state as a baseline for comparison. The specificity of the grading results in an understanding of whether the criteria is below normal, normal or above normal for the individual. This can present as less than normal health, normal health and optimal health. The three levels of *saṁhanana* include:

alpa	results in reduced strength in any form for an individual compared to their normal, healthy state
madhya	results in a moderate amount of strength which should be considered normal and healthy for an individual
uttama	results in an increased amount of strength which should be considered above normal for an individual

Charaka also explains that the proper

analysis of *saṁhanana* is required for a complete clinical assessment as a component of the *daśhavidha parīkṣha* framework. Although Suśhruta and Vāgbhaṭa do not emphasize the term *saṁhanana*, they also recognize a similar assessment under the headings of *deha* and even *bala*, to some extent, within the contexts of their own similar assessment frameworks.

तस्मादातुरंपरीक्षेतप्रकृतितश्च, विकृतितश्च, सारतश्च, संहननतश्च, प्रमाणतश्च, सात्म्यतश्च, सत्त्वतश्च, आहारशक्तितश्च, व्यायामशक्तितश्च, वयस्तश्चेति, बलप्रमाणविशेषग्रहणहेतोः || ९४

च. वि. ८lj e

Tasmādāturaṁ parīkṣheta prakṛtitaśhcha, vikṛtitaśhcha, sārataśhcha, saṁhananataśhcha, pramāṇataśhcha, sātmyataśhcha, sattvataśhcha, āhāraśhaktitaśhcha, vyāyāmaśhaktitaśhcha, vayastaśhcheti, balapramāṇaviśheṣhagrahaṇahetoḥ || 94

Cha. Vi. 8/94

Tasmād (Therefore), āturaṁ (any unhealthy individual) parīkṣheta (should be assessed based on their) prakṛtitaśhcha (prakṛti, or normal baseline constitution), vikṛtitaśhcha (vikṛti, or deviation from normal baseline), sārataśhcha (dhātu sāra, or quality supportive tissues), saṁhananataśhcha (saṁhananata, or properly formed physical body), pramāṇataśhcha (pramāṇa, or measuresments of the physical body), sātmyataśhcha (or their customary ways of living a healthy life), sattvataśhcha (sattva, or their mental tendencies), āhāraśhaktitaśhcha (āhāraśhakti, or their capacity to injest and digest food), vyāyāmaśhaktitaśhcha (*vyāyāmaśhakti*, or their capacity to perform physical work), vayastaśhcheti (and vaya, or their age and predicted lifespan), bala pramāṇa (in terms of each one's graded measurement of strength [ie, low, medium, high] viśheṣha grahaṇa ([and] to understand the specific) hetoḥ (causative factors for deviation from normal health).

In this overview of the *daśhavidha parīkṣha* framework, Charaka clearly includes *saṁhanana* as a major component. While each of these are assessed individually, they ultimately are all combined to provide a complete clinical picture of the current state of health or deviation for the individual. Information from each one can be used to help understand the others.

Charaka also makes a small reference to the importance of strong, healthy *saṁhanana* as a specific factor in the maintenance of overall health and higher resistance to disease. This is explained while discussing the two undesirable states of *sthūla* (overweight) and *kṛśha* (underweight), which are both prone to disease. In this context, he states that proper *saṁhanana* is ideal.

सममांसप्रमाणस्तु समसंहननो नरः|
दृढेन्द्रियो विकाराणां न बलेनाभिभूयते || १८
क्षुत्पिपासातपसहः शीतव्यायामसंसहः|
समपक्ता समजरः सममांसचयो मतः || १९

च. सू. २१।१८-१९

Samamāṁsapramāṇastu samasaṁhanano naraḥ | Dṛḍhendriyo vikārāṇāṁ na balenābhibhūyate || 18
Kṣhutpipāsātapasahaḥ śhītavyāyāmasaṁsahaḥ | Samapaktā samajaraḥ samamāṁsachayo mataḥ || 19

Cha. Sū. 21/18-19

Sama (Normal, complete development) māṁsa (of the muscular structures, muscular system and muscles) pramāṇastu (is measurable as) sama (normal, properly developed) saṁhanano (saṁhanana) naraḥ (in human beings). Dṛḍha ([Along with] firm, strong) indriyo (sense organs in all functions and manifestations) abhibhūyate ([these two] are superior) balena (in providing the strength [needed to]) vikārāṇāṁ na (not experience disease).

Sahaḥ (Those who are endowed with these strengths) saṁsahaḥ (can easily cope with) kṣhut (hunger), pipāsa (thirst), ātapa (sun), śhīta (cold), vyāyāma ([and] physical work). Mataḥ (They are understood [to have]) sama (normal, healthy) paktā (processes of digestion), sama (normal, healthy) jaraḥ (processes of ageing), sama (and normal, healthy) māṁsachayo (growth of muscular structures).

TEST YOURSELF

Learn, review and memorize key terms from this section.

saṁhanana

bālya avastha

madhya avastha

vṛddha avastha

pramāṇa

sama

alpa

madhya

uttama

daśhavidha parīkṣha

deha

bala

Chapter 21: Review

ADDITIONAL READING

Read and review the references listed below to expand your understanding of the concepts in this chapter. Write down the date that you complete your reading for each. Remember that consistent repetition is the best way to learn. Plan to read each reference at least once now and expect to read it again as you continue your studies.

References marked with (skim) can be read quickly and do not require commentary review.

CLASSICS		1st read	2nd read
Charaka	Cha. Sū. 21/18-19 Cha. Vi. 8/94 Cha. Vi. 8/116		
Suśhruta			
Aṣhṭāṅga Hṛdaya			
Bhāva Prakāśha			

JOURNALS & CURRENT RESOURCES

Journal article: *A Conceptual Study of Samhanana as a Measuring Tool*, Waghulade Hemangini Sanjay

Journal article: *An Observational Study of Samhanana as a Measuring Tool*, Waghulade Hemangini Sanjay

QUESTIONS & ANSWERS

Record your questions for this chapter here for further research and discussion.

Question:

Answer:

Question:

Answer:

Question:

Answer:

SELF-ASSESSMENT

1. *Saṁhanana* is described as
   a. Act of striking the body together
   b. Compactness of physical body
   c. Stable well-formed shape
   d. Well developed *dhātus* through proper nourishment
   e. All of the above

2. Assessment of *saṁhanana* helps to determine
   a. Current stage of life
   b. Development of the *dhātus*
   c. Level of compact development
   d. Strength and muscularity
   e. All of the above

3. An individual's ability to achieve a higher level of *saṁhanana* is based on
   a. Current stage of life
   b. Gender
   c. Proper nourishment
   d. Proper exercise
   e. None of the above

4. Which stage of life is capable of achieving the highest level of *saṁhanana*?
   a. *Bālya avastha*
   b. *Madhya avastha*
   c. *Vṛddha avastha*
   d. A and B
   e. B and C

5. Which stage of life is capable of declining to the lowest level of *saṁhanana*?
   a. *Bālya avastha*
   b. *Madhya avastha*
   c. *Vṛddha avastha*
   d. A and B
   e. A and C

6. How is *saṁhanana* measured?
   a. *Alpa, madhya, uttama*
   b. *Avara, madhyama, uttama*
   c. *Bālya, madhya, vṛddha*
   d. All of the above
   e. None of the above

7. Charaka states the assessment of *saṁhanana* is based upon
   a. *Prakṛti*
   b. An individual's state of health
   c. *Dhātu sāra*
   d. The *daśhavidha parīkṣha*
   e. All of the above

8. Suśhruta and Vāgbhaṭa don't mention *saṁhanana*, but it is recognized within their frameworks of *parīkṣha* as
   a. *Avastha*
   b. *Deha* and *bala*
   c. *Dhātu sāra*
   d. *Prakṛti*
   e. All of the above

9. Which of the following aid the assessment of *saṁhanana* according to Charaka?
   a. Age and predicted lifespan
   b. Capacity to ingest and digest food
   c. Capacity to perform physical work
   d. *Sattva*, or mental tendency
   e. All of the above

10. Charaka states that proper saṁhanana allows an individual to
    a. Digest food well
    b. Maintain their physical proportions as kṛśha (underweight)
    c. Have strong *indriya* and well-developed *māṁsa*
    d. All of the above
    e. None of the above

CRITICAL THINKING

1. How can *saṁhanana* be explained by "striking the body together?" Use any analogy to elaborate your answer.
2. When measuring or assessing *saṁhanana*, it should always be compared against the same individual as the baseline. Explain why this is important and the potential effect in a clinical setting.
3. Do you recognize a high level of *saṁhanana* in any famous individual? How is that person usually described?
4. The three levels of *saṁhanana* assessment include *alpa*, *madhya* and *uttama*. Are these three sufficient or are more assessment levels required? Explain your perspective.

Chapter 22 : Nidrā (Sleep)

KEY TERMS

divā	kṛśha	rātri jāgaraṇa	svāpa
divā svapna	manas	sattva	svapna
hṛdaya	nidrā	śhayana	tamas
jāgaraṇa	rajas	sthūla	trayopastambha
jñānendriya	rātri	svabhāva	triguṇa
karmendriya			

The concept of sleep is well-understood and well-defined in the Āyurvedic classics. It is one of the primary factors in sustaining health according to Vāgbhaṭa who includes it as one of the *trayopastambha* (the three supports of vitality). He states:

आहारशयनाब्रह्मचर्यैर्युक्त्या प्रयोजितैः ।
शरीरं धायते नित्यमागारमिव धारनैः ॥ ५२

अ. हृ. सू. ७।५२

Āhārāśhayanābrahmacharyairyuktyā prayojitaiḥ |
Śharīraṁ dhāyate nityamāgāramiva dhāranaiḥ || 52

AH Sū. 7/52

Āhārā (Food, dietary intake), śhayana (sleep, rest, laying down), abrahmacharyair (not following a lifestyle of a brahmacharya) yuktyā (properly) prayojitaiḥ (applied) dhāyate (protect) śharīraṁ (the body) nityam āgāramiva (just as a house must be constantly) dhāranaiḥ (held up [by three supports).

Sleep is a primary requirement for maintenance and support of normal health.

Following this statement, Vāgbhaṭa then elaborates on aspects of sleep including normal physiology, types and effects. Charaka discusses similar details about sleep and specifically includes his explanation within the context of *sthūla* and *kṛśha*, two disorders characterized by over-nourishment and under-nourishment in Cha. Sū. 21/35-59. This contextual placement indicates the importance of sleep as a factor in the nourishment and growth of the body. Suśhruta discusses the topic in the context of *garbha śhārīra* in Su. Śhā. 4/33-56.

PARIBHĀṢHĀ AND PARYĀYA

Sleep is described classically using a number of terms. Review each to understand their contextual meanings, implications and interpretations appropriately.

Nidrā is one of the most commonly used terms to denote sleep. The Monier-Williams dictionary defines it as:

nidrā	to fall asleep, sleep, slumber
	sleep, slumber, sleepiness, sloth

The term derives from the Sanskrit *dhātu* √ *drā* prefixed with *ni-*. These can be understood as:

√ drā	to run, make haste
	to run hither and thither
	to sleep

ni- down, back, in, into, within

may also indicate negation

As a complete term, *nidrā* indicates inactivity or going into a state of sleep.

Vāgbhaṭa also uses the term *śhayana* to indicate sleep. The Monier-Williams dictionary defines this as:

śhayana lying down, resting, sleeping

the act of lying down or sleeping, rest, repose, sleep

a bed, couch, sleeping-place

Svapna is another common term used to indicate sleep:

svapna sleep, sleeping

sleepiness, drowsiness

sleeping too much, sloth, indolence

dreaming, a dream

The key distinction with *svapna* is that it can refer to the dream state of sleep.

Definition #1: Suśhruta's perspective

Suśhruta defines *nidrā* through a simile to highlight the importance of its universal effect on all human beings.

निद्रां तु वैष्णवीं पाप्मानमुपदिशन्ति, सा स्वभावत एव सर्वप्राणिनोऽभिस्पृशति ।

सु. शा. ४।३३

Nidrāṁ tu vaiṣhṇavīṁ pāpmānamupadiśhanti, sā svabhāvata eva sarvaprāṇino ' bhispṛśhti |

Su. Śhā. 4/33

Tu (Thus), nidrāṁ (sleep) upadiśhanti (is taught to be) vaiṣhṇavīṁ (like the incarnation of *Viṣhṇu*), pāpma (for which bad deeds, or sins) anam (cause one to pray). Sā svabhāvata eva (Likewise, by its very nature, [sleep]) abhispṛśhti (affects, influence) sarva (all) prāṇino (living beings).

Suśhruta's simile is made in reference to the universal nature of deities' effects over all living beings and creatures. He states that all must account for their sins and bad actions before such deity without exception. In this same way, sleep is unavoidable or inescapable, and exerts its effects over all living beings.

Definition #2: Charaka's perspective

Nidrā is defined by Charaka through a description of its functions and outcomes seen through clinical assessment.

निद्रायत्तं सुखं दुःखं पुष्टिः कार्श्यं बलाबलम् | वृषता क्लीबता ज्ञानमज्ञानं जीवितं न च || ३६

च. सू. २१।३६

Nidrāyattaṁ sukhaṁ duḥkhaṁ puṣhṭiḥ kārśhyaṁ balābalam | Vṛṣhatā klībatā jñānamajñānaṁ jīvitaṁ na cha || 36

Cha. Sū. 21/36

Nidrā (Sleep) yattaṁ (properly engaged in [produces]) sukhaṁ (happiness) duḥkhaṁ (or unhappiness), puṣhṭiḥ (promotion of healthy growth) kārśhyaṁ (or reduction), bala (physical strength) abalam (or lack of strength), vṛṣhatā (virility) klībatā (or impotency), jñānam (intelligence) ajñānaṁ (or absence of intelligence) cha (and) jīvitaṁ (life) na (or absence of it).

Definition #3: Vāgbhaṭa's perspective

Vāgbhaṭa reiterates Charaka's statements.

निद्रायत्तं सुखं दुःखं पुष्टिः कार्श्यं बलाबलम् ॥ ५३

वृषता क्लीबता ज्ञानमज्ञानं जीवितं न च ।

अ. हृ. सू. ७।५३

Nidrāyattaṁ sukhaṁ duḥkhaṁ pushṭiḥ kārśhyaṁ balābalam || 53
Vṛshatā klībatā jñānamajñānaṁ jīvitaṁ na cha |

AH Sū. 7/53

Yattaṁ (Engaging properly in) nidrā (sleep) na cha (or not [produces]) sukhaṁ (happiness, contentment) duḥkhaṁ ([or] unhappiness, discontentment), pushṭiḥ (growth, increase, nourishment, plumpness [of the body]) kārśhyaṁ ([or] emaciation, wasting, reduction [of the body]), bala (physical strength) abalam ([or] absence of physical strength), vṛshatā (virility) klībatā ([or] impotency), jñānam (intelligence) ajñānaṁ ([or] absence of intelligence) jīvitaṁ ([and] life).

The results of proper and improper sleep are summarized as:

Proper sleep	Improper sleep
Sukha Happiness, contentment	*Duḥkha* Unhappiness, discontentment
Pushṭi Growth, increase, nourishment, plumpness of the body	*Kārśhya* Emaciation, wasting, reduction of the body
Bala Physical strength	*Abala* Absence of physical strength
Vṛshatā Virility	*Klībatā* Impotency
Jñāna Intelligence	*Ajñāna* Absence of intelligence
Jīvita Life, vitality	*Na* Absence of life

TEST YOURSELF

Learn, review and memorize key terms from this section.

nidrā

___

śhayana

___

svapna

___

BHEDA

Sleep is categorized based on its occurrence during the night or day, and separately according to its cause of onset. All classical authors differentiate sleeping at night versus the day because of its effects on the body and normal health. While each type may be indicated appropriately in certain situations, the general recommendation is that one should accustom themselves to sleeping at night only.

These two types of sleep occur during *rātri* (nighttime) or *divā* (daytime). By default, any reference to sleep using the terms *nidrā*, *śhayana* or *svapna* should be understood to imply nighttime. Sleeping for any length of time during the day is always referred to as *divā svapna*, where *divā* specifically indicates day.

Rātri and divā svapna

Charaka discusses the difference effects that each of these types of sleep imparts. He states:

रात्रौ जागरणं रूक्षं स्निग्धं प्रस्वपनं दिवा |
अरूक्षमनभिष्यन्दि त्वासीनप्रचलायितम् || ५०

च. सू. २१।५०

Rātrau jāgaraṇaṁ rūkṣhaṁ snigdhaṁ
prasvapanaṁ divā |
Arūkṣhamanabhiṣhyandi
tvāsīnaprachalāyitam || 50

Cha. Sū. 21/50

Rātrau (During the nighttime), jāgaraṇaṁ (staying awake [causes]) rūkṣhaṁ (dryness); snigdhaṁ (unctuousness) prasvapanaṁ ([is caused by] sleeping, napping) divā (during the daytime). Arūkṣham (Non-dryness [and]) anabhiṣhyandi (non-blockage of the channels of the body) tu (however, [are caused by]) āsīna (sitting) prachalāyitam (and just nodding off).

Vāgbhaṭa reiterates the same statement.

रत्रौ जागरणं रूक्षं, स्निग्धं प्रस्वपनं दिवा ॥ ५५
अरूक्षमनभिष्यन्दि त्वासीनप्रचलायितम् ।

अ. हृ. सू. ७।५५

Ratrau jāgaraṇaṁ rūkṣhaṁ, snigdhaṁ
prasvapanaṁ divā || 55
Arūkṣhamanabhiṣhyandi
tvāsīnaprachalāyitam |

AH Sū. 7/55

Ratrau (During the night) jāgaraṇaṁ (staying awak) rūkṣhaṁ (causes dryness), snigdhaṁ (unctuousness) prasvapanaṁ (is produced by napping) divā (during the day). 55

Arūkṣham (Neither dryness) anabhiṣhyandi (nor blockage of the channels) tu (however, [are caused by]) āsīna (sitting) prachalāyitam (and just nodding off).

The opposite effects of *nidrā* and *divā svapna* are fundamentally related to the normal physiological activities of the human body and its variances between night and day. The heart has a key role to play in this which will be discussed in the following section.

Differences during the night and day cause the channels of the human body to be in various physiological states. With normal activity in the daytime, channels are open and flowing easily. Sleeping during the daytime impedes this normal flow and predisposes to the collection of circulating *doṣhas* in susceptible areas of the body, particularly on the micro level.

At night, in normal, healthy physiology, the bodily channels close. By remaining awake during these times, any physical or mental activity increases the force of movement through all channels which results in higher pressure. This has an immediate effect on *vāta doṣha*, causing it to increase and resulting in an increase of one of its primary *guṇas*, *rūkṣha*.

This entire concept of staying awake at night, causing *vāta prakopa* and resulting in *rūkṣhatva* is referred to as *jāgaraṇa* or *rātri jāgaraṇa*.

These fundamental principles can be seen in the effect of sleeping during the day on *kapha doṣha*. In normal, healthy physiology, the body is expected to be active during the day. To provide adequate energy for these activities, the channels are open, easily flowing and carrying nutritive fluid. By sleeping during the day, especially in a horizontal position, the circulatory system naturally slows and becomes prone to stasis. The contents of the fluid settle because of lack of movement resulting in the accumulation of material or *doṣhas* throughout the body. This increases *kapha*'s primary *guṇa*, *snigdha*.

Five types of sleep based on onset

Suśhruta discusses five causes for the onset of sleep. These are stated directly as categories, without any delineation with regard to healthy or unhealthy types. That understanding should be implied, however, once the descriptions are clear.

तत्र यदा संज्ञावहानि स्रोतांसि तमोभूयिष्टः श्लेष्मा प्रतिपद्यते तदा तामसी नाम निद्रा सम्भवत्यनवबोधिनी, सा प्रलयकाले; तमोभूयिष्ठानामहःसु निशासु च भवति, रजोभूयिष्ठानामनिमित्तं, सत्त्वभूयिष्ठानामर्धरात्रे; क्षीणश्लेष्मणामनिलबहुलानां मनःशरीराभितापवतां च नैव, सा वैकारिकी भवति ॥ ३३

सु. शा. ४।३३

Tatra yadā saṁjñāvahāni srotāṁsi tamobhūyiṣhṭaḥ śhleṣhmā pratipadyate tadā tāmasī nāma nidrā sambhavatyanavabodhinī, sā pralayakāle; tamobhūyiṣhṭhānāmahaḥsu niśhāsu cha bhavati, rajobhūyiṣhṭhānāmanimittaṁ, sattvabhūyiṣhṭhānāmardharātre; kṣhīṇaśhleṣhmaṇāmanilabahulānāṁ manaḥśharīrābhitāpavatāṁ cha naiva, sā vaikārikī bhavati || 33

Su. Śhā. 4/33

Tatra (And so), yadā (whenever) tamo-bhūyiṣhṭaḥ śhleṣhmā (abundant, or overflowing tamas and kapha) pratipadyate (reach) saṁjñāvahāni srotāṁsi (the channels of consciousness) tadā (then) tāmasī (the tāmasī [type of sleep]) nāma (as it is called) sambhavati (causes) nidrā (sleep) anavabodhinī (permanently, from which one does not awake). Sā pralaya-kāle (This occurs at the time of *pralaya*, ie, the end of life, or end of the world); tamo-bhūyiṣhṭhānāmahaḥsu (when tamas is abundant), niśhāsu cha (during both the night and day) bhavati ([sleep] occurs), rajo-bhūyiṣhṭhānām (when rajas is abundant), animittaṁ ([sleep occurs] for no reason), sattva-bhūyiṣhṭhānām (when sattva is abundant [sleep occurs]), ardha (halfway) rātre (in the night); kṣhīṇa-śhleṣhmaṇām (when kapha is deficient), anila-bahulānāṁ (vāta is excessive), manaḥ-śharīra ābhitāpavatāṁ cha (and/or there is disease in the mind or body), naiva (none of these types [of sleep]), sā vaikārikī (or abnormal [types of sleep]) bhavati (manifest).

These five types are summarized as:

Nidrā bheda	Nearest English explanation
Tāmasī	Increased *tamas* and *kapha* reach the *saṁjñāvaha srotas* and the individual never awakens, as occurs during *pralaya*.
Tamas	Due to abundance of *tamo guṇa*, sleep occurs anytime during night or day.
Rajas	Due to abundance of *rajo guṇa*, sleep occurs for no reason.
Sattva	Due to abundance of *sattva*, sleep occurs halfway through the night.
Vaikārikī	Due to: - *Kṣhīṇa-śhleṣhma* - *Anila-bahulā* - *Manaḥ-śharīra ābhitāpavatā* Sleep is absent or abnormal.

Seven types of sleep based on onset

Charaka describes seven causes for the onset of sleep. Out of these, one is considered normal and healthy. The seven include:

तमोभवा श्लेष्मसमुद्भवा च मनःशरीरश्रमसम्भवा च | आगन्तुकी व्याध्यनुवर्तिनी च रात्रिस्वभावप्रभवा च निद्रा || ५८

च. सू. २१|५८

Tamobhavā śhleṣhmasamudbhavā cha manaḥśharīraśhramasambhavā cha | Āgantukī vyādhyanuvartinī cha rātrisvabhāvaprabhavā cha nidrā || 58

Cha. Sū. 21/58

Tamo-bhavā (Due to factors predominated by *tamas*), śhleṣhma-samudbhavā (factors that produce *kapha* [*doṣha*]), cha (and) manaḥ-śharīra-śhrama sambhavā (factors that result in exhaustion of the mind or physical body) cha (and) āgantukī (external causes), vyādhi-anuvartinī cha (and their subsequent diseases or effects), rātri-svabhāva-prabhavā cha (and [due to] the special effect of the nature of the night) nidrā (sleep [occurs]).

These seven types are summarized as:

Nidrā bheda	Nearest English explanation
Tamas	Inertia, one of the *triguṇas*
Śhleṣhma-samudbhavā	Factors that produce *kapha doṣha*
Manaḥ-śhrama sambhavā	Factors that result in exhaustion of the mind
Śharīra-śhrama sambhavā	Factors that result in exhaustion of the physical body
Āgantukī	External causes
Vyādhi-anuvartinī	Diseases (caused subsequently by any of the preceding; or subsequent effects of any disease)
Rātri-svabhāva-prabhavā	The special effect of the nature of the night

Of these seven, sleep which is caused due to *rātri-svabhāva-prabhavā* is considered the only normal, healthy type of sleep. He explains this as:

रात्रिस्वभावप्रभवा मता या तां भूतधात्रीं प्रवदन्ति तज्ज्ञाः | तमोभवामाहुरघस्य मूलं शेषाः पुनर्व्याधिषु निर्दिशन्ति || ५९

च. सू. २१|५९

Rātrisvabhāvaprabhavā matā yā tāṁ bhūtadhātrīṁ pravadanti tajjñāḥ | Tamobhavāmāhuraghasya mūlaṁ śheṣhāḥ punarvyādhiṣhu nirdiśhanti || 59

Cha. Sū. 21/59

Rātri-svabhāva-prabhavā (Sleep caused by the special effect of the nature of the night) matā (is known as) yā tāṁ (the best type). Pravadanti (It is also called) bhūtadhātrīṁ (*bhūtadhātrī*, or that which supports or nurses the building blocks of life) tajjñāḥ (amongst those familiar with the term). Tamo-bhavām ([Sleep caused due to] factors predominated by *tamas*) āhuraghasya mūlaṁ ([is] the root of all evil, sinful, dangerous behaviors) nirdiśhanti ([the other types] are seen) śheṣhāḥ (in specific) punarvyādhiṣhu (manifestations of diseases).

TEST YOURSELF

Learn, review and memorize key terms from this section.

rātri

____

divā

____

divā svapna

____

tamas

____

rajas

____

sattva

____

jāgaraṇa

____

rātri jāgaraṇa

____

NORMAL SLEEP PROCESS

The normal process of sleep is largely regulated by *manas* and the *triguṇas*, *tamas*, *rajas* and *sattva*. These components, along with chetanā, primarily reside in hṛdaya and move throughout the body via a special conduit of exudative channels mentioned by Suśhruta in the context of the normal processes of sleep, called the *saṁjñāvaha srotas*. Because the heart is the main home location for all of these components, Suśhruta explains its role through a simile.

Role of hṛdaya in sleep

पुण्डरीकेण सदृशं हृदयं स्यादधोमुखम् ।
जाग्रतस्तद्विकसति स्वपतश्च निमीलति ॥ ३२

सु. शा. ४।३२

Puṇḍarīkeṇa sadṛśhaṁ hṛdayaṁ syādadhomukham | Jāgratastadvikasati svapataśhcha nimīlati ||

Su. Śhā. 4/32

Hṛdayaṁ (The heart [is]) sadṛśhaṁ (just like) puṇḍarīkeṇa (a lotus blossom) syād-adhomukham (positioned facing downward). Jāgratastad (While awake), vikasati (it is open), svapataśhcha (and when asleep), nimīlati (it is closed).

This simile reinforces the concepts of opened versus closed during day and night and the direct impact of these states on the heart's functions.

Suśhruta then elaborates on the normal processes of sleep. The role of *tamas* is critical to induce a state of healthy sleep.

हृदयं चेतनास्थानमुक्तं सुश्रुत ! देहिनाम् ।
तमोऽभिभूते तस्मिंस्तु निद्रा विशति देहिनम् ॥ ३४

सु. शा. ४।३४

Hṛdayaṁ chetanāsthānamuktaṁ Suśhruta! Dehinām | Tamo ' bhibhūte tasminstu nidrā niśhati dehinam || 34

Su. Śhā. 4/34

Hṛdayaṁ (The heart) chetanā-sthāna (is the primary location for chetanā) muktaṁ ([and] the source from where *chetanā* flows), Suśhruta (Suśhruta)! Tamo ([When] the effect of *tamas*) abhibhūte (overpowers) dehinām (the physical body), tasminstu (in that moment) nidrā (sleep) niśhati (occurs through the night) dehinam (in the body).

Role of triguṇa in sleep

In addition to *tamas*, *sattva* plays a key role in that it is responsible for awakening the individual from sleep. The cycles of sleeping and waking are so inherent in nature that they have also been explained as *svabhāva*.

निद्राहेतुस्तमः, सत्त्वं बोधने हेतुरुच्यते ।
स्वभाव एव वा हेतुर्गरीयान् परिकीर्त्यते ॥ ३५

सु. शा. ४।३५

Nidrāhetustamaḥ, sattvaṁ bodhane heturuchyate | Svabhāva eva vā heturgarīyān parikīrtyate || 35

Su. Śhā. 4/35

Nidrā (Sleep) hetus (is caused by) tamaḥ (tamas), sattvaṁ (sattva) heturuchyate (is known as the cause for) bodhane (awakening). Svabhāva eva vā (Or even nature itself) parikīrtyate (is said to be) heturgarīyān (the most important reason).

Normal physiology of sleep

Charaka describes the normal physiological process of sleep. He states that the *jñānendriya* cease to interact with their desired objects via their regular, active inputs while *karmendriya* cease to express their normal functions. Combined with the abundance of *tamas*, the mind is able to be subdued into a state of sleep.

यदा तु मनसि क्लान्ते कर्मात्मानः
क्लमान्विताः | विषयेभ्यो निवर्तन्ते तदा
स्वपिति मानवः || ३५

च. सू. २१।३५

Yadā tu manasi klānte karmātmānaḥ klamānvitāḥ | Viṣhayebhyo nivartante tadā svapiti mānavaḥ || 35

Cha. Sū. 21/35

Yadā (Whenever) tu manasi klānte (the mind becomes fatigued or exhausted), karmātmānaḥ ([and] the controlling center for stimulating action) klamānvitāḥ (becomes tired and vacant) viṣhayebhyo (and the objects of both sense and action organs) nivartante (are disengaged from interaction) tadā (then) svapiti (sleep) mānavaḥ (comes over the mind).

State of suspended animation

Suśhruta explains an additional interesting state where even though the individual appears to be awake, the *ātma* is inactive. This occurs when the *jñānendriya* and *karmendriya* become increasingly overwhelmed by *tamas*. Even though the *jñānendriya* continue to interact with their desired objects via active inputs and the *karmendriya* continue to express their normal functions, the *bhūtātma* is inactive, or asleep.

करणानां तु वैकल्ये तमसाऽभिप्रवर्धिते ।
अस्वपन्नपि भूतात्मा प्रसुप्त इव चोच्यते ॥ ३७

सु. शा. ४।३७

Karaṇānāṁ tu vaikalye tamasā ' bhipravardhite | Asvapannapi bhūtātmā prasupta iva chochyate || 37

Su. Śhā. 4/37

Karaṇānāṁ (When the "doers," ie, the sense and action organs of the body) tu vaikalye (become confused, weakened, frail) tamasā (because of tamas) abhipravardhite (more and more), asvapannapi (then, even when not asleep), bhūtātmā (the soul, or inherent intelligence of the primary building blocks of life) prasupta iva (become inactive, fall asleep, are closed or quiet) cha uchyate (and so it is told).

Dreams

Svāpa, or dreams and the state of dreaming, are explained by Suśhruta. He states that while the present, living body is asleep, the mind disengages and is able to experience all good and bad memories via the soul.

पूर्वदेहानुभूतांस्तु भूतात्मा स्वपतः प्रभुः ।
रजोयुक्तेन मनसा गृह्णात्यर्थाञ्शुभाशुभान् ॥ ३६

सु. शा. ४।३६

Pūrvadehānubhūtāṁstu bhūtātmā svapataḥ prabhuḥ | Rajoyuktena manasā gṛhṇātyarthāñśhubhāśhubhān || 36

Su. Śhā. 4/36

Pūrva deha (Prior to the physical body) ānubhūtāṁstu (and its experiences), bhūtātmā (the soul) prabhuḥ (maintains authority) svapataḥ (to experience dreams) manasā (through the mind) rajo-yuktena (combined with rajas), gṛhṇāti (it accesses) arthaāñ (all things) śhubha-aśhubhān (good and bad).

General recommendations for sleep

Classically, normal, healthy sleep is always intended to occur at night as a regular part of routine and living. Any deviation from this is considered abnormal and unhealthy. Sleeping during the daytime has specific rules, regulations, indications and contra-indications to ensure that it does not cause a deviation from normal health. These details will be covered in Volume 3 (Svastha Vṛtta).

यथाकालमथो निद्रां रात्रौ सेवेत सात्म्यतः ।
असात्म्याज्जागरादर्धं प्रातः
स्वप्यादभुक्तवान् ॥ ६५

अ. हृ. सू. ७।६५

Yathākālamatho nidrāṁ rātrau seveta sātmyataḥ | Asātmyājjāgarādardhaṁ prātaḥ svapyādabhuktavān || 65

AH Sū. 7/65

Yathākālamatho nidrāṁ rātrau seveta sātmyataḥ | Asātmyājjāgarādardhaṁ prātaḥ svapyādabhuktavān

TEST YOURSELF

Learn, review and memorize key terms from this section.

hṛdaya ______

manas ______

triguṇa ______

svabhāva ______

jñānendriya ______

karmendriya ______

svāpa ______

OUTCOMES

The purpose of sleep is to support normal health and maintain correct *dhātu sāmyata*. Proper outcomes of sleep and their opposites can be understood through many general *lakṣhaṇas* that indicate common states of normal or abnormal health as seen previously in this chapter through the definitions.

Charaka describes the outcomes in the context of *sthūla* and *kṛśha*. Both of these are abnormal states of *dhātus* which are predominant in excessive and deficient growth. Sleep is explained in detail within the context of *sthūla* and *kṛśha* because it is a primary factor in producing either of these states. Proper sleep routines and habits are required to manage and correct both of these conditions.

अकालेऽतिप्रसङ्गाच्च न च निद्रा निषेविता |
सुखायुषी पराकुर्यात् कालरात्रिरिवापरा || ३७

सैव युक्ता पुनर्युङ्क्ते निद्रा देहं सुखायुषा |
पुरुषं योगिनं सिद्ध्या सत्या बुद्धिरिवागता || ३८

च. सू. २१।३७-३८

Akāle ' tiprasaṅgāchcha na cha nidrā niṣhevitā | Sukhāyuṣhī parākuryāt kālarātririvāparā || 37

Saiva yuktā punaryuṅkte nidrā dehaṁ sukhāyuṣhā | Puruṣhaṁ yoginaṁ siddhyā satyā buddhirivāgatā || 38

Cha. Sū. 21/36-38

Niṣhevitā (It is observed that) akāle ([sleeping] at the wrong time), ati-prasaṅgāch-cha (or [sleeping] too much) na cha nidrā (or not sleeping) parākuryāt (takes away) sukha (happiness) āyuṣhī ([and] longevity, vitality), kālarātrir ivāparā (just like the night before the end of the world). 37

Saiva (In the same way), nidrā (sleep) yuktā (done correctly) punaryuṅkte (according to the instructions provided), sukhāyuṣhā ([provides] happiness and longevity, vitality) dehaṁ (to the body) siddhyā (just as the power) satyā (of truth) buddhirivāgatā puruṣhaṁ (creates a particular type of knowledge for individuals) yoginaṁ (who adhere to *yoga*).

Vāgbhaṭa reiterates much of Charaka's explanations of proper and improper sleep and its results.

अकालेऽतिप्रसङ्गाच्च न च निद्रा निषेविता || ५४

सुखायुषि पराकुर्यात् कालरात्रिरिवापरा ।

अ. हृ. सू. ७।५४

Akāle ' tiprasaṅgāchcha na cha nidrā niṣhevitā || Sukhāyuṣhi parākuryāt kālarātritivāparā |

AH Sū. 7/54

Niṣhevitā (It is observed that) akāle ([sleeping] at the wrong time), ati-prasaṅgāch-cha (or [sleeping] too much) na cah nidrā (or not sleeping) parākuryāt (takes away) sukha (happiness) āyuṣhī ([and] longevity, vitality), kālarātrir ivāparā (just like the night before the end of the world).

TEST YOURSELF

Learn, review and memorize key terms from this section.

sthūla

____

kṛśha

____

Chapter 22: Review

ADDITIONAL READING

Read and review the references listed below to expand your understanding of the concepts in this chapter. Write down the date that you complete your reading for each. Remember that consistent repetition is the best way to learn. Plan to read each reference at least once now and expect to read it again as you continue your studies.

References marked with (skim) can be read quickly and do not require commentary review.

CLASSICS		1st read	2nd read
Charaka	Cha. Sū. 21/25-59		
Suśhruta	Su. Śhā. 4/33-56		
Aṣhṭāṅga Hṛdaya	AH Sū. 7/53-68		
Bhāva Prakāśha			

JOURNALS & CURRENT RESOURCES

Concept of Swapna (Dream): An Ayurvedic Perspective, Dr. Kanchan Chowdhury, et al.
TRAYOPASTHAMBAS: THREE SUPPORTIVE PILLARS OF AYURVEDA, Bagde A. B., et al.

QUESTIONS & ANSWERS

Record your questions for this chapter here for further research and discussion.

Question:

Answer:

Question:

Answer:

Question:

Answer:

SELF-ASSESSMENT

1. Which of the following is a result of proper *nidrā*?
   a. *Bala*
   b. *Jñāna*
   c. *Puṣhṭi*
   d. *Sukha*
   e. All of the above

2. The term *nidrā* indicates going into a state of sleep. What does *svapna* indicate?
   a. Dream state
   b. Drowsiness
   c. Lying down
   d. Resting
   e. All of the above

3. Staying awake throughout the night can be considered
   a. *Kapha śhamana*
   b. *Rātri jāgaraṇa*
   c. *Rūkṣhatva*
   d. *Vāta prakopa*
   e. All of the above

4. Charaka states sleeping during *divā* causes
   a. Accumulation of the *doṣhas*
   b. *Vāta śhamana*
   c. *Kapha prakopa*
   d. *Snigdhatva*
   e. All of the above

5. Which type of sleep do Suśhruta and Charaka both describe?
   a. Exhaustion of the body
   b. Exhaustion of the mind
   c. *Rajas*
   d. *Tamas*
   e. *Sattva*

6. Why does Charaka state *rātri-svabhāva-prabhavā* is the best type of *nidrā*?
   a. It is *bhūtadhātrī*
   b. It is normal, healthy sleep
   c. It is caused by the special nature of the night
   d. It supports life and prevents diseases
   e. All of the above

7. Suśhruta states the primary location for *chetanā* is?
   a. All over the body
   b. *Hṛdaya*
   c. *Manas*
   d. *Sattva*
   e. All of the above

8. How does Charaka describe the normal physiology of *nidrā*?
   a. Combined abundance of *tamas*
   b. *Jñānendriya* cease to interact with their objects
   c. *Karmendriya* cease to express their functions
   d. The senses and action organs disengage from interaction
   e. All of the above

9. How does Suśhruta explain *svāpa*?
   a. Dreams are experienced by both *manas* and *rajas*
   b. *Manas* disengages from the body and experiences memories via the soul
   c. Memories from the soul, both good and bad
   d. Soul maintains authority over dreams
   e. All of the above

10. Charaka states proper sleep routines and habits are required to manage
    a. *Dhātu sāmyata*
    b. *Kṛśha*
    c. *Sthūla*
    d. B and C
    e. All of the above

CRITICAL THINKING

1. How could the causes for the different types of *nidrā* possibly be distinguished in a clinical setting? Use any one of the seven types and explain how you might try to assess its influence on an individual.

2. Why has Charaka explained *nidrā* in the context of *kṛśha* and *sthūla*? How could this influence recommendations for healthy sleep habits?

3. Explain the roles of *sattva*, *rajas* and *tamas* in the process of sleep.

4. Review Suśhruta's analogy of the heart and its role in sleep. Draw this analogy to represent an individual's state of being awake versus being asleep.

5. Do the classical Āyurvedic explanations of sleep apply to nocturnal animals? Explain your reasoning.

Chapter 23 : Manas, indriya, sattva-rajas-tamas

KEY TERMS

agni
ākāśha
anutva
ap
artha
ātma
āyu
chakṣhu
chetaḥ
chetanā
chintya
ekatva
gandha
ghrāṇa
guda
hasta
hṛdaya
indriya
indriya adhiṣhṭhāna
indriya artha
indriya buddhi
indriya dravya
jñānendriya
karmendriya
manas
mano guṇa
mano karma
mano viṣhaya
manovahā srotas
pāda
pañcha pañchaka
pṛthvi
rajas
rasa
rasana
rūpa
śhabda
samjñāvahā srotas
śhārīra
sattva
sparśha
sparśhana
śhrotra
tamas
tri-guṇa
ubhayātmaka
ubhayendriya
upastha
vāk
vāyu

Manas is an extensive and complex concept in classical Āyurveda. It is one of the major components responsible for maintaining and actualizing human life. While it is not directly attached to the human body in the same physical way that the *dhātus* are, it pervades the entire body and constantly moves through it. *Manas* is responsible for bringing the intentions of *ātma* to life. It coordinates all of the physical body's interactions with the outside world.

Manas is one of several key components that are involved in coordination of thoughts, understanding and actions. In classical explanations, its components and functions exist in a very extensive fashion throughout the texts. Here, these components and actions are being organized in the best way possible to maintain their true representation and allow them to be understood in a step-by-step, logical fashion.

While it is challenging to delineate these tightly woven concepts, this chapter will focus on *manas*, *indriya* and the *tri-guṇa* only in order to lay a clear foundation for additional concepts. In the Chapters 24 and 26, the complete picture of *manas*, *indriya*, and the remaining key components will be explained. These components, including *buddhi* (innate intelligence), *ahaṅkāra* (self-identify), *chetanā* (consciousness) and *ātma* (the soul), are responsible for creating active, conscious life beyond the logical control of *manas*.

Manas is produced as one of the outputs of *sṛṣhṭi utpatti*. Because of its generation as part of that process, its manifested outcome is strongly influenced by that sequence of events. Throughout this chapter, keep in mind that the *tri-guṇas* are the unifying concepts between *manas*, *ātma* and *śhārīra*. All components within the processes of *sṛṣhṭi utpatti* will be explained in detail in Chapter 26.

PARIBHĀṢHĀ AND PARYĀYA

The concept of *manas* has been elaborated and discussed throughout much of Vedic literature. In the context of Āyurveda, Charaka provides the most information in several chapters through the entire treatise.

Definition

Charaka provides several statements that provide insight as definitions for manas.

अतीन्द्रियं पुनर्मनः ... || ४

च. सू. ८।४

Atīndriyaṁ punarmanaḥ ... || 4

Cha. Sū. 8/4

Atīndriyaṁ (Beyond the *indriyas* [senses]) punarmanaḥ (is the mind, as stated before).

The simplicity of this statement likely assumes that the reader is already familiar with the concepts of *manas* from related branches of Vedic sciences and philosophies. This reference intends to remind the reader that manas is a key component of *āyu* but it is beyond the physical level of the *śharīra* where the *indriya* reside.

Because of the relationship between *manas* and the *indriya*, the *śharīra* is capable of experiencing the world around it and interacting with it.

मनःपुरःसराणीन्द्रियाण्यर्थग्रहणसमर्थानि भवन्ति || ७

च. सू. ८।७

Manaḥpuraḥsarāṇīndriyāṇyarthagrahaṇasamarthāni bhavanti || 7

Cha. Sū. 8/7

Manaḥ-puraḥ (Being in front of *manas*), sarāṇīndriyāṇy (the active senses) bhavanti (are) artha-grahaṇa (able to grasp their objects) samarthāni (in the correct way).

The presence of *manas* is required for normal functioning of *indriya*.

मनसस्तु चिन्त्यमर्थः | तत्र मनसो मनोबुद्धेश्च त एव समानातिहीनमिथ्यायोगाः प्रकृतिविकृतिहेतवो भवन्ति || १६

च. सू. ८।१६

Manasastu chintyamarthaḥ | Tatra manaso manobuddheśhcha ta eva samānātihīnamithyāyogāḥ prakṛtivikṛtihetavo bhavanti || 16

Cha. Sū. 8/16

Manas-astu (It is the responsibility of the mind) chintyam-arthaḥ (to think, deliberate, question, imagine, reflect upon or consider anything). Tatra (And so), manaso (when the mind) manobuddheśhcha (and the intellectual functions of the mind) bhavanti (are) samāna (correctly), ati (excessively), hīna (deficiently), mithyā (or improperly) yogāḥ (associated) ta eva (with their objects), prakṛti-vikṛti-hetavo (they become the cause for normal and abnormal states [of health]).

These three references provide a basic introduction to *manas*, its relationship with *indriya*, and the importance of its proper function for normal health.

Synonyms

Charaka mentions two synonyms for *manas*, *sattva* and *chetaḥ*.

सत्त्वसञ्ज्ञकं, 'चेतः' इत्याहुरेके,

च. सू. ८।४

Sattvasañjñakaṁ, 'chetaḥ' ityāhureke,

Cha. Sū. 8/4

Sattva-sañjñakaṁ (It is known as *sattva*), 'chetaḥ' ityāhureke (and also known by some as *chetaḥ*).

Sattva is an important synonym for *manas* as it connects the features and actions of *manas* to the *tri-guṇas*. Charaka states that *sattva* is

तत्र शुद्धमदोषमाख्यातं कल्याणांशत्वात् ... || ३६

च. शा. ४।३६

Tatra śhuddhamadoṣhamākhyātaṁ kalyāṇāṁśhatvāt ... | 4

Cha. Śhā. 4/36

Tatra (And so), śhuddham (the *śhuddha* [type of *manas*, ie, *sattva*]) adoṣham-ākhyātaṁ (is said to be free of *doṣha*) kalyāṇāṁ-śhatvāt (due to its composition of benevolence).

Cetaḥ is an equally important synonym for *manas*. It refers to *chittaṁ*, or the activation of consciousness. This is a key component of the generation of life which will be discussed in Chapters 24 and 26.

TEST YOURSELF

Learn, review and memorize key terms from this section.

indriya

manas

artha

chintya

sattva

chetaḥ

ROLE OF MANAS IN ĀYU

Manas is one of the four main components in *āyu*. It connects *ātma* to the physical body.

Recall that Charaka defines *āyu* as:

शरीरेन्द्रियसत्त्वात्मसंयोगो ... | ४२

च. सू. १।४२

Śharīrendriyasattvātmasaṁyogo ... | 42

Cha. Sū. 1/42

Śharīra (*Śharīra*, the physical body), indriya (*indriya*, the senses), sattva (*sattva*, or *manas*, the mind and) ātma (*ātma*, the soul) saṁyogo (in a combined state constitute *āyu*, or life).

These four are the most basic components required to support life. *Manas* plays a key role in this by connecting the *śhārīra* and its *indriya* to the *ātma*.

Manas is also included as one of the *adhyātma dravya-guṇa saṅgraha*. This group includes the *manas*, *mano-artha*, *buddhi* and *ātma*. This group will be discussed in Chapter 24.

Ultimately, *manas* is responsible for processing all information received from the *jñānendriya* and controlling the output of actions through the *karmendriya*. Because of this unique position over both types of *indriya*, *manas* is also referred to as *ubhayātmaka*, or *ubhayendriya*. Suśhruta mentions this in Su. Śhā. 1/4 by stating:

उभयात्मकं मनः ... || ४

सु. शा. १।४

Ubhayātmakaṁ manaḥ ... || 4

Su. Śhā. 1/4

Manaḥ (*Manas*) ubhaya-ātmakaṁ (acts as the controller of both [types of *indriya*]).

Because of this unique position that *manas* has over the *indriya* and essentially the physical body, it is often compared to a chariot in a simile. The horses are likened to the *indriya*, the chariot is considered the *śharīra*, and the chariot-driver is *manas*. When *manas* is in control of the *indriya*, the individual experiences a smooth, comfortable ride. However, when the *indriya*, or horses, take control of the reigns, anything can happen.

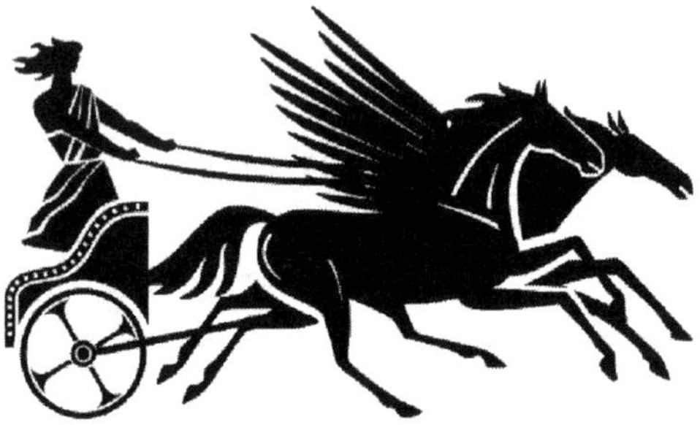

TEST YOURSELF

Learn, review and memorize key terms from this section.

manas

āyu

śhārīra

indriya

sattva

ātma

ubhayātmaka

ubhayendriya

jñānendriya

karmendriya

MANO STHĀNA

The location of *manas* is somewhat controversial. According to various authors, it is located in the heart or brain. Additionally, *manas* is said to travel throughout the body wherever *chetanā* exists.

Charaka and Suśhruta make reference to special *srotases* which allow *manas* to move throughout the body. In the context of the disorder *unmāda*, Charaka states that the pathology occurs in the *manovahā srotas*. Suśhruta describes the *samjñāvahā srotas* as the transportation system for *manas* in the physiology of sleep.

Charaka does mention the heart as being the main location for *manas* by referring to it through its synonyms.

Importance of the hṛdaya

In the 30th chapter of *Sūtra-sthāna*, Charaka explains the importance of *hṛdaya* as the major home location for the important components of life.

षडङ्गमङ्गं विज्ञानमिन्द्रियाण्यर्थपञ्चकम् |
आत्मा च सगुणश्चेतश्चिन्त्यं च हृदि संश्रितम्
|| ४

च. सू. ३०।४

Ṣhaḍaṅgamaṅgaṁ
vijñānamindriyāṇyarthapañchakam |
Ātmā cha saguṇaśhchetaśhchintyaṁ
cha hṛdi saṁśhritam || 4

Cha. Sū. 30/4

Ṣhaḍ-aṅgam (The six limbs of the body), aṅgaṁ (all of the bodily parts and organs), vijñānam (consciousness), indriyāṇy-artha-pañchakam (all of the *indriya*, their objects and five types of components), ātmā cha (and the soul) sa-guṇaśh (along with all of its qualities, ie the *ātmāguṇa*), chetaśh (as well as *chetaḥ*, or *manas*) chintyaṁ cha (and [its object or responsibility] thinking) saṁśhritam (all reside) hṛdi (in the heart).

Both *manas* and its main responsibility, *chintya*, are stated to be located in the heart. The additional components listed here must also be taken into consideration when considering the role of the heart in health and life.

To highlight the importance of the heart, Charaka goes on to explain its role in the body using a simile.

प्रतिष्ठार्थं हि भावानामेषां हृदयमिष्यते|
गोपानसीनामागारकर्णिकेवार्थचिन्तकैः || ५
तस्योपघातान्मूर्च्छायं भेदान्मरणमृच्छति | ६

च. सू. ३०|५-६

Pratiṣhṭhārthaṁ hi bhāvānāmeṣhāṁ
hṛdayamiṣhyate |
Gopānasīnāmāgārakarṇikevārthachinta
kaiḥ || 5
Tasyopaghātānmūrchchhāyaṁ
bhedānmaraṇamṛchchhati | 6

Cha. Sū. 30/5-6

Pratiṣhṭhārthaṁ hi (As the foundation for all these things [mentioned previously]), hṛdayamiṣhyate (the heart acts as) bhāvānāmeṣhāṁ (the house). Gopānasīnāmāgāra (Just as a house is protected or supported by) karṇikeva (its central girder), ārthachintakaiḥ (so does the heart support the mind, thoughts, etc [mentioned above]). || 5

Tasya upaghātān (And so if it [the heart] sustains any injury or damage), mūrchchhāyaṁ bhedān (it causes incurable loss of consciousness), maraṇa (death) mṛchchhati (or passing away).

Finally, Charaka summarizes and reemphasizes the key components supported by the heart.

यद्धि तत् स्पर्शविज्ञानं धारि तत्तत्र संश्रितम्
|| ६

च. सू. ३०|६

Yaddhi tat sparśhavijñānaṁ dhāri
tattatra saṁśhritam || 6

Cha. Sū. 30/6

Yaddhi tat (And that [heart]) tattatra saṁśhritam (is the primary location for) sparśha-vijñānaṁ (the knowledge or perception of touch sensation) dhāri (and life, ie, āyu).

TEST YOURSELF

Learn, review and memorize key terms from this section.

manas
___

chetanā
___

manovahā srotas
___

samjñāvahā srotas
___

hṛdaya
___

chintya

MANO GUṆA

Manas is known and understood to behave in specific ways based on its composition of *guṇas*. There are two types of classifications that explain its *guṇas*.

First, the creation of *manas* and the reason for its specific imprint of behaviors in any individual is largely based on its composition of the *tri-guṇas* at the moment when life is produced. The output or result of this is completely individualized as it is based on a cumulative result of *karma* and any influences during gestation.

Second, *manas* is understood through two specific *guṇas* that are generally considered universal principles. These explain certain behaviors and apparent actions of *manas* as they are seen in the majority of people.

Tri-guṇas

Recall that the *tri-guṇas* consist of *sattva*, *rajas* and *tamas*. The proportion of each of these in an individual produces certain mental behaviors, actions and characteristic tendencies.

Charaka describes the *tri-guṇas* as three general types of *sattva*, or *manas*.

त्रिविधं खलु सत्त्वं- शुद्धं, राजसं, तामसमिति| तत्र शुद्धमदोषमाख्यातं कल्याणांशत्वात्, राजसं सदोषमाख्यातं रोषांशत्वात्, तामसमपि सदोषमाख्यातं मोहांशत्वात् | ... || ३६

च. शा. ४।३६

Trividhaṁ khalu sattvaṁ - śhuddhaṁ, rājasaṁ, tāmasamiti | Tatra śhuddhamadoṣhamākhyātaṁ kalyāṇāṁśhatvāt, rājasaṁ sadoṣhamākhyātaṁ roṣhāṁśhatvāt, tāmasamapisadoṣhamākhyātaṁ mohāṁśhatvāt | ... || 36

Cha. Śhā. 4/36

Trividhaṁ (The three types) khalu (that are told) sattvaṁ (of *sattva* [ie, *manas*] are) - śhuddhaṁ (*śhuddha*, or pure *sattva*), rājasaṁ (*rājasa*, or predominated by action), tāmasamiti (and *tāmasa*, or predominated by inertia). Tatra (And so), śhuddham (the *śhuddha*, or pure type) adoṣham-ākhyātaṁ (is said to be free of *doṣha*) kalyāṇāṁśhatvāt (due to its high proportion of benevolence), rājasaṁ (the *rājasa*, or active type), sadoṣham-ākhyātaṁ (is said to be associated with *doṣha*) roṣhāṁśhatvāt (due to its high proportion of anger, rage, wrath, passion and fury), tāmasamapi (and the *tāmasa* type) sadoṣham-ākhyātaṁ (is said to be associated with *doṣha*) mohāṁśhatvāt (due to its high proportion of confusion, delusion, foolishness, inability to discriminate and error).

Suśhruta provides a more elaborate description of the characteristics seen in each of the three types.

सात्त्विकास्तु - आनृशंस्यं संविभागरुचिता तितिक्षा सत्यं धर्म आस्तिक्यं ज्ञानं बुद्धिर्मेधा स्मृतिर्धृतिरनभिषङ्गश्च; राजसास्तु - दुःखबहुलताऽटनशीलताऽधृतिरहङ्कार आनृतिकत्वमकारुण्यं दम्भो मानो हर्षः कामः क्रोधश्च; तामसास्तु - विषादित्वं नास्तिक्यमधर्मशीलता बुद्धेर्निरोधोऽज्ञानं दुर्मेधस्त्वमकर्मशीलता निद्रालुत्वं चेति ॥ १८

सु. शा. १।१८

Sāttvikāstu - ānṛśhaṁsyaṁ saṁvibhāgaruchitā titikṣhā satyaṁ dharma āstikyaṁ jñānaṁ buddhirmedhā smṛtirdhṛtiranabhiṣhaṅgaśhcha; rājasāstu - duḥkhabahulatā ' ṭanaśhīlatā ' dhṛtirahaṅkāra ānṛtikatvamakāruṇyaṁ dambho mano harṣhaḥ kāmaḥ krodhaśhcha; tāmasāstu - viṣhāditvaṁ nāstikyamadharmaśhīlatā buddhernirodho ' jñānaṁ durmedhastvamakarmaśhīlatā nidrālutvaṁ cheti || 18

Su. Śhā. 1/18

Sāttvikāstu (In *sāttvika* types of people, it is seen that they are) - ānṛśhaṁsyaṁ (kind, benevolent, compassionate), saṁvibhāga-ruchitā (mindfully aware of how they share and proportion the things which they like), titikṣhā (patient), satyaṁ (truthful), dharma (committed to their responsibilities), āstikyaṁ (believers in a higher power), jñānaṁ (knowledgeable), buddhir (well-connected to their innate intelligence and able to discriminate and act accordingly), medhā (wise), smṛtir (having a strong memory), dhṛtir (courageous, self-controlled), anabhiṣhaṅgaśhcha (and free from attachments); rājasāstu (in *rājasika* types of people, it is seen that they are) - duḥkha-bahulatā (very discontent, always dissatisfied), aṭana-śhīlatā (having the character trait of always wanting to move around), adhṛtir (unsteady, unable to control) ahaṅkāra (their sense of individuality), ānṛtikatvam (addicted to lying, being untruthful, or misrepresenting the truth), akāruṇyaṁ (harsh, cruel), dambho (fraudulent, deceitful, hypocritical), mano harṣhaḥ (always seeking ways to please their mind), kāmaḥ (lustful, passionate, sensual), krodhaśhcha (angry, wrathful); tāmasāstu (in *tāmasika* types of people, it is seen that they are) - viṣhāditvaṁ (full of grief or despair, despondent), nāstikyam (atheists), adharma-śhīlatā (having the character trait of always avoiding their responsibilities), buddher-nirodho (blocking their innate intelligence), ajñānaṁ (prone to ignorance), durmedhastvam (prone to lack of wisdom), akarma-śhīlatā (having the character trait of laziness, avoiding work and activities), nidrālutvaṁ cheti (and always sleepy or drowsy).

All three, *sattva*, *rajas* and *tamas*, are always present and required to function together as a whole to produce a proper state of health. Their proportion can be identified based on the recurrent characteristics and behaviors seen in an individual. Based on these repetitive behaviors, the predominance of a specific *tri-guṇa*, or type of *manas* can be determined.

यद्गुणं चाभीक्ष्णं पुरुषमनुवर्तते सत्त्वं तत्सत्त्वमेवोपदिशन्ति मुनयो बाहुल्यानुशयात् || ६

च. सू. ८।६

Yadguṇaṁ chābhīkṣhṇaṁ puruṣhamanuvartate sattvaṁ tatsattvamevopadiśhanti munayo bāhulyānuśhayāt || 6

Cha. Sū. 8/6

Yad-guṇaṁ (That *guṇa*, or characteristic) cha-abhīkṣhṇaṁ (which is constantly, repeatedly) puruṣham-anuvartate (demonstrated or present in the individual's) sattvaṁ (*sattva* [ie, *mānasika prakṛti*]) tat-sattvam-eva-upadiśhanti (is said to be that type of *sattva*) munayo bāhulyānuśhayāt (which is predominant in him, according to the experts).

The qualities and characteristics of each of the *tri-guṇa* can be reviewed in the following tables.

Sattva guṇa (śhuddha) with nearest English equivalent	Cha. Śhā. 4/36	Su. Śhā. 1/18
Adoṣham-ākhyātaṁ kalyāṇāṁśhatvāt Said to be free of doṣha due to its high proportion of benevolence	✓	
Ānṛśhaṁsya Kind, benevolent, compassionate		✓
Saṁvibhāga-ruchitā Mindfully aware of how they share and proportion the things which they like		✓
Titikṣhā Patient		✓
Satya Truthful		✓
Dharma Committed to their responsibilities		✓
Āstikya Believers in a higher power		✓
Jñāna Knowledgable		✓
Buddhi Well-connected to their innate intelligence and able to discriminate and act accordingly		✓
Medhā Wise		✓
Smṛti Having a strong memory		✓
Dhṛti Courageous, self-controlled		✓
Anabhiṣhaṅga Free from attachments		✓

Rājasa guṇa with nearest English equivalent	Cha. Śhā. 4/36	Su. Śhā. 1/18
Sadoṣham-ākhyātaṁ roṣhāṁśhatvāt Said to be associated with *doṣha* due to its high proportion of anger, rage, wrath, passion and fury	✓	
Duḥkha-bahulatā Very discontent, always dissatisfied		✓
Aṭana-śhīlatā Having the character trait of always wanting to move around		✓
Adhṛti ahaṅkāra Unsteady, unable to control their sense of individuality		✓
Ānṛtikatva Addicted to lying, being untruthful, or misrepresenting the truth		✓
Akāruṇya Harsh, cruel		✓
Dambho Fraudulent, deceitful, hypocritical		✓
Mano harṣhaḥ Always seeking ways to please their mind		✓
Kāmaḥ Lustful, passionate, sensual		✓
Krodha Angry, wrathful		✓

Tāmasa guṇa with nearest English equivalent	Cha. Śhā. 4/36	Su. Śhā. 1/18
Sadoṣham-ākhyātaṁ mohāṁśhatvāt Said to be associated with doṣha due to its high proportion of confusion, delusion, foolishness, inability to discriminate and error	✓	
Viṣhāditva Full of grief or despair, despondent		✓
Nāstikya Atheists		✓
Adharma-śhīlatā Having the character trait of always avoiding their responsibilities		✓
Buddher-nirodho Blocking their innate intelligence		✓
Ajñāna Prone to ignorance		✓
Durmedhastva Prone to lack of wisdom		✓
Akarma-śhīlatā Having the character trait of laziness, avoiding work and activities		✓
Nidrālutva Always sleepy or drowsy		✓

Mano guṇas

The *mano guṇas* are two specific features of *manas* that are described in order to explain certain behaviors of *manas*. These may appear to function in a way that is contradictory to the actual behavior.

स्वार्थेन्द्रियार्थसङ्कल्पव्यभिचरणाच्चानेकमेकस्मिन् पुरुषे सत्त्वं,
रजस्तमःसत्त्वगुणयोगाच्च; न चानेकत्वं,
नह्येकं ह्येककालमनेकेषु प्रवर्तते ;
तस्मान्नैककाला सर्वेन्द्रियप्रवृत्तिः || ५

च. सू. ८।५

Svārthendriyārthasaṅkalpavyabhicharaṇāchchānekamekasmin puruṣhe sattvaṁ, rajastamaḥsattvaguṇayogāchcha; na chānekatvaṁ, nahyekaṁ hyekakālamanekeṣhu pravartate; tasmānnaikakālā sarvendriyapravṛttiḥ || 5

Cha. Sū. 8/5

Ekamekasmin puruṣhe (In a single individual), svārthendriya (their own *indriya*), artha-saṅkalpa (variations in the objects of perception), vyabhicharaṇāchchān sattvaṁ (uncertainty causing the mind to change), rajas (and *rajas*), tamaḥ (*tamas*) sattva (and *sattva*) guṇa (*guṇa*) yogāchcha (combinations) na chānekatvaṁ (might make it appear that the mind is not just one entity). Nahyekaṁ (But this is not true, and the mind is only one) hyekakālamanekeṣhu pravartate (as there is only contact with one object at a time); tasmānnaikakālā sarvendriyapravṛttiḥ (not all of the indriya are in contact with their objects all of the time).

Due to the speed of the mind, it may appear that more than one activity is occurring at the same time. However, Charaka emphasizes here that it is not the case. Instead, the mind is only able to process one thing at a time.

In a similar yet more concise reference, *manas* is stated to have two specific *guṇas* - *aṇutva* and *ekatva*.

अणुत्वमथ चैकत्वं द्वौ गुणौ मनसः स्मृतौ || १९

च. शा. १।१९

Aṇutvamatha chaikatvaṁ dvau guṇau manasaḥ smṛtau || 19

Cha. Śhā. 1/19

Aṇutvam (Minuteness, or atomic nature) atha chaikatvaṁ (and singularity, or oneness) dvau guṇau (are the two characteristics) manasaḥ (of *manas*) smṛtau (that must be known).

TEST YOURSELF

Learn, review and memorize key terms from this section.

mano guṇa

tri-guṇa

sattva

rajas

tamas

anutva

ekatva

MANO KARMA

The main action of *manas* is to think, as defined by Charaka ("*Manasastu chintyamarthaḥ,*" Cha. Sū. 8/16). Additionally, manas is responsible for several key functions that allow for various types of mental processing.

इन्द्रियाभिग्रहः कर्म मनसः स्वस्य निग्रहः|
ऊहो विचारश्च, ततः परं बुद्धिः प्रवर्तते || २१

च. शा. १।२१

Indriyābhigrahaḥ karma manasaḥ svasya nigrahaḥ | Ūho vichāraśhcha tataḥ paraṁ buddhiḥ pravartate || 21

Cha. Śhā. 1/21

Indriyābhigrahaḥ (Taking and maintaining control of the *indriya*), karma (is the action and responsibility) manasaḥ (of *manas*) svasya nigrahaḥ ([along with] restraint of the self), ūho (deduction), vichāraśhcha (and contemplation). Tataḥ (Beyond this) paraṁ (the absolute) buddhiḥ (power of the innate intelligence) pravartate (begins).

Manas is responsible for specific actions and processes of thought up to a certain point. Beyond that, the individual's *buddhi*, or innate intelligence takes over. This is one of the products generated through *sṛṣhṭi utpatti* which will be discussed in Chapter 26.

In order for *manas* to be able to accomplish these actions, it must be in direct contact with the *indriya*. Without that contact, information cannot be gathered, processed and acted upon. Charaka explains this connection using the specific technical term, *sannikarṣha*, which derives from classical Vedic philosophies.

लक्षणं मनसो ज्ञानस्याभावो भाव एव च|
सति ह्यात्मेन्द्रियार्थानां सन्निकर्षे न वर्तते ||
१८
लक्षणं मनसो ज्ञानस्याभावो भाव एव च | ...
१९

च. शा. १।१८

Lakṣhaṇaṁ manaso jñānasyābhāvo bhāva eva cha | Sati hyātmendriyārthānāṁ sannikarṣhe na vartate || 18
Vaivṛttyānmanaso jñānaṁ sānnidhyāttachcha vartate | ... 19

Cha. Śhā. 1/18

Lakṣhaṇaṁ (Characteristics) jñānasyābhāvo (may not be known) bhāva eva cha (or even might be known) manaso (by the mind) sati hyātmendriyārthānāṁ (depending on the *ātma*'s ability) sannikarṣhe (to connect with the objects of the *indriya*); na vartate (otherwise, it does not occur). Vaivṛttyānmanaso (When the mind is not interrupted) jñānaṁ (the knowledge, understanding, or processing of information) sānnidhyāttachcha vartate (approximates and can occur).

This explanation highlights the key connecting role that the *manas* plays in receiving information through the *indriya* so that it can be enacted upon correctly. When *manas* is able to concentrate and fully connect with the *indriya*, the quality of the information received is higher. And when *manas* is unable to focus and connect with the *indriya*, the information may not be received at all, or may be false or misunderstood.

Mano viṣhaya

When *manas* engages in action, it focuses its processes of thinking on specific objects. These are known as the *mano viṣhaya*.

चिन्त्यं विचार्यमूह्यं च ध्येयं सङ्कल्प्यमेव च |
यत्किञ्चिन्मनसो ज्ञेयं तत् सर्वं ह्यर्थसञ्ज्ञकम्
|| २०

च. शा. १।२०

Chintyaṁ vichāryamūhyaṁ cha
dhyeyaṁ saṅkalpyameva cha |
Yatkiñchinmanaso jñeyaṁ tat sarvaṁ
hyarthasañjñakam || 20

Cha. Śhā. 1/20

Chintyaṁ (Thinking), vichāryam (choosing), ūhyaṁ (predicting), cha (and) dhyeyaṁ (meditating), saṅkalpyameva cha (and willfully intending) yat kiñchinmanaso jñeyaṁ (and whatever can be known by the mind) tat sarvaṁ hyarthasañjñakam (are all to be considered its objects [of perception]).

Each of these terms carries a specific, significant meaning. Review these terms along with their definitions and roots.

Mano viṣhaya	Definitions and nearest English explanation
Chintya Thinking	From √ *chint*, derived from the Sanskrit *dhātu* √ *chit* *Chintya* means to be thought about or imagined, to be considered or reflected or meditated upon, to be deliberated about, questionable. *Chint* means to think, have a thought or idea, reflect, consider, to think about, reflect upon, direct the thoughts towards. *Chit* means to perceive, fix the mind upon, attend to, be attentive, observe, take notice of, to understand, comprehend, know.
Vichārya Choosing	Chakrapāṇi defines *vichāra* as: ÏÞ¸ lÐΣ° ΨΣǿdı ΨlÞ™l ÏÞ¯ ÿœøµ p̱ (¸ 7 p- ¸ . ¼l. b_cb) Vichāro heyopādeyāvayā vikalpanam | Cha. Śhā. 1/21 (Cakr.) *Vicāra* refers to the ability to make the correct choice from various options.
Ūhya Predicting	Chakrapāṇi defines *ūhya* as: ç ° l | ½Σ̧ øl¾løˈÈǿÏÞž ÿœµ p̱ (¸ 7 p- ¸ . ¼l. b_cb) Ūhyā ālochanājñānaṁ nirvikalpam | Cha. Śhā. 1/21 (Cakr.) *Ūhyā* refers to the ability to utilize knowledge outside of direct observation, which is not dependent on the senses.
Dhyeya Meditating	*Dhyeya* (from √ *dhyai*) means to be meditated on, fit for meditation, to be pondered or imagined. *Dhyai* means to think of, imagine, contemplate, meditate on, call to mind, recollect (with *manasā*, *chetasā*, *dhiyā*, *hṛdaya*, etc). *Dhyeya* extends beyond the realm of *manas* alone and is considered an action of *ahaṅkāra* and *buddhi* (see Chapters 24 and 26).
Saṅkalpya Willfully intending	*Saṅkalpya* (from *saṁkalpa*) means a conception or idea or notion formed in the mind or heart, especially will, volition, desire, purpose, definite intention or determination or decision or wish for, sentiment, conviction, persuasion. *Saṅkalpya* extends beyond the realm of *manas* alone and is considered an action of *ahaṅkāra* and *buddhi* (see Chapters 24 and 26).

TEST YOURSELF

Learn, review and memorize key terms from this section.

mano karma

---

mano viṣhaya

INDRIYA

One of *manas*' primary *karmas* is *indriyābhigrahaḥ*, taking and maintaining control of the *indriya* (Cha. Śhā. 1/21). As the *ubhayendriya*, or main controller of both the *jñānendriya* and *karmendriya*, *manas* maintains a unique and important position in the functional processing of information and all actions that ensue.

Charaka introduces the process of how information is received through the *indriya* and then reviewed by *manas*. Logical consideration of the information is made by *manas* itself, while the determination of how to act upon it generally includes additional components such as *ahaṅkāra* and *buddhi*.

इन्द्रियेणेन्द्रियार्थो हि समनस्केन गृह्यते| कल्प्यते मनसा तूर्ध्वं गुणतो दोषतोऽथवा || २२

च. शा. १।२२

Indriyeṇendriyārtho hi samanaskena gṛhyate | Kalpyate manasā tūrdhvaṁ guṇato doṣhato ' thavā || 22

Cha. Śhā. 1/22

Indriyeṇa (Thus, the *indriya*) samanaskena (always) gṛhyate (grasp) indriyārtho hi (their own objects) kalpyate (with the interaction) manasā (of the mind). Tūrdhvaṁ (Initially), guṇato (the *guṇas* [are perceived]); doṣhato (while the understanding of the *doṣhas*) athavā (follows later).

The mind initially receives information about the overall characteristics and features of any situation. To process this information and determine its good or bad features, right or wrong applications, etc, it takes some amount of time. The remaining processes of thinking, considering, hypothesizing and choosing the desired course of action do not happen instantaneously.

All authors accept the existence of five *jñānendriya* consistently. Charaka lists these as:

एकैकाधिकयुक्तानि खादीनामिन्द्रियाणि तु| पञ्च कर्मानुमेयानि येभ्यो बुद्धिः प्रवर्तते || २४

च. शा. १।२४

Ekaikādhikayuktāni khādīnāmindriyāṇi tu | Pañcha karmānumeyāni yebhyo buddhiḥ pravartate || 24

Cha. Śhā. 1/24

Ekaikādhikayuktāni (Each one of the *indriya* contains a predominance of one of each) khādīnāmindriyāṇi tu (of *kha* [ie, *ākāśha*] etc). Pañcha karmānumeyāni (Each of the five has its own specific actions) yebhyo buddhiḥ pravartate (which are the result of their respective *buddhi*).

The explanation provided here describes the core connections between the *indriya*, their primary *mahābhūta* and their respective *buddhi*. The connections are created during the process of *sṛṣhṭi utpatti* and produce the unique composition of each individual at the level of their *indriya*.

Jñānendriya

The five *jñānendriya* include the five senses that are capable of receiving information of the surrounding world based on the intentions and direction of *manas*.

तत्र चक्षुः श्रोत्रं घ्राणं रसनं स्पर्शनमिति पञ्चेन्द्रियाणि || ८

च. सू. ८।८

Tatra chakṣhuḥ śhrotraṁ ghrāṇaṁ rasanaṁ sparśhanamiti pañchendriyāṇi || 8

Cha. Sū. 8/8

Tatra (And so), chakṣhuḥ (*chakṣhu*, the eye [producing the sense of vision]), śhrotraṁ (*śhrotra*, the ear [producing the sense of hearing]), ghrāṇaṁ (*ghrāṇa*, the nose [producing the sense of smell]), rasanaṁ (*rasana*, the tongue [producing the sense of taste]), sparśhanamiti (and *sparśhana*, the skin [producing the sense of touch]) pañchendriyāṇi (are the five [*jñāna*] *indriya*).

Each of the *jñānendriya* also contains a predominance of a specific *mahābhūta* that allows it to function in its own particular way.

महाभूतानि खं वायुरग्निरापः क्षितिस्तथा | शब्दः स्पर्शश्च रूपं च रसो गन्धश्च तद्गुणाः || २७

च. शा. १।२७

Mahābhūtāni khaṁ vāyuragnirāpaḥ kṣhitistathā | Śhabdaḥ sparśhaśhcha rūpaṁ cha raso gandhaśhcha tadguṇāḥ || 27

Cha. Śhā. 1/27

Mahābhūtāni (The *mahābhūtas* include) khaṁ (*ākāśha*), vāyur (*vāyu*), agnir (*agni*), āpaḥ (*ap*), kṣhitistathā (and *pṛthvi*). Śhabdaḥ (*śhabda*, or sound), sparśhaśhcha (*sparśha*, or touch), rūpaṁ (*rūpa*, or vision) cha raso (*rasa*, or taste) gandhaśhcha (and *gandha*, or smell) tadguṇāḥ (are each of their *guṇas*).

In the order described above, each of the *mahābhūtās* is associated to a specific *guṇa*. Recall from Chapter 3 that these are also the *viśheṣha guṇas* attributed to each *mahābhūtā*.

The *viśheṣha guṇa* is the specific quality accessible to that *bhūta* alone and is determined by each *bhūta*'s unique connection to a single sense. This relationship is based on the order of generation of the *bhūtas* during the formation of *pañcha tanmātras* (see Chapter 26).

These *guṇas* represent the attributes found in any *dravya* that is predominant in a specific *mahābhūta*. Every *dravya* contains a composition of all *mahābhūtas* with a certain predominance. Therefore, the *viśheṣha guṇas* must also exist in a proportionate manner. Charaka explains this as:

तेषामेकगुणः पूर्वो गुणवृद्धिः परे परे | पूर्वः पूर्वगुणश्चैव क्रमशो गुणिषु स्मृतः || २८

च. शा. १।२८

Teṣhāmekaguṇaḥ pūrvo guṇavṛddhiḥ pare pare | Pūrvaḥ pūrvaguṇaśhchaiva kramaśho guṇiṣhu smṛtaḥ || 28

Cha. Śhā. 1/28

Teṣhām (Of the five [*mahābhūtas* listed previously, following the same order]) eka-guṇaḥ pūrvo (the first one has one *guṇa*) guṇa-vṛddhiḥ (and one *guṇa* is added) pare pare (with each of the succeeding ones [ie, each succeding *bhūta*]). Pūrvaḥ pūrvaguṇaśhchaiva (Each prior one is added to the next one) kramaśho (consecutively) guṇiṣhu (in that which has the *guṇa*) smṛtaḥ (is how it is known).

This concept of *guṇa-vṛddhi* applies to both *dravya* and the *indriya*. Note that the application of cumulative increase of each *bhūta* with its preceding *bhūta* is stated to be based on a mathematical rule. However, the classics do not specify an exact formula for this. There are several factors to consider based on the *bhūta*'s composition, mass, *guṇa* and *karma*. This progression occurs because a *bhūta* maintains the major "leader" position in the overall proportion and is the predominant one.

तत्रानुमानगम्यानां
पञ्चमहाभूतविकारसमुदायात्मकानामपि
सतामिन्द्रियाणां तेजश्चक्षुषि, खं श्रोत्रे, घ्राणे
क्षितिः, आपो रसने,स्पर्शनेऽनिलो
विशेषेणोपपद्यते| तत्र यद्यदात्मकमिन्द्रियं
विशेषात्तत्तदात्मकमेवार्थमनुगृह्णाति,
तत्स्वभावाद्विभुत्वाच्च || १४

च. सू. ८।१४

Tatrānumānagamyānāṁ
pañchamahābhūtavikārasamudāyātmak
ānāmapi satāmindriyāṇāṁ
tejaśhchakṣhuṣhi, khaṁ śhrotre, ghrāṇe
kṣhitiḥ, āpo rasane, sparśhane ' nilo
viśheṣheṇopapadyate | Tatra
yadyadātmakamindriyaṁ
viśheṣhāttattadātmakamevārthamanugṛ
hṇāti, tatsvabhāvādvibhutvāchcha || 14

Cha. Sū. 8/14

Tatra (And so), anumāna-gamyānāṁ (being known through *anumāna*, or inference), pañcha-mahābhūta (the five *mahābhūta*) vikāra (in their manifestations) samudāyātmakānāmapi (and combinations) satāmindriyāṇāṁ (comprise the *indriya* of which), tejaśhchakṣhuṣhi (*tejas* is predominant in the eyes), khaṁ śhrotre (*ākāśha* is predominant in the ears), ghrāṇe kṣhitiḥ (*pṛthvi* is predominant in the nose), āpo rasane (*ap* is predominant in the tongue), sparśhane anilo (and *vāyu* is predominant in the skin) viśheṣheṇa upapadyate (and each exists especially in these locations). Tatra (And so), yadyad ātmakamindriyaṁ (each *indriya* inherently) anugṛhṇāti (grasps) viśheṣhāttattad (the specific information) ātmakamevārtham (based on its main, inherent constituent [ie, the *mahābhūta* which is predominant]), tat (that [is due to]) svabhāvād (the nature of) vibhutvāchcha (the ubiquitous presence of all components).

Based on the preceding descriptions, the *indriya* and all of their related components are summarized in the following table.

Jñānendriya	Mahābhūtā	Guṇa	Guṇa-vṛddhi
Śhrotra	Ākāśha	Śhabda	Ākāśha Śhabda
Sparśhana	Vāyu	Sparśha	Vāyu + Ākāśha Sparśha + Śhabda
Cakṣhu	Agni	Rūpa	Agni + Vāyu + Ākāśha Rūpa + Sparśha + Śhabda
Rasana	Ap	Rasa	Ap + Agni + Vāyu + Ākāśha Rasa + Rūpa + Sparśha + Śhabda

Ghrāṇa	Pṛthvi	Gandha	Pṛthvi + Ap + Agni + Vāyu + Ākāśha Gandha + Rasa + Rūpa + Sparśha + Śhabda

Karmendriya

The *karmendriya* include the five organs of action that are capable of producing effects based on the intentions and direction of manas.

हस्तौ पादौ गुदोपस्थं वागिन्द्रियमथापि च |
कर्मेन्द्रियाणि पञ्चैव पादौ गमनकर्मणि ||
२५
पायूपस्थं विसर्गार्थं हस्तौ ग्रहणधारणे |
जिह्वा वागिन्द्रियं वाक् च सत्या
ज्योतिस्तमोऽनृता || २६

च. शा. १।२५-२६

Hastau pādau gudopasthaṁ vāgindriyamathāpi cha | Karmendriyāṇi pañchaiva pādau gamanakarmaṇi || 25
Pāyūpasthaṁ visargārthaṁ hastau grahaṇadhāraṇe | Jihvā vāgindriyaṁ vāk ca satyā jyotistamo ' nṛtā || 26

Cha. Śhā. 1/25-26

Hastau (The two hands), pādau (the two feet), guda (the anus), upasthaṁ (the genitals), vāk (and the tongue) indriyamathāpi cha karmendriyāṇi pañchaiva (are the five action organs). Pādau (The two feet) gamana-karmaṇi (provide the action of going, walking, movement) pāya (the anus) ūpasthaṁ (and the genital organ) visargārthaṁ (provide the action of passing excretory materials), hastau (the two hands) grahaṇa-dhāraṇe (grasp and also hold, or support), jihvā (the tongue) vāg-indriyaṁ (produces the sense of speech), vāk cha (as well as speech itself), satyā (which when true promotes) jyotis (brightness, intelligence, especially innate intelligence) tamo anṛtā (or ignorance, errors, mental confusion when false).

The *pañcha karmendriya* are not associated with *mahābhūtas* but have primary *karma* instead. Review these in the following table.

Karmendriya Action organs	Karma Primary actions
Hastau The two hands	*Grahaṇa-dhāraṇe* Grasp and also hold, or support
Pādau The two feet	*Gamana-karmaṇi* Provide the action of going, walking, movement
Guda or *pāyu* The anus	*Visargārtha* Provide the action of passing excretory materials
Upastha The genital organ	*Visargārtha* Provide the action of passing excretory materials

Vāk The tongue	*Vāg-indriyaṁ, vāk ca satyā jyotistamo anṛtā* Produces the sense of speech as well as speech itself, which when true promotes brightness, intelligence, (especially innate intelligence) or ignorance, errors, mental confusion when false

TEST YOURSELF

Learn, review and memorize key terms from this section.

indriya

ubhayendriya

jñānendriya

karmendriya

śhrotra

sparśhana

chakṣhu

rasana

ghrāṇa

ākāśha

vāyu

agni

ap

pṛthvi

śhabda

sparśha

rūpa

rasa

gandha

hasta

pāda

guda

upastha

vāk

PAÑCHA PAÑCHAKA

The complexities of the *pañcha jñānendriya* are detailed and clarified through the framework of the *pañcha pañchaka*. This structure includes five aspects of the *jñānendriya* and explains how each component functions in the process of gathering information to send to *manas*.

इह खलु पञ्चेन्द्रियाणि, पञ्चेन्द्रियद्रव्याणि,
पञ्चेन्द्रियाधिष्ठानानि, पञ्चेन्द्रियार्थाः,
पञ्चेन्द्रियबुद्धयो
भवन्ति,इत्युक्तमिन्द्रियाधिकारे || ३

च. सू. ८।३

Iha khalu pañchendriyāṇi,
pañchendriyadravyāṇi,
pañchendriyādhiṣhṭhānāni,
pañchendriyārthāḥ,
pañchendriyabuddhayo bhavanti,
ityuktamindriyādhikāre || 3

Cha. Sū. 8/3

Iha khalu (In this school of practice), pañcha-indriyāṇi (the five *indriya*, or five senses), pañcha-indriya dravyāṇi (the five *indriya dravya*, or five predominant elements of the senses), pañcha-indriya adhiṣhṭhānāni (the five *indriya adhiṣhṭhāna*, or five locations of the senses), pañcha-indriya arthāḥ (the five *indriya artha*, or five objects of the senses), pañcha-indriya buddhayo (and the five *indriya buddhi*, or five sensory processing centers) bhavanti (are) ityuktam (thus known as) indriyādhikāre (the controllers of the senses).

Charaka reiterates these components in the context of describing *śhārīra* in Cha. Śhā. 7/7.

Following their initial introduction, each of the components of the *pañcha pañchaka* are identified and listed. Detailed explanations are not provided in the same references. Instead, it is expected that the reader be familiar with the terminology used in the framework to understand the application of concepts.

The *pañcha-indriya*, or five senses, include:

तत्र चक्षुः श्रोत्रं घ्राणं रसनं स्पर्शनमिति
पञ्चेन्द्रियाणि || ८

च. सू. ८।८

Tatra chakṣhuḥ śhrotraṁ ghrāṇaṁ
rasanaṁ sparśhanamiti pañcendriyāṇi ||
8

Cha. Sū. 8/8

Tatra (And so), chakṣhuḥ (the eyes), śhrotraṁ (the ears), ghrāṇaṁ (the nose), rasanaṁ (the tongue) sparśhanamiti (and the skin) pañcendriyāṇi (are the *pañcha-indriya*, or five senses).

These five physical structures represent the organs that house the senses.

The *pañcha-indriya dravya*, or the five predominant elements of the senses, include:

पञ्चेन्द्रियद्रव्याणि- खं वायुर्ज्योतिरापो
भूरिति || ९

च. सू. ८।९

Pañchendriyadravyāṇi - khaṁ
vāyurjyotirāpo bhūriti || 9

Cha. Sū. 8/9

Pañchendriyadravyāṇi (The *pañcha-indriya dravya*, or the five predominant elements of the senses include) khaṁ (*ākāśha*), vāyur (*vāyu*), jyotir (*tejas*), āpo (*ap*) bhūriti (and *pṛthvi*).

Each *bhūta* is the predominant *bhūta* found in its corresponding *indriya*. It is the particular bhūta that can be received through that one *indriya*.

The *pañcha-indriya adhiṣhṭhāna*, or the five locations of the senses, include:

पञ्चेन्द्रियाधिष्ठानानि- अक्षिणी कर्णौ
नासिके जिह्वा त्वक् चेति || १०

च. सू. ८।१०

Pañchendriyādhiṣhṭhānāni - akṣhiṇī
karṇau nāsike jihvā tvak cheti || 10

Cha. Sū. 8/10

Pañchendriyādhiṣhṭhānāni (The *pañcha-indriya adhiṣhṭhāna*, or the five locations of the senses, include) - akṣhiṇī (the eyes), karṇau (both ears), nāsike (the nose), jihvā (the tongue), tvak ceti (and the skin).

The *pañcha-indriya artha*, or five objects of

the senses, include:

पञ्चेन्द्रियार्थाः- शब्दस्पर्शरूपरसगन्धाः || ११

च. सू. ८।११

Pañchendriyārthāḥ - śhabdasparśharūparasagandhāḥ || 11

Cha. Sū. 8/11

Pañcha-indriya-arthāḥ (The *pañcha-indriya artha*, or the five objects of the senses, include) – śhabda (sound), sparśha (touch), rūpa (sight), rasa (taste), gandhāḥ (and smell).

The *pañcha-indriya buddhi*, or five sensory processing centers, include:

पञ्चेन्द्रियबुद्धयः - चक्षुर्बुद्ध्यादिकाः ताः पुनरिन्द्रियेन्द्रियार्थसत्त्वात्मसन्निकर्षजाः क्षणिका निश्चयात्मिकाश्च इत्येतत्पञ्चपञ्चकम् || १२

च. सू. ८।१२

Pañchendriyabuddhayaḥ - chakṣhurbuddhyādikāḥ tāḥ punarindriyendriyārthasattvātmasannikarṣhajāḥ kṣhaṇikā niśhchayātmikāśhcha ityetat pañchapañchakam || 12

Cha. Sū. 8/12

Pañchendriyabuddhayaḥ (The five sensory processing centers include) - chakṣhur-buddhyādikāḥ (the *chakṣhu-buddhi*, or the vision processing center), tāḥ punar (and the remaining *indriyas* along with their own *indirya buddhi*). Sannikarṣhajāḥ (Due to their close proximity or contact with) indriya (the sense), indriya artha (the object of the sense), sattva (the mind), ātma (and the soul), kṣhaṇikā (momentary) niśhchayātmikāśhcha (but definitive contacts are produced), ityetat (and these are known as) pañchapañchakam (the five-component framework of the senses).

Indriya Senses	Indriya dravya Predominant elements of the senses	Indriya adhiṣhṭhāna Locations of the senses	Indriya artha Objects of the senses	Indriya buddhi Sensory processing centers
Cakṣhu The eyes	*Agni* Fire	*Akṣhiṇī* The eyes	*Rūpa* Sight	*Cakṣhu-buddhi* Vision processing center
Śhrotra The ears	*Ākāśha* Space	*Karṇau* Both ears	*Śhabda* Hearing	*Śhrotra-buddhi* Hearing processing center
Ghrāṇa The nose	*Pṛthvi* Earth	*Nāsika* The nose	*Gandha* Smell	*Ghrāṇa-buddhi* Smell processing center
Rasana The tongue	*Ap* Water	*Jihvā* The tongue	*Rasa* Taste	*Rasaṇa-buddhi* Taste processing center
Sparśhana The skin	*Vāyu* Air	*Tvak* The skin	*Sparśha* Touch	*Sparśhana-buddhi* Touch processing center

TEST YOURSELF

Learn, review and memorize
key terms from this section.

pañcha
pañchaka

---

indriya

---

indriya
dravya

---

indriya
adhiṣhṭhāna

---

indriya artha

---

indriya
buddhi

Chapter 23: Review

ADDITIONAL READING

Read and review the references listed below to expand your understanding of the concepts in this chapter. Write down the date that you complete your reading for each. Remember that consistent repetition is the best way to learn. Plan to read each reference at least once now and expect to read it again as you continue your studies.

References marked with (skim) can be read quickly and do not require commentary review.

CLASSICS		1st read	2nd read
Charaka	Cha. Sū. 8/ Cha. Śhā. 1/		
Suśhruta	Su. Śhā. 1/		
Aṣhṭāṅga Hṛdaya			
Bhāva Prakāśha			

JOURNALS & CURRENT RESOURCES

QUESTIONS & ANSWERS

Record your questions for this chapter here for further research and discussion.

Question:

Answer:

Question:

Answer:

Question:

Answer:

SELF-ASSESSMENT

1. What are the core functions of *manas* as stated by Charaka?
   a. *Manas* thinks, questions, imagines, or considers anything
   b. *Manas* and *indriya* are the ultimate controllers of *śharīra*
   c. *Indriya* can act on their own through their *indriya buddhi*
   d. *Manas* is capable of performing multiple tasks simultaneously
   e. None of the above

2. Which synonym of *manas* indicates it is free of *doṣhas*?
   a. *Artha*
   b. *Chetaḥ*
   c. *Chintya*
   d. *Indriya*
   e. *Sattva*

3. What acts as the controller of *jñānendriya* and *karmendriya*?
   a. *Manas*
   b. *Ubhayātmaka*
   c. *Ubhayendriya*
   d. A and C
   e. All of the above

4. Where does Charaka state *manas* is located?
   a. *Hṛdaya*
   b. *Manovahā srotas*
   c. *Samjñāvahā srotas*
   d. Where *chetanā* exists
   e. All of the above

5. *Sattva guṇa* is *śhuddha*. Which of the following describes *śhuddha*?
   a. Connected to innate intelligence
   b. Kind, benevolent, compassionate
   c. Truthful, with a high sense of responsibility
   d. Wise and knowledgeable
   e. All of the above

6. Charaka states *manas* is *anutva* and *ekatva*. What does this mean?
   a. Capable of atomic and single processing
   b. *Mano guṇas*
   c. *Tri-guṇa*
   d. A and B
   e. All of the above

7. *Mano viṣhaya* refers to which of the following?
   a. *Chintya*
   b. *Dhyeya*
   c. *Saṅkalpya*
   d. *Ūhya* and *vichārya*
   e. All of the above

8. The concept of *guṇa-vṛddhi* applies to which of the following?
   a. *Dravya*
   b. *Indriya*
   c. *Mahābhūtas*
   d. A and B
   e. All of the above

9. Which of the following *pañcha pañchaka* relates to the *adhiṣhṭhāna* of *chakṣhu indriya*?
   a. *Indriya adhiṣhṭhāna akṣhiṇī*
   b. *Indriya adhiṣhṭhāna jihvā*
   c. *Indriya adhiṣhṭhāna karṇau*
   d. *Indriya adhiṣhṭhāna nāsika*
   e. *Indriya adhiṣhṭhāna tvak*

10. Which of the following *pañcha pañchaka* relates to the *dravya* of *rasana indriya*?
    a. *Indriya dravya agni*
    b. *Indriya dravya ākāśha*
    c. *Indriya dravya ap*
    d. *Indriya dravya pṛthvi*
    e. *Indriya dravya vāyu*

CRITICAL THINKING

1. Review the *mano viṣhaya*. Explain a practical example of each and how *manas* produces each type.

2. Choose any *indriya* from the *pañcha pañchaka* and draw its components and process in detail. Label its steps in functional order.

3. Describe the positive and negative effects of the *mano guṇas*. How can the negative effects of each be offset by the others?

4. Consider the Sanskrit *dhātu* of the term *chintya*. Is this *dhātu* related to the term *chitta*? What is the significance of this relationship?

5. Explain *indriyābhigraha* and its possible impacts on mental health.

Chapter 24 : Ātma

KEY TERMS

adhyātma dravya-guṇa saṅgraha	hṛdaya	pañcha pañchaka	smṛti
ahaṅkāra	indriya buddhi	paramātma	smṛti bhraṁśha
ātma	jīvātma	puruṣha	sṛṣhṭi utpatti
avyakta	jñāna	rajas	tamas
buddhi	Kārya-Kāraṇa siddhānta	rājasika	tāmasika
chetanā	mahat	rāśhi-puruṣha	tri-guṇa
dhṛti	manas	sattva	
	mokṣha	sāttvika	

The components of *āyu* that extend beyond the *śharīra* and *manas* enter into a rather controversial realm according to various systems of medical sciences. In many traditional streams and cultures, the inclusion of these components is considered inseparable from understanding life in a fully holistic manner, and they are required for proper treatment at all stages and with all available means. In other cultures, these concepts may be considered solely philosophical, unscientific, and inappropriate in medical practice.

Āyurveda takes a fully holistic approach and considers life, health and all of its supportive mechanisms to be within the scope of its practice. By utilizing the mechanisms of the scientific Āyurvedic framework including methods of *pramāṇa*, *siddhānta*, *parīkṣhā* and others, the case is made in the classics for the existence of these intangible components.

Because of the difficulty in directly perceiving them, observing them, and having the ability to control them in specific, repeatable circumstances, they are considered invalid according to the current definition of science. It is important to remember that in order to acknowledge these components as a fundamental part of the Āyurvedic framework, one must consider their existence, characteristics, behaviors and other features through the Āyurvedic system itself.

This chapter will focus on the *ātma*, the individual's persistent spirit that persists across multiple manifestations of life. Additionally, the components which work directly and indirectly with *ātma* will also be explained here. These components originate from the group of *aṣhṭa prakṛti* as explained in *sṛṣhṭi utpatti* (see Chapter 26).

ĀTMA

Ātma is often referred to in the classics using various terms depending on context. Charaka and Suśhruta distinguish *ātma* in different manifestations as well. The depth of explanation of *ātma* originates from the Vedic philosophical systems that provide the basis for understanding the extensive processes through *sṛṣhṭi utpatti*, *sthiti* and *laya* (see Chapter 26).

Paryāya

The most common and important synonyms of *ātma* are detailed below. Review them to understand the contexts in which *ātma* is described.

Purușha

Charaka refers to *ātma* as *purușha* throughout Cha. Śhā. 1/. He explains that *purușha* is *ātma* when considering the true nature of the individual. This true nature is the permanent, continuous and on-going state of consciousness which is the *ātma*.

The term *purușha* is also used to refer to the individual as the current manifestation of *ātma* embodied in human form. In this way, the individual is the focus of the practical application of the science of Āyurveda, and so he is also known as *karma purușha* or *chikitsā purușha*. In this context, it is always the human body which is the subject of treatment. *Ātma* is the observer.

Avyakta

In the explanation of *sṛșhṭi utpatti*, *ātma* originates from a state of *avyakta*, which is the unmanifest realm. Suśhruta explains this clearly with an analogy.

सर्वभूतानां कारणमकारणं सत्त्वरजस्तमोलक्षणमष्टरूपमखिलस्य जगतः सम्भवहेतुरव्यक्तं नाम । तदेकं बहूनां क्षेत्रज्ञानामधिष्ठानं समुद्र इवौदकानां भावानाम् ॥ ३

सु. शा. १।३

Sarvabhūtānāṁ kāraṇamakāraṇaṁ sattvarajastamolakṣhaṇamaṣhṭarūpama khilasya jagataḥ sambhavaheturavyaktaṁ nāma | Tadekaṁ bahūnāṁ kṣhetrajñānāmadhiṣhṭhānaṁ samudra ivaudakānāṁ bhāvānām ||

Su. Śhā. 1/3

Sarva-bhūtānāṁ kāraṇam (As the cause for all *bhūtas* [ie, basic elements of life]), akāraṇaṁ (yet having no cause [for itself]) sattva-rajas-tamo lakṣhaṇam (and having the characteristics of *sattva*, *rajas* and *tamas*), aṣhṭa-rūpam (along with eight forms or manifestation), akhilasya jagataḥ sambhava hetur (and being the cause for the creation of the whole world), avyaktaṁ nāma (it is called *avyakta*). Tad-ekaṁ (This one) bahūnāṁ kṣhetra jñānām (is known to be the field or source of many others) adhiṣhṭhānaṁ samudra iva (just as the ocean is the place or home) audakānāṁ bhāvānām (of many types of aquatic species).

The concept of *avyakta* is that it is distinct and separate from the material world which is based on the *bhūtas*. Although it has no cause for itself, it is the direct cause for manifestation of the material world and all of its constituents. The characteristics and features of *sattva*, *rajas* and *tamas* pervade through *avyakta* and into the material world by way of the eight forms that manifest during the process of *sṛșhṭi utpatti*.

Sattva

Sattva is another important synonym for *ātma*. Out of the *tri-guṇa*, *sattva* represents pure clarity and the truth of the genuine *ātma*. *Sattva* in its association at the *ātma* level is unaffected by *rajas* and *tamas* until it is impelled into its manifestation through the actions of *prakṛti* and *purușha*.

Understanding ātma

The classics describe *atma* through its actions and results because only these can be directly observed by normal human senses. To explain the existence of *ātma*, Charaka bases much of his logic on the *Kārya-Kāraṇa siddhānta*. His position is that something in addition to the physical body must exist that causes life to be produced. Additionally, something must be responsible for experiencing the good and bad outcomes of all actions performed.

अहङ्कारः फलं कर्म देहान्तरगतिः स्मृतिः |
विद्यते सति भूतानां कारणे देहमन्तरा || ५२

च. शा. १।५२

Ahaṅkāraḥ phalaṁ karma dehāntaragatiḥ smṛtiḥ | Vidyate sati bhūtānāṁ kāraṇe dehamantarā || 52

Cha. Śhā. 1/52

Ahaṅkāraḥ (*Ahaṅkāra*, or self-identification) smṛtiḥ (is the one known to) phalaṁ (enjoy the fruitful outcomes), karma (engage in actions), dehāntaragatiḥ (and go from within one body to the next). Vidyate (It exists, even as) sati bhūtānāṁ (the *bhūtas* [ie, the manifestation of life] are destroyed) kāraṇe dehamantarā (to be the cause for continuity of the internal self).

Here, Charaka refers to *ātma* through one of its eight forms, the *ahaṅkāra*. This form is mainly responsible for the self-identification that occurs during each manifestation of life, but it is also closely connected to the state of *avyakta*. Beyond the individual life, *ahaṅkāra* also provides continuity of certain inclinations, behaviors and other traits through its tendency to maintain certain proportions of *sattva*, *rajas* and *tamas* and their respective behaviors.

Ātma, in its manifested form of human life, is permanently attached to its eight forms, *manas* and *śharīra*. Through this attachment, it is able to engage *manas*, and in certain situations influence the manner in which *manas* interacts with the *indriya*, and ultimately the physical world. This involvement is completely dependent upon the stability and health of the connection between all these components. It is largely influenced by the proportion of *sattva* available to execute the appropriate decisions resulting in action or inaction in each situation.

आत्मा ज्ञः करणैर्योगाज् ज्ञानं त्वस्य प्रवर्तते | करणानामवैमल्यादयोगाद्वा न वर्तते || ५४

पश्यतोऽपि यथाऽऽदर्शे सङ्क्लिष्टे नास्ति दर्शनम् | तत्त्वं जले वा कलुषे चेतस्युपहते तथा || ५५

च. शा. १।५४-५५

Ātmā jñaḥ karaṇairyogāj jñānaṁ tvasya pravartate |
Karaṇānāmavaimalyādayogādvā na vartate || 54
Paśhyato ' pi yathādarśhe saṅkliṣhṭe nāsti darśhanam | Tattvaṁ jale vā kaluṣhe cetasyupahate tathā || 55

Cha. Śhā. 1/54-55

Ātmā jñaḥ (*Ātma*'s intellectual knowledge) tvasya pravartate (arises from the) karaṇairyogāj jñānaṁ (intellectual knowledge obtained through connection with its products [ie, *manas*, *indriya*]). Karaṇānām avaimalyād ayogād vā (Without this connection, or without these same products), na vartate (nothing [ie, no knowledge] arises).

Paśhyato api (Even when conspicuous), yathādarśhe (if these recognizable components) saṅkliṣhṭe (are damaged or not functioning properly), nāsti darśhanam (nothing [ie, no knowledge]) will be perceived). Tattvaṁ ([This happens] just as) kaluṣhe (dirt) jale vā (makes water cloudy), cetasyupahate tathā ([thus] chetaḥ is scattered about).

Here, Charaka emphasizes the importance of the connection from *ātma* all the way through *manas* and the *indriya* in order to gain true *jñāna*. The involvement of *ātma* through the entire process is required to generate truthful knowledge because of the influence and presence of *sattva guṇa*.

Existence of ātma

The existence of *ātma* is explained by Charaka through logical statements and analogies primarily found in Cha. Śhā. 1/.

These analogies provide important insight because it is impossible for normal human senses to see or perceive *ātma* directly. It is important to note that even at the time of these writings, Charaka was fully aware of other philosophical doctrines that did not accept the existence of *ātma*. His explanations clearly seek to maintain the position of Āyurveda and its inclusion of *ātma* in its foundational theories.

Suśhruta succinctly explains why *ātma* cannot be directly seen or perceived.

न शक्यश्चक्षुषा द्रष्टुं देहे सूक्ष्मतमो विभुः ।
दृश्यते ज्ञानचक्षुर्भिस्तपश्चक्षुर्भिरिव च ॥ ५०

सु. शा. ५।५०

Na śhakyaśhchakṣhuṣhā draṣhṭuṁ dehe sūkṣhmatamo vibhuḥ | Dṛṣhyate jñānachakṣhurbhistapaśhchakṣhurbhireva cha || 50

Su. Śhā. 5/50

Na (It is not) śhakyaśh (possible) chakṣhuṣhā (for the eyes [ie, the sense of vision]) draṣhṭuṁ (to see, examine or investigate) dehe (within the body) sūkṣhma-tamo (that which is the most subtle or minute) vibhuḥ (and eternal [ie, the *ātma*]). Dṛṣhyate (Seeing [the *ātma*]) jñāna chakṣhurbhis ([is possible when] the eyes, or sense of vision] are capable of that level of knowledge) tapaśh chakṣhurbhireva cha (and deep meditation allows the eyes to visualize it).

Because of the constraints on knowing and observing *ātma* directly, Charaka provides a detailed explanation that includes *lakṣhaṇas* indicative of *ātma*'s presence in the human body. This explanation takes place as a dialogue between Agniveśha who asks Punarvasu Ātreya how to recognize the presence of *ātma*.

प्राणापानौ निमेषाद्या जीवनं मनसो गतिः |
इन्द्रियान्तरसञ्चारः प्रेरणं धारणं च यत् ||
७०

देशान्तरगतिः स्वप्ने पञ्चत्वग्रहणं तथा |
दृष्टस्य दक्षिणेनाक्ष्णा सव्येनावगमस्तथा ||
७१

इच्छा द्वेषः सुखं दुःखं प्रयत्नश्चेतना धृतिः |
बुद्धिः स्मृतिरहङ्कारो लिङ्गानि परमात्मनः ||
७२

यस्मात् समुपलभ्यन्ते लिङ्गान्येतानि जीवतः
| न मृतस्यात्मलिङ्गानि तस्मादाहुर्महर्षयः ||
७३

शरीरं हि गते तस्मिञ् शून्यागारमचेतनम् |
पञ्चभूतावशेषत्वात् पञ्चत्वं गतमुच्यते || ७४

च. शा. १।७०-७४

Prāṇāpānau nimeṣhādyā jīvanaṁ manaso gatiḥ | Indriyāntarasañchāraḥ preraṇaṁ dhāraṇaṁ cha yat || 70

Deśhāntaragatiḥ svapne pañchatvagrahaṇaṁ tathā | Dṛṣhṭasya dakṣhiṇenākṣhṇā savyenāvagamastathā || 71

Ichchhā dveṣhaḥ sukhaṁ duḥkhaṁ prayatnaśhchetanā dhṛtiḥ | Buddhiḥ smṛtirahaṅkāro liṅgāni paramātmanaḥ || 72

Yasmāt samupalabhyante liṅgānyetāni jīvataḥ | Na mṛtasyātmaliṅgāni tasmādāhurmaharṣhayaḥ || 73

Śharīraṁ hi gate tasmiñ śhūnyāgāramachetanam | Pañchabhūtāvaśheṣhatvāt pañchatvaṁ gatamucyate || 74

Cha. Śhā. 1/71-74

Prāṇa-apānau (The presence of both *prāṇa* and *apāna*, which control intake and output), nimeṣhādyā (blinking of the eyes, or the urge to blink especially in response to stimuli), jīvanaṁ (the presence of jīva, or life) manaso gatiḥ (the going of the mind [from one place to another in the mind]), indriyāntara-sañchāraḥ (internal communication and transfer of information between the *indriya*), preraṇaṁ (the inspiration, initiation or impetus) dhāraṇaṁ cha (and the ability to hold and maintain concentration over) yat (them [ie, the *manas* and *indriya*]),

Deśha-antaragatiḥ svapne (While dreaming, being able to go to other places), pañchatvagrahaṇaṁ tathā (even the ability to comprehend death), dṛshṭasya dakṣhiṇenākṣhṇā savyenāvagamastathā (and that what is seen in the right eye is also known by the left),

Ichchhā (Desires), dveṣhaḥ (aversions), sukhaṁ (happiness, contentment), duḥkhaṁ (discontent), prayatnaśh (effort), chetanā (consciousness), dhṛtiḥ (self-determination), buddhiḥ (innate intelligence), smṛtir (memory), ahaṅkāro (and self-identification) liṅgāni (are the signs and indications) paramātmanaḥ (of the presence of the *paramātma* [manifested as *jīvātma* within the individual]).

Yasmāt (Because) liṅgānyetāni (of these signs and indications), sam-upalabhyante (it should be known that) jīvataḥ (life is present). Na mṛtasyātmaliṅgāni (These signs and indications are not present in a dead body), tasmād (therefore) āhurmaharṣhayaḥ (this is considered to prove the existence [of *ātma* in a living body]).

Śharīraṁ hi (The body itself) gate tasmiñ śhūnyāgāram (becomes empty when it [*ātma*] goes out, or leaves) achetanam (and it becomes void of consciousness). Pañchabhūtāvaśheṣhatvāt (Only the five *bhūtas* remain) pañchatvaṁ gatamucyate (and the body is said to be in a state of *pañchatva*).

Punarvasu Ātreya provides a very clear, specific list of *lakṣhaṇas* to identify the presence of *ātma*. See also Cha. Sū. 11/6-33, BP Pū. 2/33 for similar explanations. Review the *lakṣhaṇas* in the following table.

Jīva (ātma) lakṣhaṇas	Signs of life indicating the presence of *ātma* Nearest English explanation
Prāṇa-apānau	The presence of both *prāṇa* and *apāna*, which control intake and output
Nimeṣhādyā	Blinking of the eyes, or the urge to blink especially in response to stimuli
Jīvana	The presence of *jīva*, or life
Manaso gatiḥ	The going of the mind [from one place to another in the mind]
Indriyāntara-sañchāraḥ	Internal communication and transfer of information between the *indriya*
Preraṇa	Inspiration, initiation or impetus
Dhāraṇa cha yat	The ability to hold and maintain concentration over the *manas* and *indriya*
Deśha-antaragatiḥ svapne	While dreaming, being able to go to other places
Pañchatvagrahaṇa tathā	The ability to comprehend death
Dṛṣhṭasya dakṣhiṇenākṣhṇā savyenāvagamastathā	That what is seen in the right eye is also known by the left
Ichchhā	Desires
Dveṣha	Aversions
Sukha	Happiness, contentment
Duḥkha	Discontent
Prayatna	Effort
Chetanā	Consciousness
Dhṛti	Self-determination
Buddhi	Innate intelligence
Smṛti	Memory
Ahaṅkāra	Self-identification

Charaka additionally states that these *lakṣhaṇas* are only present because of *ātma*'s interactions with *manas* and *indriya*. This only occurs on the level of *jīvātma* where the *ātma* is attached to a specific *deha*. At the level of *avyakta*, no *lakṣhaṇas* are available to indicate its presence.

Ātma activates manas

Ātma plays a critical role in the activation of *manas* to receive inputs and information through the *indriya* and engage the physical body into actions. While *manas* is ultimately the deciding factor in the actions, *ātma*, and its related components of *buddhi*, *ahaṅkāra*, *smṛti* and *dhṛti* have the capacity to be strongly influential.

Charaka explains the distinction in these entities by stating that *manas* is *achetana* and *kriyavat* (able to perform actions), whereas *ātma* is *chetana* yet unable to directly perform actions. *Ātma* is ultimately responsible for the actions performed, however, because it initiates *manas* and the *indriya* to perform all activities. It is ultimately responsible for these actions as it is the permanent, persisting observer of the current manifestation of life.

अचेतनं क्रियावच्च मनश्चेतयिता परः |
युक्तस्य मनसा तस्य निर्दिश्यन्ते विभोः
क्रियाः || ७५

चेतनावान् यतश्चात्मा ततः कर्ता निरुच्यते |
अचेतनत्वाच्च मनः क्रियावदपि नोच्यते ||
७६

च. शा. १।७५-७६

Achetanaṁ kriyāvachcha manaśhchetayitā paraḥ | Yuktasya manasā tasya nirdiśhyante vibhoḥ kriyāḥ || 75

Chetanāvān yataśhcātmā tataḥ kartā niruchyate | Achetanatvāchcha manaḥ kriyāvadapi nochyate || 76

Cha. Śhā. 1/75-76

Achetanaṁ (Lacking consciousness), kriyāvachcha (but capable of action), manaśh-chetayitā (is how *manas* is to be perceived). Paraḥ (On the other hand), yuktasya (it should be understood that) manasā tasya (while it [*ātma*] is in contact with *manas*) nirdiśhyante (they [*manas* and *indriya*] are directed) vibhoḥ (by the eternal [*ātma*]) kriyāḥ (in their actions).

Chetanāvān (By having consciousness), yataśhchātmā (the *ātma*) tataḥ (thus) niruchyate (is said to be) kartā (the doer). Achetanatvāchcha (Being without consciousness), manaḥ (the mind) na-uchyate (is not said to be) kriyāvadapi (the one ultimately responsible for action).

The specific differences between *ātma* and *manas* are summarized in the following table.

Inherent attribute	*Manas*	*Ātma*
Presence of *chetanā*	None	Present
Role in producing *kriyā* (action)	Produces action directly	Produces action indirectly through initiating *manas* and the *indriya*
Level of responsibility in the production of *kriyā* (action)	Not responsible for actions produced	Ultimately responsible for all actions

Ātma bheda

For the purposes of understanding *ātma* in the context of therapeutic application, it is considered to be of two main types. As Suśhruta described in Su. Śhā. 1/3, the same concept of *avyakta* can be understood in two forms. One of which is completely beyond the scope of human perception. It is responsible for the generation of the second type which contains the multitude forms seen in manifested life.

Charaka provides a very similar explanation on this and specifically names each type of *ātma*. He describes the two as *paramātma* and *rāśhi-puruṣha*.

प्रभवो न ह्यनादित्वाद्विद्यते परमात्मनः |
पुरुषो राशिसञ्ज्ञस्तु मोहेच्छाद्वेषकर्मजः || ५३

च. शा. १।५३

Prabhavo na hyanāditvādvidyate paramātmanaḥ | Puruṣho rāśhisañjñastu mohechchhādveṣhakarmajaḥ || 53

Cha. Śhā. 1/53

Prabhavo na (Its special feature is that) paramātmanaḥ (the *paramātma*, or infinite soul) hyan-āditvād-vidyate (is known as having no beginning). Puruṣho rāśhisañjñastu (The *rāśhi-puruṣha* is known as having a specific beginning) karmajaḥ (due to its results of previous actions which produce) moha (delusion), ichchhā (desires), dveṣha (and aversions).

This statement clarifies the major distinctions between *paramātma* and *rāśhi-puruṣha*. *Paramātma* is eternal and has no beginning or end whereas *rāśhi-puruṣha* takes a specific manifestation as a life form to experience the results of its previous actions due to its attachment or association with *rajas* and *tamas*. Physical manifestation results in *rāśhi-puruṣha* having a distinct beginning and end in the timeframe of any single manifestation. This appearance of impermanence occurs only on the physical level of the *bhūtas*.

This concept is explained further to highlight the *Kārya-Kāraṇa siddhānta*, or the application of the law of cause and effect.

अनादिः पुरुषो नित्यो विपरीतस्तु हेतुजः |
सदकारणवन्नित्यं दृष्टं हेतुजमन्यथा || ५९

च. शा. १।५९

Anādiḥ puruṣho nityo viparītastu hetujaḥ | Sadakāraṇavannityaṁ dṛṣhṭaṁ hetujamanyathā || 59

Cha. Śhā. 1/59

Anādiḥ (Having no beginning) puruṣho nityo (is the eternal *puruṣha* [ie, *paramātma*]). Viparītastu (The opposite one of that) hetujaḥ (is born due to its causative factors [ie, being impelled by *rajas* and *tamas*]). Sad-akāraṇavan-nityaṁ (Those things being of absolute truth and having no cause are eternal); dṛṣhṭaṁ (that which can be seen) hetujam-anyathā (has a specific cause and is known to be otherwise [ie, temporary]).

The differences between the two types of *ātma* are further explained in Cha. Śhā. 1/80-85 and Su. Śhā. 1/9.

Rāśhi-puruṣha is also known as *jīvātma*. Bhāvamiśhra provides a succinct explanation of jīvātma in BP Pū. 2/32.

एवं चतुर्विंशतिभिस्तत्त्वैः सिद्धे वपुर्गृहे ।
जीवात्मा नियतेर्निघ्रो वसति स्वान्तदूतवान्
|| ३१

भा. प्र. पू. २।३१

Evaṁ chaturviṁśhatibhistattvaiḥ siddhe vapurgṛhe | Jīvātmā niyaternighno vasati svāntadūtavān || 32

BP Pū. 2/31

Evaṁ (Thus), jīvātmā (the *jīvātma*, or individual soul), chaturviṁśhatibhis-tattvaiḥ (composed of the 24 *tattva*) gṛhe siddhe (resides in the house produced as) vapur (the body), niyater (and is eternal) nighno (yet dependent upon) vasati (this dwelling place) svāntadūtavān (along with its own internal messenger [ie, *manas*]).

Jīvātma is the persistent and eternal component of a temporary living being and the responsible witness to all actions, outcomes and experiences that the individual undergoes during their course of life. Recognition of these events primarily occurs through the *jīvātma*'s connection with *manas*.

Adhyātma dravya-guṇa saṅgraha

The *adhyātma dravya-guṇa saṅgraha* is the group of components associated with *ātma* that include *manas*, its objects, *buddhi*, *ātma* and *chetanā*. The name of the group directly indicates that which is at the front of, or along with *ātma*. These components are significant because they are responsible as a group for the actualization of the *ātma*'s intentions and their effects have the ability to steer one towards a predominance of the *tri-guṇa*.

मनो मनोर्थो बुद्धिरात्मा
चेत्यध्यात्मद्रव्यगुणसङ्ग्रहः
शुभाशुभप्रवृत्तिनिवृत्तिहेतुश्च, द्रव्याश्रितं
चकर्म; यदुच्यते क्रियेति || १३

च. सू. ८|१३

Mano manortho buddhirātmā chetyadhyātmadravyaguṇasaṅgrahaḥ śhubhāśhubhapravṛttinivṛttihetuśhcha, dravyāśhritaṁ cha karma; yaduchyate kriyeti || 13

Cha. Sū. 8/13

Mano (*Manas*, the mind), manortho (*mano-artha*, the objects of the mind), buddhir (*buddhi*, innate intellect), ātmā (*ātma*, the soul), chety (and *chetanā*, consciousness) adhyātma-dravya-guṇa-saṅgrahaḥ (are the *adhyātma-dravya-guṇa-saṅgraha*, or group of components associated with *ātma*). Śhubha-aśhubha (That which is favorable or unfavorable), pravṛtti-nivṛtti (and initiation or avoidance of actions) hetuśhcha (are due to) dravyāśhritaṁ (these dravya [ie, the entire group]). Cha (And) karma (actions) yad (of these same components) uchyate (are to be considered) kriyeti (in the context of therapy as well).

Within this entire group, *ātma* is ultimately the one responsible for actions. It is the controller of *manas* and the *indriya*, and responsible for the outcome of their actions. See Cha. Sū. 8/4 for an additional explanation.

Transmigration of ātma

The transmigration of *ātma* into a physical body is described in detail in Cha. Sa. 2/31-38 and Cha. Śhā. 2/44. Vāgbhaṭa provides a short explanation along with several helpful analogies in AH Śhā. 1/2-4.

Chetanā adhiṣhṭhāna

Chetanā is one of the indicators of the presence of *ātma*. Its locations in the body are specifically mentioned as all parts except those which do not experience or feel pain. The primary, central location of *chetanā* is the heart.

हृदयं चेतनाधिष्ठानमेकम् || ८

च. शा. ७।८

Hṛdayaṁ chetanādhiṣhṭhānamekam || 8

Cha. Śhā. 7/8

Hṛdayaṁ (The heart) chetanā-adhiṣhṭhānam-ekam (is the main location of *chetanā*).

See Cha. Sū. 30/7 for a similar explanation.

वेदनानामधिष्ठानं मनो देहश्च सेन्द्रियः | केशलोमनखाग्रान्नमलद्रवगुणैर्विना || १३६

च. शा. १।१३६

Vedanānāmadhiṣhṭhānaṁ mano dehaśhcha sendriyaḥ | Keśhalomanakhāgrānnamaladravaguṇai rvinā || 136

Cha. Śhā. 1/136

Vedanānāmadhiṣhṭhānaṁ (The locations where pain and happiness can be felt) mano dehaśhcha (are where the mind is present in the body) sendriyaḥ (along with the *indriya*). Keśha (The hair on the head), loma (the hair on the body), nakha-āgra (the tips of the nails), anna (consumed food), mala (waste materials), drava (and waste fluids) guṇairvinā (are without these characteristics [ie, incapable of sensation]).

See also BP Pū. 3/327.

Responsibilities of ātma

The main purpose for *ātma* taking birth into a physical human body is to act as the observer and initiator of all actions, as well as receive the results of previous actions. Any actions which are performed by the individual become the responsibility of *ātma*. By the principle of cause and effect, all actions have outcomes which must also be fulfilled by the same *ātma*.

न हि कर्म महत् किञ्चित् फलं यस्य न भुज्यते | क्रियाघ्नाः कर्मजा रोगाः प्रशमं यान्ति तत्क्षयात् || ११७

च. शा. १।११७

Na hi karma mahat kiñchit phalaṁ yasya na bhujyate | Kriyāghnāḥ karmajā rogāḥ praśhamaṁ yānti tatkṣhayāt || 117

Cha. Śhā. 1/117

Na hi karma mahat (There is no major action) yasya na (which itself is not) bhujyate (made use of) kiñchit phalaṁ (as some type of beneficial outcome). Kriyāghnāḥ (Therapeutic intervention to reduce) karmajā rogāḥ (diseases due to previous actions) praśhamaṁ (produce a restoration to normal health) yānti tatkṣhayāt (only when the effects of the action itself are reduced).

See also Cha. Śhā. 1/116-117.

Attachment of ātma

The *ātma* is compelled to take birth in a specific life form and physical body based on its previous actions and responsibilities to fulfill the outcomes of those actions. In its unattached form, *ātma* has certain abilities that are not generally present in its attached form. It may behave more in line with *paramātma* by means of association. While manifested as *jīvātma*, it is bound by its attachments based on *rajas* and *tamas*.

स सर्वगः सर्वशरीरभृच्च स विश्वकर्मा स च विश्वरूपः | स चेतनाधातुरतीन्द्रियश्च स नित्ययुक् सानुशयः स एव || ३२

च. शा. २।३२

Sa sarvagaḥ sarvaśharīrabhṛchcha sa viśhvakarmā sa cha viśhvarūpaḥ | Sa chetanādhāturatīndriyaśhcha sa nityayuk sānuśhayaḥ sa eva [16] || 32

Cha. Śhā. 2/42

Sa (It [*ātma*] can) sarvagaḥ (go in all places), sarvaśharīrabhṛchcha (and be carried in all [any types of] bodies), sa (it) viśhvakarmā (can accomplish or create anything [ie, is capable of doing any type of action]), sa cha (and it) viśhvarūpaḥ (can take on any form). Sa (It) chetanādhātur (is *chetanā-dhātu*, the source and support of consciousness), atīndriyaśhcha (and it goes beyond the senses), sa (it) nityayuk (is always active) sānuśhayaḥ sa eva (and it becomes attached as a consequence of actions).

Detachment, rebirth and mokṣha

During the course of the individual's lifespan, the *ātma* remains attached to the physical form in order to fulfill its responsibilities. At the time of detachment, *ātma* disassociates itself from its connections through *manas* and the *indriya*. Depending on its remaining responsibilities incurred due to its actions, it may associate in another subsequent form. When its attachments to *rajas* and *tamas* are nullified and its responsibilities are complete, it is not compelled to associate in any physical form.

पुरुषः प्रलये चेष्टैः पुनर्भावैर्वियुज्यते || ६७

अव्यक्ताद्व्यक्ततां याति व्यक्तादव्यक्ततां पुनः | रजस्तमोभ्यामाविष्टश्चक्रवत् परिवर्तते || ६८

येषां द्वन्द्वे परा सक्तिरहङ्कारपराश्च ये | उदयप्रलयौ तेषां न तेषां ये त्वतोऽन्यथा || ६९

च. शा. १|६७-gj

Puruṣhaḥ pralaye cheṣhṭaiḥ punarbhāvairviyujyate || 67

Avyaktādvyaktatām̐ yāti vyaktādavyaktatām̐ punaḥ | Rajastamobhyāmāviṣhṭaśhchakravat parivartate || 68

Yeṣhām̐ dvandve parā saktirahaṅkāraparāśhcha ye | Udayapralayau teṣhām̐ na teṣhām̐ ye tvato ' nyathā || 69

Cha. Śhā. 1/67-69

Puruṣhaḥ (*Puruṣha* [ie, the manifestation of life embodied in the 24 *tattva*, and ultimately *jīvātma*]) pralaye (at its time of *pralaya*, or death), cheṣhṭaiḥ punarbhāvair-viyujyate (again breaks away from all of the components that allowed its actions).

Avyaktād-vyaktatām̐ yāti (All of these components vacillate between states of unmanifest and manifest) vyaktād-avyaktatām̐ punaḥ (and go back and forth to manifest and unmanifest again and again). Rajas-tamobhyām (Both *rajas* and *tamas*) āviṣhṭaśhchakravat (are subject to this cycle) parivartate (and to repeat it).

Yeṣhām̐ dvandve (The pair of these) parā (as well as) saktir-ahaṅkāra-parāśhcha ye (the power of self-identification) udaya (create the consequence of) pralayau teṣhām̐ (their own death) na teṣhām̐ ye (yet those who are not [under the consequence of *rajas*, *tamas* and *ahaṅkāra*]) tvato anyathā (experience otherwise).

The process of death and detachment, along with subsequent rebirth is said to be experienced by *ātma* when it is bound by attachment to *rajas* and *tamas* and influenced by *ahaṅkāra*. When these components no longer exert an influence on the *ātma*, it is not compelled to experience rebirth. This state is considered *mokṣha*.

तदेतच्छरीरं सङ्ख्यातमनेकावयवं दृष्टमेकत्वेन सङ्गः, पृथक्त्वेनापवर्गः| तत्र प्रधानमसक्तं सर्वसत्तानिवृत्तौ निवर्तते इति || १८

च. शा. ७|१८

Tadetachchharīraṁ saṅkhyātamanekāvayavaṁ dṛshṭamekatvena saṅgaḥ, pṛthaktvenāpavargaḥ | Tatra pradhānamasaktaṁ sarvasattānivṛttau nivartate iti || 18

Cha. Śhā. 7/18

Tadetac-charīraṁ (And so the physical body) saṅkhyātam-aneka-avayavaṁ (is organized in an enumerable way and it consists of multiple parts and components). Dṛshṭamekatvena (When seen as a whole), saṅgaḥ (it is considered *saṅga*, or a complete assemblage to which there is attachment). Pṛthaktvena (When separated), apavargaḥ (it is considered to be abandoned, absolved or detached). Tatra (Of all of this), pradhānam (the chief, or primary component [ie, *ātma*]) asaktaṁ (is unattached [to the *saṅga*]), sarva sattānivṛttau (and when it turns away from all existence) nivartate iti (it escapes [from the cycle of rebirth]).

TEST YOURSELF

Learn, review and memorize key terms from this section.

ātma

sṛshṭi utpatti

purusha

avyakta

sattva

Kārya-Kāraṇa siddhānta

manas

rajas

tamas

jñāna

paramātma

rāśhi-purusha

jīvātma

adhyātma dravya-guṇa saṅgraha

buddhi

chetanā

tri-guṇa

hṛdaya

mokṣha

BUDDHI

Buddhi is one of the eight forms or representations of *ātma* in its manifestation of the 24 *tattva*. It most closely represents the innate intelligence that is experienced by an individual when they "know" something but may not understand how they know it. *Buddhi* is able to open a window to the true knowledge that *ātma* provides. *Buddhi* is likely intuition.

A healthy and properly functioning *buddhi* produces *jñāna*, or intellectual knowledge, which is truthful, accurate and uninfluenced by embellishments. It is often factual information and the individual may not be able to immediately explain its source.

Buddhi is also referred to as *mahat*, which is the first of the eight forms of *ātma* to be generated out of *avyakta*. Suśhruta explains this in Su. Śhā. 1/4.

Charaka describes the actions of *buddhi* as that which extends beyond the realm of *manas* and *indriya*.

... ततः परं बुद्धिः प्रवर्तते || २१

च. शा. १।२१

... tataḥ paraṁ buddhiḥ pravartate || 21

Cha. Śhā. 1/21

Tataḥ paraṁ (And beyond that [functioning of *manas* and *indriya*]) buddhiḥ (*buddhi*, or innate intelligence) pravartate (commences).

Because of the close proximity between *buddhi* and *ātma*, *buddhi* has a prominent role to play in responding to processed information and directing *manas* to act.

जायते विषये तत्र या बुद्धिर्निश्चयात्मिका|
व्यवस्यति तया वक्तुं कर्तुं वा बुद्धिपूर्वकम्
|| २३

च. शा. १।२३

Jāyate viṣhaye tatra yā buddhirniśhchayātmikā | Vyavasyati tayā vaktuṁ kartuṁ vā buddhipūrvakam || 23

Cha. Śhā. 1/23

Jāyate (It comes from) viṣhaye (contact with the objects of the *indriya*) tatra yā (thus allowing) buddhir (*buddhi*) niśhchayātmikā (to obtain a certain result of knowledge). Vyavasyati (It considers this knowledge), buddhipūrvakam (and then afterwards *buddhi* influences) tayā (this individual) vaktuṁ (to speak) kartuṁ vā (or act).

Buddhi is also present within each of the *indriya*. These *indriya buddhi* are listed in the *pañcha pañchaka* and are responsible for converting the information received from the *indriya* into a form that can be understood by *manas*.

भेदात् कार्येन्द्रियार्थानां बह्व्यो वै बुद्धयः
स्मृताः | आत्मेन्द्रियमनोर्थानामेकैका
सन्निकर्षजा || ३३

च. शा. १।३३

Bhedāt kāryendriyārthānāṁ bahvyo vai buddhayaḥ smṛtāḥ | Ātmendriyamanorthānāmekaikā sannikarṣhajā || 33

Cha. Śhā. 1/33

Bhedāt (Different types) kāry-endriyārthānāṁ bahvyo (of produced *indriya* identify their specific objects) vai buddhayaḥ (through their own type of *buddhi*) smṛtāḥ (is explained [in this science]). Ātma (The *ātma*, or individual soul), indriya (*indriya*, or senses), manortha (and *mano-artha*, or objects of the mind) anāmekaikā (each have their own way) sannikarṣhajā (of producing contact with their respective objects).

See also BP Pū. 2/11.

Smṛti

Smṛti may be considered an ancillary component to *ātma* and its eight forms, and it is closely connected to *buddhi*. *Smṛti* includes everything that can be remembered and it normally remains within the realm of memories related to the current manifestation of life.

When functioning in a normal, healthy state, *smṛti* is responsible for maintaining, accessing and recalling accurate memories. However, when improperly influenced by *rajas* or *tamas*, these memories can be easily skewed, resulting in an individual's perspective being misunderstood and often misrepresented. This state of invalid *smṛti* is referred to as *smṛti bhraṁśha*, which literally means the deviation, decline or decay of memory.

तत्त्वज्ञाने स्मृतिर्यस्य रजोमोहावृतात्मनः | भ्रश्यते स स्मृतिभ्रंशः स्मर्तव्यं हि स्मृतौ स्थितम् || १०१

च. शा. १।१०१

Tattvajñāne smṛtiryasya rajomohāvṛtātmanaḥ | Bhraśhyate sa smṛtibhraṁśhaḥ smartavyaṁ hi smṛtau sthitam || 101

Cha. Śhā. 1/101

Tattva-jñāne (The components responsible for *jñāna*) smṛtiryasya (are deranged by *smṛti*) bhraśhyate (when it [*smṛti*] falls) rajo-mohāvṛt-ātmanaḥ (under the control of abnormal *rajas* or *tamas*). Sa smṛtibhraṁśhaḥ (This is known as *smṛti bhraṁśha*, or the deviation, decline or decay of memory). Smartavyaṁ hi (This same *smṛti* in its normal condition) smṛtau sthitam (holds all memories).

Dhṛti

Dhṛti is another ancillary component to *ātma* and its eight forms, and it is closely connected to *buddhi*. It represents the individual's self-determination and resolve to maintain character and behavior. Charaka defines *dhṛti* in a succinct statement.

नियन्तुमहितादर्थाद्धृतिर्हि नियमात्मिका || १००

च. शा. १।१००

Niyantumahitādarthāddhṛtirhi niyamātmikā || 100

Cha. Śhā. 1/100

Niyantum (That which can restrain) ahitād-arthād (from any unsuitable or unhealthy objects) dhṛtirhi (is *dhṛti*, or self-determination), niyamātmikā (which is characterized by its ability to restrain [the mind]).

An individual's ability to exert self-control and discipline over their actions, behaviors, thinking, and other mental inclinations, represents the strength of their *dhṛti*. This power of *dhṛti* has a direct impact on the state of *manas* and its ability to influence overall health. It is a main factor in establishing, maintaining and promoting the correct proportion of *sattva*, *rajas* and *tamas*. *Dhṛti* has the potential to shape and influence an individual's immediate and long-term mental state by exercising the ability to favor specific tri-guṇa over others.

TEST YOURSELF

Learn, review and memorize key terms from this section.

buddhi

____

mahat

____

jñāna
pañcha pañchaka
indriya buddhi
smṛti
smṛti bhraṁśha
dhṛti

AHAṄKĀRA

The *ahaṅkāra* of each individual represents their self-identification. It is generated from *mahat* (or *buddhi*) during the process of *sṛṣhṭi utpatti* and is produced from the same *tri-guṇas*. *Ahaṅkāra* provides the necessary functions of individuality and personality. It allows self-attachment to the individual's physical manifestation.

In its simplest form, *ahaṅkāra* can be likened to teaching a young child to know their name and where they live. At this most basic level, *ahaṅkāra* acts as a survival mechanism. The ideal scenario is that *ahaṅkāra* operate within the truthful realm of *sattva*.

However, when overcome by *rajas* and *tamas*, *ahaṅkāra* can interrupt the normal flow of *jñāna* from *ātma* through *manas* and the *indriya*. This interruption is generally plagued by the effects of *rajas* and *tamas* and often creates challenges for the individual both internally and externally.

Suśhruta and Bhāvamiśhra both define and describe *ahaṅkāra* similarly. They recognize the importance and influence of the *tri-guṇas* on the behavior of *ahaṅkāra* by classifying it as the three types. Review their explanations and consider the characteristics within the contexts of the *tri-guṇa lakṣhaṇas*.

तल्लिङ्गाच्च महतस्तल्लक्षण एवाहङ्कार उत्पद्यते; स त्रिधो वैकारिकस्तैजसो भूतदिरिति ... ॥ ४

सु. शा. १।४

Talliṅgāchcha mahatastallakṣhaṇa evāhaṅkāra utpadyate; sa tridho vaikārikastaijaso bhūtadiriti ... || 4

Su. Śhā. 1/4

Mahatastal-lakṣhaṇa (From *mahat* [ie, *buddhi*], and its own qualities) utpadyate (is thus produced) evāhaṅkāra (*ahaṅkāra*, self-identification), tal-liṅgāchcha (having the very same qualities [of *tri-guṇa*]), sa tridho (which is of three types) vaikārikas (*sāttvika*), taijaso (*rājasika*) bhūtadiriti (and *tāmasika*).

महतस्त्रिगुणाज्जातोऽहङ्कारस्त्रिगुणान्वितः । सात्त्विको राजसश्चापि तामसश्चेति स त्रिधा ॥ १२

भा. प्र. पू. २।१२

Mahatastriguṇājjāto ' haṅkārastriguṇānvitaḥ | Sāttviko rājasaśhchāpi tāmasaśhcheti sa tridhā ||

BP Pū. 2/12

Mahatas-triguṇājjāto (*Mahat* [ie, *buddhi*] which is composed of the *tri-guṇa*) ahaṅkāras-triguṇānvitaḥ (generates *ahaṅkāra*, which is also composed of the *tri-guṇa*). Sāttviko (*Sāttvika*), rājasaśhchāpi (*rājasika*) tāmasaśhcheti (and *tāmasika*) sa tridhā (are known as its three types).

TEST YOURSELF

Learn, review and memorize key terms from this section.

ahaṅkāra

---

tri-guṇa

---

sāttvika

---

rājasika

---

tāmasika

Chapter 24: Review

ADDITIONAL READING

Read and review the references listed below to expand your understanding of the concepts in this chapter. Write down the date that you complete your reading for each. Remember that consistent repetition is the best way to learn. Plan to read each reference at least once now and expect to read it again as you continue your studies.

References marked with (skim) can be read quickly and do not require commentary review.

CLASSICS		1st read	2nd read
Charaka	Cha. Sū. 8/3-16 Cha. Sū. 11/6-33 Cha. Sū. 30/17-33 Cha. Śhā. 1/ Cha. Śhā. 2/ Cha. Śhā. 7/5		
Suśhruta	Su. Śhā. 1/ Su. Śhā. 5/50		
Aṣhṭāṅga Hṛdaya	AH Śhā. 1/2-4		
Bhāva Prakāśha	BP Pū. 2/ BP Pū. 3/327		

JOURNALS & CURRENT RESOURCES

QUESTIONS & ANSWERS

Record your questions for this chapter here for further research and discussion.

Question:

Answer:

Question:

Answer:

Question:

Answer:

SELF-ASSESSMENT

1. Which of the following are described in Charaka's definition of *ātma*?
   a. Continuous state of consciousness
   b. Observer
   c. *Purușha*
   d. A and B
   e. All of the above

2. Which of the following is described in Suśhruta's definition of *ātma*?
   a. Characteristics of *sattva, rajas* and *tamas*
   b. Cause for all the *bhūtas* but not of itself
   c. Originates from a state of *avyakta*
   d. B and C
   e. All of the above

3. Define the meaning of *avyakta.*
   a. *Bhūtas*
   b. *Sattva, rajas* and *tamas*
   c. *Sṛșhṭi utpatti*
   d. Unmanifested realm
   e. All of the above

4. Which component of *ātma* generates truthful knowledge?
   a. *Ahaṅkāra*
   b. *Buddhi* (*Mahat*)
   c. *Sattva guṇa*
   d. A and B
   e. B and C

5. Define the meaning of *ahaṅkāra.*
   a. *Manas* interacting with *indriya*
   b. Purity, clarity and truth
   c. *Purușha*
   d. *Sattva*
   e. Self-identification

6. According to Suśhruta what allows *ātma* to be visualized?
   a. Blinking of the eyes
   b. Concentration of manas and indriya
   c. Deep meditation
   d. Dream state
   e. What is seen in the right eye is also known by the left

7. What can influence the decisions of *manas*?
   a. *Ahaṅkāra*
   b. *Buddhi*
   c. *Dhṛti*
   d. *Smṛti*
   e. All of the above

8. Which of the following describes *jīvātmā*?
   a. Anādi
   b. Impelled by *rajas* and *tamas*
   c. Observer and initiator of all actions
   d. A and B
   e. B and C

9. What is the significance of the *adhyātma dravya-guṇa saṅgraha*?
   a. Able to direct predominance of the *tri-guṇa*
   b. Actualizes *ātma's* intentions
   c. Includes *manas*, *buddhi, ātma* and *chetanā*
   d. A and C
   e. All of the above

10. What can be trained to help improve individual character and behavior?
    a. 24 *tattva*
    b. *Ahaṅkāra*
    c. *Buddhi*
    d. *Dhṛti*
    e. *Smṛti*

CRITICAL THINKING

1. Draw a diagram of the components mentioned in this chapter and how they interact with each other. What is the classical name of the group that holds most of these components?

2. Explain at least three terms or phrases that you have learned so far which can refer to *puruṣha*.

3. How is the *chetanā-achetanā siddhānta* applied in this chapter?

4. *Buddhi*'s main responsibility is to produce *jñāna*. How can this be used to explain the similar term, *vijñāna*? What does *vijñāna* indicate, especially in names of fields of study within Āyurveda, such as Roga Vijñāna?

5. Consider the role of *ahaṅkāra* in the generation of *jñāna*. How can its influence be positive or negative?

Chapter 25 : Mṛtyu (Death)

KEY TERMS

akāla mṛtyu	āyu	kālaja mṛtyu	rişhṭa lakṣhaṇas
akālaja mṛtyu	daiva	mṛtyu	sthāyi
ariṣhṭa lakṣhaṇas	guṇa sampat	prakṛti	svabhāva
asthāyi	Indriya-sthāna	prakṛti sampat	vikṛti
ātma sampat	kāla mṛtyu	puruṣhakāra	yuga

Mṛtyu (death) is part of life that everyone eventually faces. Classically, the topic of *mṛtyu* appears in many contexts. For a healthcare professional, death is significant in that it requires a shift from targeted management to palliative care and end-of-life support. In traditional Āyurvedic practice, impending signs of death, or *ariṣhṭa lakṣhaṇas*, are analyzed carefully to guide proper management. Classical literature generally recommends that a professional refrain from attempting to treat any individual exhibiting such signs. This was intended to safeguard the professional's reputation and properly assist the individual by setting appropriate expectations.

Mṛtyu is considered as a normal phase of life, which is ideally experienced upon completion of a full lifespan lasting approximately 100 years. Death which occurred prior to this could be considered premature and may be explained due to various factors.

While explaining the reality of life, Punarvasu Ātreya describes the nature of death.

... न हि कश्चिन्न म्रियत इति समक्रियः ... | २८

च. शा. ६।२८

... Na hi kaśhchinna mriyata iti samakriyaḥ ... | 28

Cha. Śhā. 6/28

Na hi (By no means) kaśhchinna ([will] anyone) mriyata ([avoid] death) iti (thus) samakriyaḥ (is the correct outcome [of life]).

While the goals of Āyurveda clearly prioritize maintenance of health and disease management, the reality of inevitable death must also be considered appropriately.

Each of these concepts will be explored in more detail in this chapter. Note that the classics are replete with *ariṣhṭa lakṣhaṇas* which will not be covered here as they may be reviewed in each treatise.

PARIBHĀṢHĀ AND PARYĀYA

The term *mṛtyu* is translated as "death" or "dying" in the Monier-Williams dictionary. Charaka provides a definition which is much more specific within the scope of practice of Āyurveda.

प्रमाणमायुषस्त्वर्थेन्द्रियमनोबुद्धिचेष्टादीनां विकृतिलक्षणैरुपलभ्यतेऽनिमित्तैः, अयमस्मात् क्षणान्मुहूर्ताद्दिवसात्त्रिपञ्चसप्तदशद्वादशाहात् पक्षान्मासात् षण्मासात् संवत्सराद्वा स्वभावमापत्स्यत इति;

च. सू. ३०।२५

Pramāṇamāyuṣhastvarthendriya manobuddhicheṣhṭādīnāṁ vikṛtilakṣhaṇairupalabhyate ' nimittaiḥ, ayamasmātkṣhaṇānmuhūrtāddivasāt tripañchasaptadaśhadvādaśhāhāt pakṣhānmāsāt ṣhaṇmāsāt saṁvatsarādvāsvabhāvamāpatsyata iti;

Cha. Sū. 30/25

Pramāṇam (Measurement, length) āyuṣhastvartha (of lifespan is based on) indriya (the sense and action organs), mano (the state of the mind), buddhi (the state of intelligence), cheṣhṭādīnāṁ (and activities, etc). Vikṛti-lakṣhaṇair (When an abnormal change in their signs, symptoms and presentation) upalabhyate (is seen) animittaiḥ (without cause or reason), svabhāvam ([this indicates] return to nature, ie, death) āpatsyata (is approaching). Iti (Thus), ayamasmāt (in this manner) kṣhaṇānmuhūrtād (the specific moment) divasāt (of the day [in a timeframe of]) tripañcha (three days), sapta (seven days), daśhadvādaśhāhāt (or ten days, or after) pakṣhān (a half month), māsāt (one month), ṣhaṇmāsāt (six months) saṁvatsarād-vā (or year [death may be predictable]).

This definition provides a comprehensive overview of the concept and its practices. The key approach to note is that the assessment of approaching death is largely seen through the lens of measuring the remaining lifespan.

Next, Charaka describes key synonyms of *mṛtyu*.

तत्र स्वभावः प्रवृत्तेरुपरमोमरणमनित्यता निरोध इत्येकोऽर्थः;

च. सू. ३०।२५

Tatra svabhāvaḥ pravṛtteruparamo maraṇamanityatā nirodha ityeko ' rthaḥ;

Cha. Sū. 30/25

Tatra (And so), iti (each) eko (one of these) arthaḥ (means death) – svabhāvaḥ (returning to nature), pravṛtter-uparamo (actions, conduct and behavior cease), maraṇam (death, deceased), anityatā (limited, transient existence), nirodha (restraint, stoppage [of life]).

Each of these synonyms indicates death as a state or in its characteristics. They are summarized as:

Mṛtyu paryāya	Nearest English explanation
Svabhāva	Return to nature
Pravṛtti uparama	Actions, conduct and behavior cease
Maraṇa	Death, deceased
Anityatā	Limited, transient existence
Nirodha	Restraint, stoppage (of life)

Suśhruta provides a succinct statement that identifies the key factors that predominate when death is approaching.

शरीरशीलयोर्यस्य प्रकृतेर्विकृतिर्भवेत् ।
तत्त्वरिष्टं समासेन, ... ॥ ३

सु. सू. ३०।३

Śharīraśhīlayoryasya prakṛtervikṛtirbhavet | Tattvariṣhṭaṁ samāsena, ... || 3

Su. Sū. 30/3

Śharīra-śhīlayoryasya ([When] the normal behavior of the physical body has ceased) prakṛter-vikṛtir-bhavet (to be in its state of *prakṛti* and becomes *vikṛti*), tattvariṣhṭaṁ (specific signs of approaching death) samāsena (become prominently evident).

TEST YOURSELF

Learn, review and memorize key terms from this section.

mṛtyu

---

svabhāva

---

prakṛti

---

vikṛti

ĀYU AS A FUNCTION OF MṚTYU

The process of dying can occur over varied lengths of time. In certain situations, the death process is clearly recognizable and occurs quickly. In philosophical respects, death can be considered as an extended process that occurs over the entire course of life. From both perspectives it is important to assess the quantum of vitality and residual lifespan as a function of the death process.

Charaka explains this approach while introducing the concept of death through its definition and synonyms. His position is that in absence of recognizable indicators of approaching death, lifespan should be considered continuous.

अतो विपरीतमप्रमाणमरिष्टाधिकारे;
देहप्रकृतिलक्षणमधिकृत्यचोपदिष्टमायुषः
प्रमाणमायुर्वेदे ||२५

च. सू. ३०।२५

Ato viparītamapramāṇamariṣhṭādhikāre;
dehaprakṛtilakṣhaṇamadhikṛtyachopadiṣhṭamāyuṣhaḥ pramāṇamāyurvede || 25

Cha. Sū. 30/25

Ato (And so), viparītam-apramāṇam ([when] the opposite, or unmeasurable) ariṣhṭādhikāre (signs of approaching death are prominent), cha (and) deha-prakṛti-lakṣhaṇam (normal features and behaviors of the body's baseline constitution) adhikṛtya (are predominant) upadiṣhṭam (it is said that) āyuṣhaḥ (the span of life) pramāṇam (is measurable (accordingly) āyurvede (in the practice of Āyurveda).

If the indicators of approaching death are not present, then the expectation is that lifespan should persist through its normal duration. Classically, this duration is estimated to be one hundred years for the current time period. Charaka explains this as:

वर्षशतं खल्वायुषः प्रमाणमस्मिन् काले ||
२९
तस्य निमित्तं प्रकृतिगुणात्मसंपत्
सात्म्योपसेवनं चेति || ३०

च. शा. ६।२९-३०

Varṣhaśhataṁ khalvāyuṣhaḥ
pramāṇamasmin kāle || 29
Tasya nimittaṁ prakṛtiguṇātmasampat
sātmyopasevanaṁ cheti || 30

Cha. Śhā. 6/29-30

Khalu (Now), varṣhaśhataṁ (one hundred years) āyuṣhaḥ-pramāṇam (is the [normal] duration of lifespan) asmin-kāle (during this time period). Tasya (That) nimittaṁ (target [is achieved through]) prakṛti, guṇa, ātma sampat (proper maintenance of *prakṛti*, *guṇa* and *ātma*) sātmya (accustomed to the individual) upasevanaṁ cheti (and regularly utilized).

Charaka emphasizes several concepts here that indicate the importance of regular effort towards habits that promote and maintain specific requirements for an individual's health. Specifically, he mentions:

Prakṛti sampat

Normal *prakṛti* where the *doṣhas* are maintained in their *prakṛta* states

Guṇa sampat

Guṇas in all forms are maintained in their normal *prakṛta* states

Ātma sampat

The *ātma* adheres to the actions which are conducive to promoting happiness, satisfaction and fulfillment of its responsibilities.

The methods to maintain and promote these three categories are explained throughout the classical texts. Adhering to such recommendations in a personalized manner provides clear, measurable health outcomes. This is a primary reason for attaining a full lifespan.

The one-hundred year lifespan is specific to the current time period known as the *Kali Yuga*. The Monier-Williams dictionary defines *yuga* as:

yuga

An age of the world, long mundane period of years of which there are four:

1. Kṛta, or satya
2. Tretā
3. Dvāpara
4. Kali

The first three have already elapsed, while the Kali, which began at midnight between the 17th and 18th of Feb. 3102 BCE, is that in which we live; the duration of each is said to be respectively 1,728,000, 1,296,000, 864,000 and 432,000 years of men, the descending numbers representing a similar physical and moral deterioration of men in each age; the four yugas comprise an aggregate of 4,320,000 years and constitute a mahā yuga, or a great yuga

Time calculations are extensively developed in classical Vedic sciences. Review the summary of the four major yugas:

Yuga	Start	Duration (years)
Kṛta, or satya	Completed	1,728,000
Tretā	Completed	1,296,000
Dvāpara	Completed	864,000
Kali	Midnight between the 17th and 18th of Feb. 3102 BCE	432,000

The understanding of *yuga* cycles on a large scale is applied in Āyurveda to further predict the variations in expected lifespan over the course of the *yuga*.

Charaka states that as the *Kali Yuga* passes, the expected lifespan of human beings decreases by one year after every 1/100th passing of the *yuga*.

संवत्सरशते पूर्णे याति संवत्सरः क्षयम् ।
देहिनामायुषः काले यत्र यन्मानमिष्यते ॥
२६

च. वि. ३।२६

Saṁvatsaraśhate pūrṇe yāti
saṁvatsaraḥ kṣhayam |
Dehināmāyuṣhaḥ kāle yatra
yanmānamiṣhyate || 26

Cha. Vi. 3/26

Saṁvatsaraśhate pūrṇe (After the completion of $1/100^{th}$ years) yāti (and even more [implied double reading]) saṁvatsaraḥ kṣhayam (one year reduces) dehinām-āyuṣhaḥ (from the body's lifespan) kāle (in this time [*Kali Yuga*]) yatra yanmānamiṣhyate (thus it is explained).

The reading of this *śhloka* is somewhat complex. Various translations have also interpreted this line as "after the passing of 100 years" instead of $1/100^{th}$. However, the entire period of the *yuga* will not be accounted for in that manner. This reference is a prime example of the need to consult specialists in related Vedic sciences for clarification.

TEST YOURSELF

Learn, review and memorize key terms from this section.

āyu

prakṛti sampat

guṇa sampat

ātma sampat

yuga

KĀLA AND AKĀLA MṚTYU

Kāla and *akāla mṛtyu* (also *kālaja* and *akālaja mṛtyu*) refer to timely and untimely death. This age-old debate finds its place in several contexts in the *Charaka Saṁhitā* as the question naturally arises whether therapeutic intervention has any relevance if lifespan is predetermined.

While discussing the causes and outcomes of epidemics, Agniveśha asks Punarvasu Ātreya how death can occur at the proper or improper time for different people. This entire discussion should be reviewed in Cha. Vi. 3/ in the full context of epidemics. The logic that supports the existence of untimely death is further explained from a very practical standpoint in Cha. Śhā. 6/28.

The determining factors for whether *kālaja mṛtyu* or *akālaja mṛtyu* are capable of effecting a stronger result in an individual's death is stated to be due to the theories of *daiva* and *puruṣhakāra*. *Daiva* is the cumulative result of previous actions of an individual's *ātma* over their entire span of manifestations or lifetimes. *Puruṣhakāra* is the cumulative result of effort made in the individual's current lifetime. These are defined by Charaka in Cha. Vi. 3/29-35.

तं भगवानुवाच – इहाग्निवेश,
भूतानामायुर्युक्तिमपेक्षते | दैवे पुरुषकारे च
स्थितं ह्यस्य बलाबलम् || २९
दैवमात्मकृतं विद्यात् कर्म यत् पौर्वदैहिकम्
| स्मृतः पुरुषकारस्तु क्रियते यदिहापरम् ||
३०
बलाबलविशेषोऽस्ति तयोरपि च कर्मणोः |
दृष्टं हि त्रिविधं कर्म हीनं मध्यममुत्तमम् ||
३१

तयोरुदारयोर्युक्तिर्दीर्घस्य च सुखस्य च | नियतस्यायुषो हेतुर्विपरीतस्य चेतरा || ३२

मध्यमा मध्यमस्येष्टा कारणं शृणु चापरम् | दैवं पुरुषकारेण दुर्बलं ह्युपहन्यते || ३३

दैवेन चेतरत् कर्म विशिष्टेनोपहन्यते | दृष्ट्वा यदेके मन्यन्ते नियतं मानमायुषः || ३४

कर्म किञ्चित् क्वचित् काले विपाके नियतं महत् | किञ्चित्त्वकालनियतं प्रत्ययैः प्रतिबोध्यते || ३५

च. वि. ३।२९-३५

Taṁ bhagavānuvācha - ihāgniveśha! Bhūtānāmāyuryuktimapekṣhate | Daive puruṣhakāre cha sthitaṁ hyasya balābalam || 29

Daivamātmakṛtaṁ vidyāt karma yat paurvadaihikam | Smṛtaḥ puruṣhakārastu kriyate yadihāparam || 30

Balābalaviśheṣho ' sti tayorapi cha karmaṇoḥ | Dṛshṭaṁ hi trividhaṁ karma hīnaṁ madhyamamuttamam || 31

Tayorudārayoryuktirdīrghasya cha sukhasya cha | Niyatasyāyuṣho heturviparītasya chetarā || 32

Madhyamā madhyamasyeṣhṭā kāraṇaṁ śhṛṇu chāparam | Daivaṁ puruṣhakāreṇa durbalaṁ hyupahanyate || 33

Daivena chetarat karma viśhiṣhṭenopahanyate | Dṛṣhṭvā yadeke manyante niyataṁ mānamāyuṣhaḥ || 34

Karma kiñchit kvachit kāle vipāke niyataṁ mahat | Kiñchittvakālaniyataṁ pratyayaiḥ pratibodhyate || 35

Cha. Vi. 3/29-35

Taṁ bhagavānuvācha (And the Lord himself [Punarvasu Ātreya] replied) – ihāgniveśha (In these circumstances, Agniveśha), bhūtānām (the foundational) āyur-yuktim (assessment of lifespan) apekṣhate (is determined based on) daive (the influence of *daiva*) puruṣhakāre cha (and *puruṣhakāra*) sthitaṁ hyasya (according to their placement) balābalam (and strength or weakness [in the individual's life]).

Daivam (*Daiva*) ātmakṛtaṁ (is that which has been performed by the *ātma*) vidyāt (and is known as) karma yat (the actions and productions) paurvadaihikam (which have been performed in previous manifestations [and have a pre-set effect or outcome that has yet to be realized]). Smṛtaḥ puruṣhakārastu (And *puruṣhakāra* is that which any individual) kriyate yadihāparam (does by their own effort).

Balābalaviśheṣho asti (According to the specific amount of strength or weakness) tayorapi (of each of these) cha karmaṇoḥ (types of karma), dṛshṭaṁ hi (what is seen as the result) trividhaṁ (can be classified as the three levels of) karma (*karma*) hīnaṁ (based on low), madhyamam (medium) uttamam (or high).

Tayor-udārayor (Having both of these in the high category) yuktir (should lead one to understand that) dīrghasya cha (their lifespan will be long) sukhasya cha (and happy or comfortable). Niyatasya-āyuṣho (However, the opposite lifespan) hetur-viparītasya cetarā (should be expected when causes [of *daiva and puruṣhakāra*] are in the opposite category [ie, low]).

Madhyamā (The middle category) madhyama-syeṣhṭā kāraṇaṁ (results in a moderate type of outcome); śhṛṇu cāparam (listen to what is stated). Daivaṁ (A *daiva*) durbalaṁ (which is weak) hyupahanyate (is overcome by) puruṣhakāreṇa (a *puruṣhakāra* [which is stronger]).

Daivena (Similarly, *daiva*) viśhiṣhṭena (is capable of) upahanyate (overcoming) cetarat karma (a low *puruṣhakāra*). | Dṛṣhṭvā (When this is seen) yadeke (certain ones [experts]) manyante (comprehend that) niyataṁ (there is a restricted or preset) mānam (length) āyuṣhaḥ (of lifespan).

Karma kiñchit (Any of these *karmas*) vipāke (are produced) kvachit kāle niyataṁ (at their specific, predetermined time), mahat (according to their strength). Kiñchit tu kāla-niyataṁ (The specific, predetermined time) pratyayaiḥ pratibodhyate (occurs due to the auspicious timing of recovering [that specific karma]).

Charaka also defines daiva as:

निर्दिष्टं दैवशब्देन कर्म यत् पौर्वदेहिकम् ... || ११६

च. शा. १।११६

Nirdiṣhṭaṁ daivaśhabdena karma yat paurvadehikam ... || 116

Cha. Śhā. 1/116

Nirdiṣhṭaṁ (The wise state that) daiva-śhabdena (the technical term *daiva* indicates) karma yat (those actions) paurva-dehikam (which have been performed in earlier lives [literally, in earlier bodies]).

See. Cha. Śhā. 2/44 for an additional explanation.

TEST YOURSELF

Learn, review and memorize key terms from this section.

kāla mṛtyu

kālaja mṛtyu

akāla mṛtyu

akālaja mṛtyu

daiva

puruṣhakāra

ARIṢHṬA (RIṢHṬA) LAKṢHAṆAS

Ariṣhṭa, or *riṣhṭa*, *lakṣhaṇas* are signs and symptoms of impending death. Knowledge of these *lakṣhaṇas* was likely researched and developed over the course of traditional Āyurvedic practice and it provides indications of impending death based on the patient's status as well as circumstantial events. Presence of *ariṣhṭa lakṣhaṇas* could indicate an advancing pathology that may be manageable, or they could signal certain death. Today, such heralding signs and symptoms may also indicate critical, low probability outcomes or incurable clinical situations depending on resources available.

Classical works record this body of knowledge in different ways. Charaka dedicates an entire *sthāna*, named *Indriya-sthāna*, to the explanation and documentation of signs and symptoms accepted at that time. Suśhruta and Vāgbhaṭa include this information within *Śhārīra-sthāna* in the context of assessing life and death.

The name of Charaka's *Indriya-sthāna* section is significant in that it intends to convey the understanding that estimating death should be done in the context of measuring lifespan. The name itself, *Indriya-sthāna*, can be interpreted in several ways. As the term *indriya* refers to the sense organs, this study of signs and symptoms of impending death focuses largely on the changes occurring in the sense organs as death approaches and normal *prakṛti* changes. These signs and symptoms are to be assessed through the clinician's own sense organs. And according to Chakrapāṇi, *indriya* may also refer to *Indra*, which include signs of manifestation of life. The study and assessment of impending death is meant to illustrate the individual's current state in context of their remaining lifespan.

Nirukti & Paribhāṣhā

The terms *ariṣhṭa* and *riṣhṭa* are both used to refer to the *lakṣhaṇas* of impending death. They derive from the Sanskrit *dhātu* √ *riṣh*.

√ *riṣh*	to be hurt or injured, receive harm, suffer wrong, perish, be lost, fail
	to injure, hurt, harm, destroy, ruin
	to fail, meet with misfortune or disaster

Classically, the term is defined as:

फलाग्निजलवृष्टीनां पुष्पधूमाम्बुदा यथा । ख्यापयन्ति भविष्यत्त्वं तथा रिष्टानि पञ्चताम् ॥ ३

सु. सू. २८।३

Phalāgnijalavṛṣhṭīnāṁ puṣhpadhūmāmbudā yathā | Khyāpayanti bhaviṣhyattvaṁ tathā riṣhṭāni pañchatām || 3

Su. Sū. 28/3

Phala (Fruit), agni (fire), jala vṛṣhṭīnāṁ (and approaching rainstorms) yathā khyāpayanti (are known to occur by the announcement of their) puṣhpa (flower), dhūma (smoke) ambudā (and clouds). Bhaviṣhyattvaṁ tathā (Likewise, the impending) riṣhṭāni (signs of death signal) pañchatām (the return to the five basic elements).

Suśhruta goes on to state that the inability to recognize *ariṣhṭa lakṣhaṇas* at the right time does not mean that they do not manifest. These signs may appear and disappear quickly, and they are often challenging to observe and assess.

तानि सौक्ष्म्यात्प्रमादाद्वा तथैवाशु व्यतिक्रमात् । गृह्यन्ते नोद्गतान्यज्ञैर्मुमूर्षोर्न त्वसम्भवात् ॥ ४

सु. सू. २८।४

Tāni saukṣhmyātpramādādvā tathaivāśhu vyatikramāt | Gṛhyante nodgatānyajñairmumūrṣhorna tvasambhavāt || 4

Su. Sū. 28/4

Tāni (Because of their) saukṣhmyāt (minuteness, subtleness) pramādād vā (or carelessness [in observation]) tathaivāśhu (or due to their) vyatikramāt (way of manifesting) gṛhyante (which requires quick grasp) nodgatānya (before they are gone) jñairmumūrṣhorna (they should be known as present) tvasambhavāt (rather than they did not manifest).

Vāgbhaṭa provides similar definitions in AH Śhā. 5/1-2 and AH Śhā. 5/132.

Bheda

Ariṣhṭa lakṣhaṇas are classified in several ways according to their practical application. Charaka's classification method listed in Cha. In. 1/3-4 contains the most comprehensive list of categories to assess. At a high level, these can be grouped under direct signs exhibited by the patient and circumstantial indicators. Charaka instructs that the signs exhibited directly by the patient should be interpreted based on the standards of practice as detailed in *Indriya-sthāna*. Circumstantial indicators should be understood based on *upadeśha*, *yukti* and *parīkṣha*.

Charaka's classification of *ariṣhṭa lakṣhaṇas* include the categories listed in the following table.

Ariṣhṭa lakṣhaṇa bheda (Cha. In. 1/3-4)	Method of interpretation	Assessment lakṣhaṇas
Puruṣha-saṁśhraya Direct signs	• *Pratyakṣha* Direct perception • *Anumāna* Inferred knowledge • *Upadeśha* Specific instructions	• *Śharīra* Physical body • *Sattva* Mental state • *Āhāra – Vihāra* Diet and lifestyle • *Vyādhi* Current state of health and disease
Puruṣha anāśhrita Circumstantial indicators	• *Upadeśha* Specific instructions • *Yukti* Application of logical thought • *Parīkṣha* Assessment	• *Dūtādhikāra* Features of the messenger • *Chautpātikaṁ chāturakulē* Signs while traveling to the patient's home and at the home

Suśhruta provides a concise, general overview of the classification of *ariṣhṭa lakṣhaṇas* that is intended to be applied in the context of surgical applications. The *lakṣhaṇas* described are specific for *pakva vraṇa*, or suppurating wounds.

गन्धवर्णरसादीनां विशेषाणां स्वभावतः ।
वैकृतं त तदाचष्टे व्रणिनः पक्वलक्षणम् ॥ ८

सु. सू. २८।८

Gandhavarṇarasādīnāṁ viśheṣhāṇāṁ svabhāvataḥ | Vaikṛtaṁ ta tadāchaṣhṭe vraṇinaḥ pakvalakṣhaṇam || 8

Su. Sū. 28/8

Gandha (Smell), varṇa (color), rasādīnāṁ (taste, etc) viśheṣhāṇāṁ svabhāvataḥ (which are abnormal, or not in their normal state) vaikṛtaṁ ta tadāchaṣhṭe (indicate a state of disease [or incurability]) vraṇinaḥ pakvalakṣhaṇam (of a suppurating wound).

Vāgbhaṭa adds one more important classification based on the stability and permanence of the presentation of *ariṣhṭa lakṣhaṇas*. Depending on their continued manifestation, the *lakṣhaṇas* could be understood to be more or less severe.

केचित्त् तद्विधेत्याहुः स्थाय्यस्थायिविभेदयः ।
दोषाणामपि बाहुल्याद्रिष्टाभासः समुद्भवेत्
॥ ३
स दोषाणां शाम्येत्स्थाय्यवश्यं तु मृत्यवे ।

अ. हृ. शा. ५।३

Kechitt tadvidhetyāhuḥ sthāyyasthāyivibhedayaḥ |
Doṣhāṇāmapi bāhulyādriṣhṭābhāsaḥ samudbhavet || 3
Sa doṣhāṇāṁ śhāmyetsthāyyavaśhyaṁ tu mṛtyave |

AH Śhā. 5/3

Kechitt (According to some), tad-vidhetyāhuḥ (these [*ariṣhṭa lakṣhaṇas*] are known as) sthāyi (stable, permanent) asthāyi (and unstable, non-permanent) vibhedayaḥ (as the types of classification). Doṣhāṇām api bāhulyād (A great increase of the *doṣhas*) samudbhavet (produces) riṣhṭā-bhāsaḥ (the manifestation of *riṣhṭa*). 3

Sa (When these) doṣhāṇāṁ (*doṣhas*), śhāmyet (return to their normal state), sthāyyavaśhyaṁ (the remaining *sthāyi* [*ariṣhṭa lakṣhaṇas*]) tu mṛtyave (definitely produce death).

Vāgbhaṭa's explanation of *sthāyi* and *asthāyi ariṣhṭa lakṣhaṇas* provides an important perspective for clinical application. The state of the *doṣhas* plays a primary role in the determination of the moment of death. When the *doṣhas* are able to be controlled, the presenting *ariṣhṭa lakṣhaṇas* become *asthāyi*, and death may be avoided. However, when the *doṣhas* take complete control of the individual, the presenting *ariṣhṭa lakṣhaṇas* become *sthāyi* resulting in the individual's death.

The specific *ariṣhṭa lakṣhaṇas* can be reviewed from the major classical treatises. They are found throughout all 12 chapters of Charaka's Indriya-sthāna, and Su. Sū. 28/ to 32/ and AH Śhā. 5/.

TEST YOURSELF

Learn, review and memorize key terms from this section.

Indriya-sthāna

---

ariṣhṭa lakṣhaṇas

---

riṣhṭa lakṣhaṇas

---

sthāyi

---

asthāyi

Chapter 25: Review

ADDITIONAL READING

Read and review the references listed below to expand your understanding of the concepts in this chapter. Write down the date that you complete your reading for each. Remember that consistent repetition is the best way to learn. Plan to read each reference at least once now and expect to read it again as you continue your studies.

References marked with (skim) can be read quickly and do not require commentary review.

CLASSICS		1st read	2nd read
Charaka	Cha. Śhā. 1/116 Cha. Śhā. 2/44 Cha. In. 1/ - 12/ (skim)		
Suśhruta	Su. Sū. 28/ to 32/ (skim)		
Aṣhṭāṅga Hṛdaya	AH Śhā. 5/ (skim)		
Bhāva Prakāśha			

JOURNALS & CURRENT RESOURCES

QUESTIONS & ANSWERS

Record your questions for this chapter here for further research and discussion.

Question:

Answer:

Question:

Answer:

Question:

Answer:

SELF-ASSESSMENT

1. Which of the following best describes *mṛtyu*?
   a. Death or dying
   b. Normal phase of life
   c. The correct outcome of life
   d. A and B
   e. All of the above

2. *Ariṣhṭa lakṣhaṇas* represent
   a. Actions, conduct and behavior cease
   b. Changes in *prakṛti*
   c. *Svabhāva*
   d. A and C
   e. All of the above

3. Why is *āyu* a function of *mṛtyu*?
   a. Lifespan is expected to continue in absence of impending death
   b. *Daiva* and *puruṣhakāra* determine span of life
   c. *Sātmya* accustomed to the individual
   d. A and B
   e. All of the above

4. Charaka states that regular practices to promote health improves
   a. *Ātma sampat*
   b. *Guṇa sampat*
   c. *Prakṛti sampat*
   d. All of the above
   e. None of the above

5. Why is the *Kali Yuga* important in *Āyurveda*?
   a. It lasts for 432,000 years
   b. It is the current *Yuga*
   c. It provides a baseline for estimated lifespan
   d. It represents a physical and moral deterioration of humankind
   e. All of the above

6. Which of the following can affect the outcome of *kālaja* or *akālaja mṛtyu*?
   a. *Daiva*
   b. *Prakṛti sampat*
   c. *Puruṣhakāra*
   d. A and C
   e. All of the above

7. Which of the following can an individual use to alter their outcome of *kālaja mṛtyu*?
   a. *Daiva*
   b. *Prakṛti sampat*
   c. *Puruṣhakāra*
   d. B and C
   e. All of the above

8. Which of the following *karmas* is least favorable to *kāla mṛtyu*?
   a. *Hīna daiva*
   b. *Madhyamā daiva*
   c. *Madhyamā puruṣhakāra*
   d. *Uttama daiva*
   e. *Uttama puruṣhakāra*

9. Charaka's explanation of *ariṣhṭa lakṣhaṇas* is found in
   a. Indriya-sthāna
   b. *Pratyakṣha*, *anumāna* and *upadeśha*
   c. *Upadeśha, yukti* and *parīkṣha*
   d. A and B
   e. All of the above

10. Suśhruta's assessment of *ariṣhṭa lakṣhaṇas* is based on surgery and described through
   a. *Gandha*, *varṇa* and *rasādīnāṁ*
   b. *Pratyakṣha*, *anumāna* and *upadeśha*
   c. *Upadeśha, yukti* and *parīkṣha*
   d. B and C
   e. All of the above

CRITICAL THINKING

1. Are the concepts of *daiva* and *purușhakāra* seen in popular culture today? If so, how?

2. Consider *ātma sampat* in the context of *ātma guṇa.* Compare and contrast, and explain how they are interrelated.

3. Choose any of the classical *arișhṭa lakșhaṇas* and cite the source. Explain how this *lakșhaṇa* could be useful in clinical practice.

4. Consider the classical *arișhṭa lakșhaṇas* and their circumstantial indicators. Could these be scientifically applicable?

5. Why is the explanation and discussion of *kālaja* and *akālaja mṛtyu* in the context of epidemics significant? Which of types of events could be included in the same type of explanation?

Chapter 26 : Sṛṣhṭi, Sthiti and Laya

KEY TERMS

ahaṅkāra	jñānendriya	manas	ṣhoḍaśha vikāra
aṣhṭa prakṛti	karmendriya	pañcha tanmātra	sṛṣhṭi
avyakta	laya	pañchaviṁśhati tattva	sṛṣhṭi utpatti
buddhi	mahābhūta	pralaya	sthiti
chaturviṁśhati tattva	mahat	rāśhi-puruṣha	ubhayendriya

The concepts of *sṛṣhṭi*, *sthiti* and *laya* provide the theoretical basis for the cycle of life in three major phases – creation, continuation and dissolution. These three phases are practically observable in all levels of life forms up to very large scales at universal level.

Early Vedic scientists recognized the commonality of this cycle of life and included its laws as primary tenets in the foundational philosophical systems of the time. These provided the basis for many advanced Vedic sciences, including Āyurveda.

Sṛṣhṭi utpatti is a concept that bridges classical Vedic philosophy and Āyurveda. Detailed descriptions of *sṛṣhṭi utpatti* can be found in various forms throughout the *ṣhaḍ darśhana*. During the development of major Āyurvedic *sampradāya* in the *Saṁhitā* period, the concept of *sṛṣhṭi utpatti* stood as one of the founding principles. Each *sampradāya* chose a specific format of this theory to implement within its own school of thought.

Within the scope of Āyurveda, *sṛṣhṭi*, *sthiti* and *laya* should be assumed to refer to the cycle of life in the scope of human existence. While they can also encompass realms beyond material existence, those discussions are best reserved for circles of philosophical study. Here, their study intends to focus on their practical application in producing, maintaining and dissolving human life in the most appropriate way possible for an individual. Each of the three concepts will be reviewed from that specific perspective.

SṚṢHṬI

Sṛṣhṭi, or *sṛṣhṭi utpatti*, refers to the production of life. There are two major descriptions of this concept that influenced the *Charaka sampradāya* and *Suśhruta sampradāya* from their inception. These two major descriptions are known as the 24 *tattva* and 25 *tattva* models.

First, review the terms *sṛṣhṭi* and *utpatti* for a thorough understanding of the phrase.

Nirukti and paribhāṣhā

The term *sṛṣhṭi* derives from the Sanskrit *dhātu* √ *sṛj*. The Monier-Williams dictionary defines *sṛj* as:

√ *sṛj*	to let go or fly, discharge, throw, cast, hurl at
	to cast or let go (a measuring line)
	to emit, pour forth, shed, cause to flow (rain, streams, etc)
	to release, set free

	(in older language only) to emit from one's self, ie create, procreate, produce, beget

When converted into the term *sṛṣhṭi*, this results in a meaning of:

sṛṣhṭi	letting go, letting loose, emission
	production, procreation, creation, the creation of the world
	nature, natural property or disposition

Utpatti is defined as:

utpatti	arising, birth, production, origin
	resurrection
	production in general, profit, productiveness
	producing as an effect or result, giving rise to, generating as a consequence

Sṛṣhṭi, or *sṛṣhṭi utpatti*, can be understood as "the production of creation," "the origin of life" or even "the origin of the universe."

Sṛṣhṭi utpatti tattva

There are two main models that influenced the understanding of the generation of life in classical Āyurveda. These are called the *chaturviṁśhati* (24) *tattva* and the *pañchaviṁśhati* (25) *tattva*. Tattva refers to the components that comprise the entire model both individually and collectively.

Charaka mentions the *chaturviṁśhati* (24) *tattva* in Cha. Śhā. 1/17 and Suśhruta discusses them in Su. Śhā. 1/4. Both authors elaborate the extensive concept throughout each of their respective chapters. Bhāvamiśhra dedicates the entire chapter of BP Pū. 2/ to the topic.

The models of *sṛṣhṭi utpatti tattva* explain the generation of life from its unmanifest state through production of all *tattva*, or generated components. In order to fully understand this model, the basic components of human life are required. Review Chapters 23, 24 and 25 for details on individual components that will be discussed throughout this chapter.

Chaturviṁśhati (24) tattva

The 24 *tattva* is a model that describes the evolution of components during the formation of life. It begins from the state of the unmanifest, or the realm of *avyakta*. From the top-most level explained in this model, *paramātma* generates an infinite number of *jīvātma* which individually engage in the process of *sṛṣhṭi utpatti* to generate a single new physical life form each.

The 24 *tattva* consist of 24 components that are grouped into two categories. The eight *prakṛti* are generated first and are responsible for producing further products. They are proximally closer to the state of *avyakta*. The 16 *vikāra* are the final products that form the physical manifestation of life and in some cases, these can be directly seen and observed.

पुनश्च धातुभेदेन चतुर्विंशतिकः स्मृतः | मनो दशेन्द्रियाण्यर्थाः प्रकृतिश्चाष्टधातुकी || १७

च. शा. १।१७

Punaśhcha dhātubhedena chaturviṁśhatikaḥ smṛtaḥ | Mano daśhendriyāṇyarthāḥ prakṛtiśhchāṣhṭadhātukī || 17

Cha. Śhā. 1/17

Punaśhcha (According to another) dhātubhedena (classification, there are) chaturviṁśhatikaḥ (24 *dhātus* [or *tattvas*]) smṛtaḥ (as explained [in this science]) - mano (the *manas*, or mind), daśha-indriyāṇi (the ten *indriya*), arthāḥ (the [five] *indriya-artha* [ie, the *pañcha-tanmātra*]), prakṛtiśhchāṣhṭa-dhātukī (and the *aṣhṭa prakṛti dhātus*, or the eight components generated from the level of *prakṛti* [or *avyakta*, the unmanifest]).

These components will be organized in tables and diagrams following the remainder of their descriptions in this section.

Pañchaviṁśhati (25) tattva

The 25 *tattva* model is distinct from the 24 *tattva* model by virtue of its perspective on the classification of one component, *puruṣha*. *Puruṣha* is an instigating component that is directly involved with *prakṛti* to propel the *avyakta* into a state of physical manifestation, thus producing life.

In the 24 *tattva* model, *puruṣha* is considered as an inherent part of *prakṛti*. However, in the 25 *tattva* model, *puruṣha* is recognized as an individual component and separate from *prakṛti*. The remainder of the *tattva* model is otherwise the same.

Aṣhṭa prakṛti and ṣhoḍaśha vikāra

The *aṣhṭa prakṛti* and *ṣhoḍaśha vikāra* are listed in detail by Charaka. Suśhruta provides similar explanations in Su. Śhā. 1/.

खादीनि बुद्धिरव्यक्तमहङ्कारस्तथाऽष्टमः |
भूतप्रकृतिरुद्दिष्टा विकाराश्चैव षोडश || ६३
बुद्धीन्द्रियाणि पञ्चैव पञ्च कर्मेन्द्रियाणि च |
समनस्काश्च पञ्चार्था विकारा इति सञ्ज्ञिताः
|| ६४

च. शा. १।६३-६४

Khādīni buddhiravyaktamahaṅkārastathā ' ṣhṭamaḥ | Bhūtaprakṛtiruddiṣhṭā vikārāśhchaiva ṣhoḍaśha || 63
Buddhīndriyāṇi pañchaiva pañcha karmendriyāṇi cha | Samanaskāśhcha pañchārthā vikārā iti sañjñitāḥ || 64

Cha. Śhā. 1/63-64

Khādīni (The five *khā*, etc [*tanmātras*]) buddhir (*buddhi*, or innate intelligence), avyaktam (*avyakta*, or the soul), ahaṅkāra (and *ahaṅkāra*, or self-identification) stathā aṣhṭamaḥ (are the eight) bhūta prakṛtir (*prakṛti*, or components generated from *prakṛti* or *avyakta*) uddiṣhṭā (that are described), vikārāśhchaiva ṣhoḍaśha (along with the 16 *vikāra*, or the final products that form the physical manifestation of life).

Buddhīndriyāṇi (The *jñānedriya*, or senses) pañchaiva (of which there are five), pañcha karmendriyāṇi cha (and the five *karmendriya*), samanaskāśhcha (along with *manas*, or the mind), pañchārthā (and the five *indriya-artha*, or objects of the senses [ie, the *mahābhūtas*]) vikārā iti sañjñitāḥ (are known as the [16] *vikāra*, or the final products that form the physical manifestation of life).

Sequence of generation

The process of *sṛṣhṭi utpatti* begins with *avyakta*. *Prakṛti* and *puruṣha* are responsible for the initiation of the sequence of events that ultimately produce life. Suśhruta explains this state as being the cause for the generation of all *bhūtas* in Su. Śhā. 1/3.

The impulse of *avyakta* to manifest into physical form during the process of *sṛṣhṭi utpatti* is inherently guided by the *tri-guṇa*, with *rajas* and *tamas* often leading the way. During the initial stages of the process, the eight *prakṛti* manifest first. *Avyakta* generates *mahat* (or *buddhi*), which produces *ahaṅkāra*, which then creates the *pañcha tanmātras*. These initial eight are all connected via the *tri-guṇa*.

Next, the 16 *vikāra* are produced out of the effects of *sattva*, *rajas* and *tamas*. *Rajas* stimulates and initiates *sattva* to generate the *pañcha jñānendriya* and the *pañcha karmendriya*, along with one *ubhayendriya*, *manas*.

Rajas then stimulates and initiates *tamas* to generate the *pañcha mahābhūtas* as single outcomes of each of the *pañcha tanmātras*.

The relationship between the *tanmātras* and the *mahābhūtas* is significant. It provides a special connection between each *tanmātra* and a single *mahābhūta* through which information can be shared. By this communication channel, the *tanmātra-bhūta* pair is able to relay specific information which can be detected by its corresponding *jñānendriya*.

The generation of the *tanmātras* follows a specific order. It begins with *śhabda tanmātra* which then produces *sparśha*, followed by *rūpa*, *rasa* and finally *gandha*. As each *tanmātra* is generated, it also produces a corresponding *mahābhūta*. The sequential generation of each *mahābhūta* follows the same rule of *guṇa-vṛddhi*. Each subsequent *bhūta* carries small portions of all previous *bhūtas* causing the total mass of the final *bhūta* to be significantly higher.

Review Cha. Śhā. 1/65-67, Su. Śhā. 1/ and BP Pū. 2/ for the classical explanations of this sequence of generation.

The process of *tanmātra* and *mahābhūta* generation is described in the table below.

Śhabda tanmātra Subtle element of sound		*Ākāśha mahābhūta* Gross element of space or ether
↓		↓
Sparśha tanmātra Subtle element of touch		*Vayū mahābhūta* Gross element of air
↓		↓
Rūpa tanmātra Subtle element of sight	⇒	*Tejo mahābhūta* Gross element of light
↓		↓
Rasa tanmātra Subtle element of taste		*Ap* or *Jala mahābhūta* Gross element of water
↓		↓
Gandha tanmātra Subtle element of smell		*Pṛthvi mahābhūta* Gross element of earth

Srṣhṭi utpatti

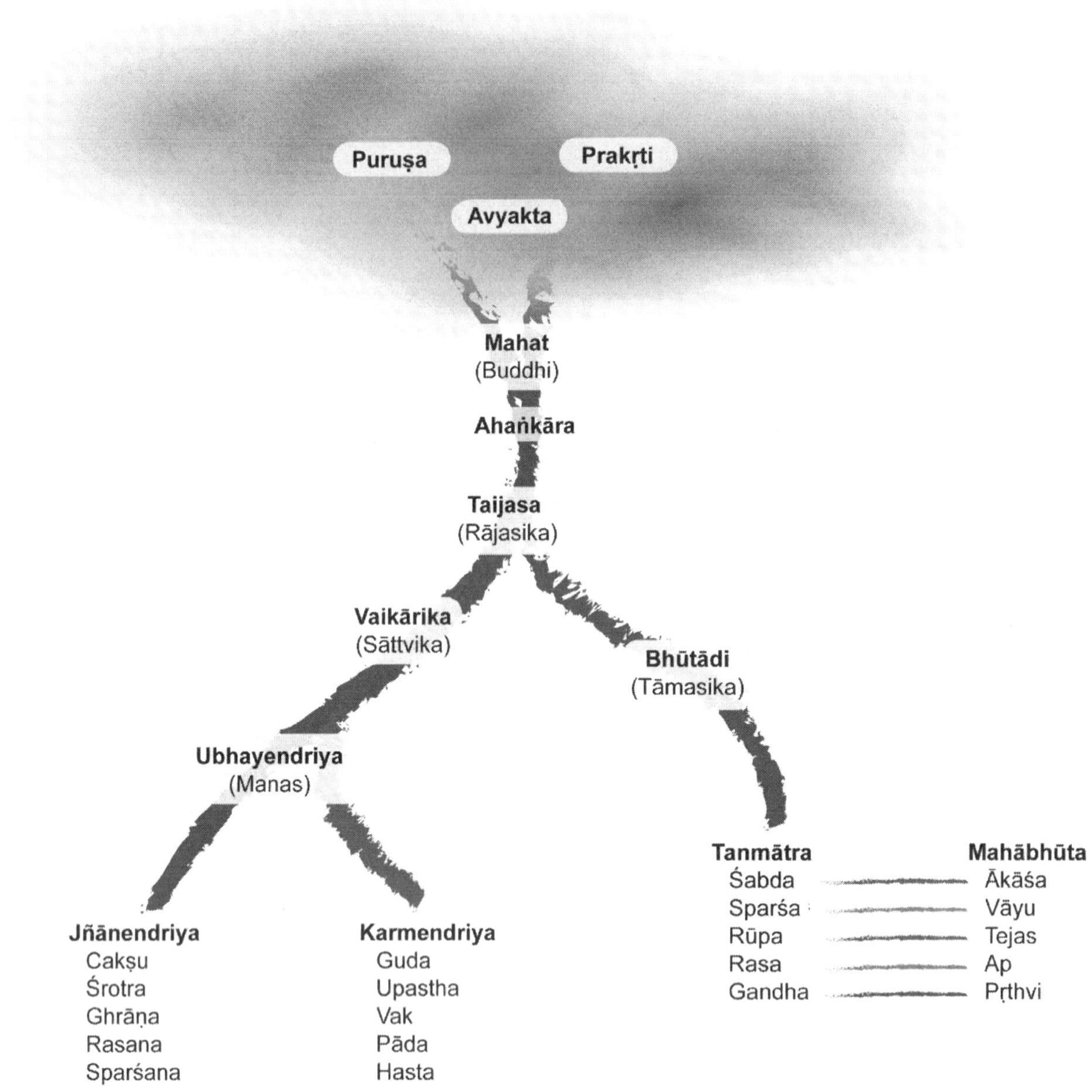

Aṣhṭa (8) *prakṛti*	*Avyakta* → *Mahat* (*Buddhi*) → *Ahaṅkāra* → *Pañcha* (5) *tanmātra*	
Ṣhoḍaśha (16) *vikāra*	1	*Ubhayendriya* (*manas*)
	5	*Jñānendriya*
	5	*Karmendriya*
	5	*Mahābhūta*

Avyakta as main controller

Of the 24 *tattva*, *avyakta* is ultimately responsible as the coordinator for the remaining. Because it is the first *tattva* to be generated, it is associated with the *tri-guṇa* in their most original state. It also is ultimately responsible to act as the witness for all actions performed by *rāśhi-puruṣha*.

बुद्धीन्द्रियमनोर्थानां विद्याद्योगधरं परम् |
चतुर्विंशतिको ह्येष राशिः पुरुषसञ्ज्ञकः || ३५

च. शा. १।३५

Buddhīndriyamanorthānāṁ vidyādyogadharaṁ param |
Chaturviṁśhatiko hyeṣha rāśhiḥ puruṣhasañjñakaḥ || 35

Cha. Śhā. 1/35

Buddhi (*Buddhi*, innate intelligence), indriya (*indriya*, the senses), mano-arthānāṁ (*mano-artha*, the objects of the mind) vidyād (are known to be) yogadharaṁ param (united and coordinated by *ātma*, the soul). Chaturviṁśhatiko hyeṣha (These 24 components together) rāśhiḥ puruṣha sañjñakaḥ (are known as *rāśhi-puruṣha*, or the individual manifestation of the soul).

Purpose of manifestation

Ātma engages in the process of *sṛṣhṭi utpatti* and embodies a physical manifestation in order to exhaust its *rajas* and *tamas* and their associated actions. This connection and attachment to *rajas* and *tamas* is the main driver for engagement. When these are completely neutralized and negated, *ātma* ceases to have a reason or cause to enter into additional physical forms.

रजस्तमोभ्यां युक्तस्य संयोगोऽयमनन्तवान्|
ताभ्यां निराकृताभ्यां तु सत्त्ववृद्ध्या निवर्तते || ३६

च. शा. १।३६

Rajastamobhyāṁ yuktasya saṁyogo ' yamanantavān | Tābhyāṁ nirākṛtābhyāṁ tu sattvavṛddhyā nivartate || 36

Cha. Śhā. 1/36

Rajas-tamobhyāṁ (Both *rajas* and *tamas*) yuktasya (are known by means of logical thought) saṁyogo (to be the cause for the conjunction [of the 24 *tattva*]) ayamanantavān (and they stretch out its mundane life). Tābhyāṁ (When both of these [*rajas* and *tamas*]) nirākṛtābhyāṁ (are free from manifesting their forms) tu sattvavṛddhyā (and *sattva* becomes increased and predominant) nivartate ([the conjunction of the 24 *tattva* and their cycle of rebirth] ceases to exists).

Along with exhausting its causative factors of *rajas* and *tamas*, the *ātma* intends to perform any additional actions, experience the beneficial outcomes of previous actions, realize a range of emotions and enjoy life and death.

अत्र कर्म फलं चात्र ज्ञानं चात्र प्रतिष्ठितम् |
अत्र मोहः सुखं दुःखं जीवितं मरणं स्वता || ३७
एवं यो वेद तत्त्वेन स वेद प्रलयोदयौ |
पारम्पर्यं चिकित्सां च ज्ञातव्यं यच्च किञ्चन || ३८

च. शा. १।३७-३८

Atra karma phalaṁ chātra jñānaṁ chātra pratiṣhṭhitam | Atra mohaḥ sukhaṁ duḥkhaṁ jīvitaṁ maraṇaṁ svatā || 37
Evaṁ yo veda tattvena sa veda pralayodayau | Pāramparyaṁ chikitsāṁ cha jñātavyaṁ yachcha kiñchana || 38

Cha. Śhā. 1/37-38

Atra (And so) karma (the actions), phalaṁ (positive results of previous actions) chātra (and even) jñānaṁ (knowledge), chātra (as well as) pratiṣhṭhitam (valuable outcomes); Atra (And) mohaḥ (delusion), sukhaṁ (happiness), duḥkhaṁ (discontent), jīvitaṁ (life), maraṇaṁ (death) svatā (and personal independence);

Evaṁ yo veda (Knowing all these) tattvena (within the context of the 24 *tattva*) sa veda (is to know) pralayodayau (both dissolution, as well as reaching the final goal [ie, release from the bonds of rebirth]). Pāramparyaṁ (In this tradition) chikitsāṁ (of therapeutic managment) cha jñātavyaṁ yachcha kiñchana (this and similar knowledge is strong).

In order to experience any of these, *ātma* must be attached to the 24 *tattva* and engaged in a physical form of life. Only with its presence can these activities take place, exhaust themselves and allow the attachments of *rajas* and *tamas* to conclude.

करणानि मनो बुद्धिर्बुद्धिकर्मेन्द्रियाणि च |
कर्तुः संयोगजं कर्म वेदना बुद्धिरेव च || ५६
नैकः प्रवर्तते कर्तुं भूतात्मा नाश्नुते फलम् |
संयोगाद्वर्तते सर्वं तमृते नास्ति किञ्चन || ५७

च. शा. १|५६-५७

Karaṇāni mano buddhirbuddhikarmendriyāṇi cha | Kartuḥ saṁyogajaṁ karma vedanā buddhireva cha || 56
Naikaḥ pravartate kartuṁ bhūtātmā nāśhnute phalam | Saṁyogādvartate sarvaṁ tamṛte nāsti kiñchana || 57

Cha. Śhā. 1/56-57

Karaṇāni (That which causes [*jñāna*] includes) mano (*manas*, the mind), buddhir (*buddhi*, innate intelligence), buddhi-karmendriyāṇi cha (and the *jñānendriya* and *karmendriya*). Kartuḥ (The one who does this [ie, *ātma*]) saṁyogajaṁ (is constantly attached to) karma (action), vedanā (sensation and pain), buddhireva cha (and innate intelligence).

Kartuṁ (The one who does these things) naikaḥ pravartate (does not exist on its own) bhūtātmā (in a state of physical manifestation) nāśhnute (nor does it obtain) phalam (the beneficial outcomes of actions [on its own]). Saṁyogād (This combination) vartate sarvaṁ tamṛte (allows the final release [from the bonds of rebirth] to take place) nāsti (and without it) kiñchana (nothing is possible).

TEST YOURSELF

Learn, review and memorize key terms from this section.

sṛṣhṭi

---

sṛṣhṭi utpatti

---

chaturviṁśhati tattva

---

pañchaviṁśhati tattva

---

aṣhṭa prakṛti

ṣhoḍaśha vikāra

avyakta

mahat

buddhi

ahaṅkāra

pañcha tanmātra

ubhayendriya

manas

jñānendriya

karmendriya

mahābhūta

rāśhi-puruṣha

STHITI

The concept of *sthiti* refers to the continuation of life. It includes all of the efforts towards maintaining, extending and fulfilling a complete lifespan. These efforts comprise the main goals of Āyurveda.

Sthiti is the second of the three phases in the cycle of life. It naturally exerts a strong sense of attachment and desire to continue the existence of life in any form.

Paribhāṣhā

The Monier-Williams dictionary defines the term *sthiti* as:

sthiti	standing upright or firmly, not falling
	standing, staying, remaining, abiding, stay, residence, sojourn in or on or at
	staying or remaining or being in any state or condition
	continuance in being, maintenance of life, continued existence (the 2nd of the three states of all created things, the 1st being utpatti, "coming into existence," and the 3rd laya, "dissolution"), permanence, duration
	duration of life
	that which continually exists, the world, earth
	maintenance, sustenance

TEST YOURSELF

Learn, review and memorize key terms from this section.

sthiti

LAYA

Laya and *pralaya* both refer to death and the process of dissolution of life. This third and final phase marks the end of the cycle of life. It is a natural part of life and deserves its own special attention, care and etiquette.

Classically in Āyurveda, death was highly respected. In many traditional Hindu cultures today, similar customs are maintained. Acceptance of this obligatory part of life is likely eased by the understanding of *ātma* and its inherent nature of continuity.

Paribhāṣhā

The Monier-Williams dictionary defines *laya* and *pralaya* as:

laya	melting, dissolution, disappearance or absorption in
	to disappear, be dissolved or absorbed
	extinction, destruction, death
	rest, repose
	place of rest, residence, house, dwelling
	mental inactivity, spiritual indifference
pralaya	dissolution, reabsorption, destruction, annihilation
	death
	the destruction of the whole world
	end
	cause of dissolution
	fainting, loss of sense or consciousness

While discussing epidemics and the loss of life that accompanies such great events, Punarvasu Ātreya explains to Agniveśha that lifespan is expected to gradually reduce over the course of large time cycles of the universe.

With the continual decrease of positive qualities of the *tri-guṇa* over time, the entire universe eventually undergoes its own process of *pralaya*.

युगे युगे धर्मपादः क्रमेणानेन हीयते |
गुणपादश्च भूतानामेवं लोकः प्रलीयते || २५
च. वि. ३।२५

Yuge yuge dharmapādaḥ krameṇānena hīyate | Guṇapādaśhcha bhūtānāmevaṁ lokaḥ pralīyate || 25

Cha. Vi. 3/25

Yuge yuge (*Yuga* after *yuga*), dharmapādaḥ (one quarter of *dharma*, or collective responsibility) krameṇānena (gradually goes on) hīyate (decreasing). Guṇapādaśhcha (And even a quarter of [beneficial] qualities and characteristics) bhūtānāmevaṁ (of all the basic elements goes on decreasing). Lokaḥ (And thus the world) pralīyate (undergoes dissolution).

TEST YOURSELF

Learn, review and memorize key terms from this section.

laya __________

pralaya __________

Chapter 26: Review

ADDITIONAL READING

Read and review the references listed below to expand your understanding of the concepts in this chapter. Write down the date that you complete your reading for each. Remember that consistent repetition is the best way to learn. Plan to read each reference at least once now and expect to read it again as you continue your studies.

References marked with (skim) can be read quickly and do not require commentary review.

CLASSICS		1st read	2nd read
Charaka	Cha. Vi. 3/25 Cha. Śhā. 1/		
Suśhruta	Su. Śhā. 1/		
Aṣhṭāṅga Hṛdaya			
Bhāva Prakāśha	BP Pū. 2/		

JOURNALS & CURRENT RESOURCES

https://www.youtube.com/watch?v=OODqrcFRtv4

http://www.iep.utm.edu/sankhya/

QUESTIONS & ANSWERS

Record your questions for this chapter here for further research and discussion.

Question:

Answer:

Question:

Answer:

Question:

Answer:

SELF-ASSESSMENT

1. Which of the following is a component of *sṛṣhṭi utpatti*?
   a. Founding principal of Ayurveda
   b. *Chaturviṁśhati* (24) *tattva*
   c. *Pañchaviṁśhati* (25) *tattva*
   d. The origin of all creation
   e. All of the above

2. What is the difference between the 24 and 25 *tattva?*
   a. *Ahaṅkāra*
   b. *Avyakta*
   c. *Buddhi*
   d. *Puruṣha*
   e. *Prakṛti*

3. Which of the following are included in the *aṣhṭa prakṛti*?
   a. *Pañcha jñānedriya, buddhi, avyakta, ahaṅkāra*
   b. *Pañcha jñānedriya, manas, indriya, ahaṅkāra*
   c. *Pañcha karmendriya, buddhi, avyakta, ahaṅkāra*
   d. *Pañcha tanmātra, avyakta, buddhi, ahaṅkāra*
   e. *Pañcha tanmātra, buddhi, manas, indriya*

4. *Sṛṣhṭi* refers to
   a. Creation of nature
   b. Maintenance of life
   c. Curative effort
   d. Destruction of the universe
   e. Purpose of life

5. Which of the following sixteen components are included in the *ṣhoḍaśha vikāra*?
   a. *Pañcha jñānedriya, pañcha karmendriya, mahābhūta, manas*
   b. *Pañcha jñānedriya, pañcha karmendriya, pañcha indriya-artha, buddhi*
   c. *Pañcha jñānedriya, pañcha tanmātra, pañcha karmendriya, manas*
   d. *Pañcha tanmātra, pañcha jñānedriya, pañcha karmendriya, avyakta*
   e. *Pañcha tanmātra, pañcha karmendriya, pañcha indriya-artha, ahaṅkāra*

6. What initiates *avyakta* to manifest into physical form during *sṛṣhṭi utpatti*?
   a. *Sattva, rajas, tamas*
   b. *Rajas*
   c. *Tamas*
   d. *Rajas, tamas*
   e. *Tri-guṇa*

7. *Rajas* stimulates and initiates *sattva* to generate
   a. *Pañcha tanmātra, pañcha mahābhūta*
   b. *Pañcha tanmātra, pañcha jñānendriya, pañcha mahābhūta*
   c. *Ubhayendriya, pañcha jñānendriya, pañcha karmendriya*
   d. *Ubhayendriya, pañcha jñānendriya, pañcha mahābhūta*
   e. *Ubhayendriya, pañcha jñānendriya*

8. *Rajas* stimulates and initiates *tamas* to generate
   a. *Pañcha tanmātra, pañcha mahābhūta*
   b. *Pañcha tanmātra, pañcha jñānendriya, pañcha mahābhūta*
   c. *Ubhayendriya, pañcha jñānendriya, pañcha karmendriya*
   d. *Ubhayendriya, pañcha jñānendriya*
   e. *Ubhayendriya, pañcha jñānendriya, pañcha tanmātra*

9. *Ātma* engages in *sṛṣhṭi utpatti* to
   a. Enjoy life and death
   b. Exhaust associated attachments of *rajas* and *tamas*
   c. Experience beneficial outcomes from previous actions
   d. Perform desired actions
   e. All of the above

10. What is the ultimate goal of *jīvātmā*?
    a. Enjoy life and death
    b. Engage in a physical form of life
    c. Experience the process of *sṛṣhṭi utpatti*
    d. Release from the bonds of rebirth
    e. All of the above

CRITICAL THINKING

1. Using the diagram of *sṛṣhṭi utpatti*, label the *aṣhṭa prakṛti* and the *ṣhoḍaśha vikāra*.

2. One of the reasons that *ātma* engages in *sṛṣhṭi utpatti* is to complete actions. Explain this in context of the purpose of Āyurveda, specifically using Charaka's explanation of the four *puruṣhārtha*. Cite the reference.

3. The special relationship between the *pañcha tanmātra* and *pañcha mahābhūta* allows individuals to interact with the material world. Choose any one example of this relationship and depict its entire process along with its appropriate *pañcha pañchaka*. Label each step and component.

4. In traditional Hindu philosophy, the relationship between *paramātmā* and *jīvātmā* is likened to one candle lighting many candles. How can this be explained in context of *sṛṣhṭi utpatti*?

5. As *sattva*, *rajas* and *tamas* create the *pañcha jñānendriya* and *pañcha karmendriya*, how can their influence be seen on these categories of senses and action organs?